Tibetan Medicine in the Contemporary World

This remarkable multi-authored volume will decisively transform conventional understanding about indigenous medical knowledge and practices of all kinds in the contemporary world.

> Margaret Lock, Professor in Social Studies in
> Medicine at McGill University

The popularity of Tibetan medicine plays a central role in the international market for alternative medicine and has been increasing and extending far beyond its original cultural area, becoming a global phenomenon. This book analyses Tibetan medicine in the twenty-first century by considering the contemporary reasons that have led to its diversity and by bringing out the common orientations of this medical system. Using case studies that examine the social, political and identity dynamics of Tibetan medicine in Nepal, India, the PRC, Mongolia, the UK and the US, the contributors to this book answer the following three, fundamental questions:

- What are the modalities and issues involved in the social and therapeutic transformations of Tibetan medicine?
- How are national policies and health reforms connected to the processes of contemporary redefinition of this medicine?
- How does Tibetan medicine fit into the present, globalized context of the medical world?

Written by experts in the field from the US, France, Canada, China and the UK, this book will be invaluable to students and scholars interested in contemporary medicine, Tibetan studies, health studies and the anthropology of Asia.

Laurent Pordié is Director of the Department of Social Sciences at the French Institute of Pondicherry and a Fellow at the Centre de Recherche 'Cultures, Santé, Sociétés' (CReCSS), Paul Cézanne University at Aix-Marseille.

Needham Research Institute Series
Series editor: Christopher Cullen

Joseph Needham's 'Science and Civilisation' series began publication in the 1950s. At first it was seen as a piece of brilliant but isolated pioneering. However, at the beginning of the twenty-first century, it is clear that Needham's work has succeeded in creating a vibrant new intellectual field in the West. The books in this series cover topics relating broadly to the practice of science, technology and medicine in East Asia, including China, Japan, Korea and Vietnam. The emphasis is on traditional forms of knowledge and practice, but without excluding modern studies which connect their topics with their historical and cultural context.

Celestial Lancets
A history and rationale of acupuncture and moxa
Lu Gwei-Djen and Joseph Needham
With a new introduction by Vivienne Lo

A Chinese Physician
Wang Ji and the Stone Mountain Medical Case histories
Joanna Grant

Chinese Mathematical Astrology
Reaching out to the stars
Ho Peng Yoke

Medieval Chinese Medicine
The Dunhuang medical manuscripts
Edited by Vivienne Lo and Christopher Cullen

Chinese Medicine in Early Communist China, 1945–1963
Medicine of revolution
Kim Taylor

Explorations in Daoism
Medicine and alchemy in literature
Ho Peng Yoke

Tibetan Medicine in the Contemporary World
Global politics of medical knowledge and practice
Edited by Laurent Pordié

Tibetan Medicine in the Contemporary World

Global politics of medical
knowledge and practice

Edited by Laurent Pordié

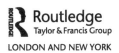

LONDON AND NEW YORK

First published 2008
by Routledge
2 Park Square, Milton Park, Abingdon, Oxon OX14 4RN

Simultaneously published in the USA and Canada
by Routledge
711 Third Avenue, New York, NY 10017

Routledge is an imprint of the Taylor & Francis Group, an informa business

First issued in paperback 2011

Typeset in Times New Roman by
Keystroke, 28 High Street, Tettenhall, Wolverhampton

British Library Cataloguing in Publication Data
A catalogue record for this book is available from the British Library

Library of Congress Cataloging in Publication Data
Tibetan medicine in the contemporary world : global politics of medical
knowledge and practice / [edited by] Laurent Pordié.
p. ; cm. – Needham Research Institute series)
Includes bibliographical references.
1. Medicine, Tibetan. I. Pordié, Laurent. II. Series.
[DNLM: 1. Medicine, Tibetan Traditional–methods–Case Reports.
2. Health Knowledge, Attitudes, Practice–Case Reports. 3. World
Health–Case Reports. WB 50.1 T553 2008]
R603.T5T54 2008
610–dc22
2007031100

ISBN10: 0–415–44789–5 (hbk)
ISBN10: 0–415–66670–8 (pbk)
ISBN10: 0–208–93254–4 (ebk)

ISBN13: 978–0–415–44789–8 (hbk)
ISBN13: 978–0–415–66670–1 (pbk)
ISBN13: 978–0–208–93254–4 (ebk)

Contents

Notes on contributors

Vincanne Adams is Professor of Medical Anthropology in the Department of Anthropology, History and Social Medicine at the University of California at San Francisco. She is the author of numerous articles and several books on medicine and social change in Nepal and Tibet, including *Tigers in the Snow and Other Virtual Sherpas* (Princeton University Press, 1996), *Doctors for Democracy* (Cambridge University Press, 1998) and *Sex in Development* (with S.L. Pigg, Duke University Press, 2005).

Yildiz Aumeeruddy-Thomas received her Ph.D. in Ethnobotany and Terrestrial Ecology from the University of Montpellier. She is a research fellow at the Centre National de la Recherche Scientifique (CNRS-CEFE) and associated with the Institut de Recherche pour le Développement (IRD). Her fields of interest are ethnoecology and ethnobotany, the relationships between local knowledge/practices and global norms, vernacular, scientific and citizen knowledge, cognitive processes and social dynamics within local territories. Her publications include the co-edited volume *Himalayan Medicinal and Aromatic Plants: Balancing Use and Conservation* (IDRC–WWF, 2005).

Chen Hua is Associate Professor at the Department of Anthropology, Zhongshan (Sun Yat-sen) University, Guangzhou, China. He has done research on medical anthropology and physical anthropology since 1982, with special emphasis on traditional medicines. His has published articles and books such as *Principles of Traditional Chinese Medicine* (in Chinese) and *An Introduction to Medical Anthropology* (in Chinese).

Sienna R. Craig is Assistant Professor of Anthropology at Dartmouth College, Hanover, New Hampshire. She earned her Ph.D. from Cornell University on the relationship between Tibetan medicine and biomedicine in contemporary Tibet, with a specific focus on clinical research and the standardization, commoditization and industrialization of Tibetan medicine production. She has conducted research on Nepal, Tibet and the greater Himalayan region. Craig is also the co-founder of Drokpa, a non-profit organization. Her works include the book *Horses like Lightning: A Passage through Mustang* (Wisdom Publications, forthcoming).

Casey Hilliard is a Ph.D. student at McGill University. Her master's thesis examined the socio-political forces contributing to the formal development of Tibetan medicine in post-socialist Mongolia. Her current research interests centre on the social, cultural and political implications of the global health and fitness industry.

Craig R. Janes is Professor and Associate Dean in the Faculty of Health Sciences at Simon Fraser University, Burnaby, British Columbia, Canada. His present research interests include the globalization of Asian medical systems, international public health, maternal and child health, social epidemiology, and the political economy of global health services reform.

Yeshi C. Lama was an anthropologist, who completed her thesis at the School of Oriental and African Studies, University of London (2002). She was posted at the WWF Nepal Programme on mountain projects and programmes that seek to conserve biodiversity and promote sustainable livelihoods. Her research interests concerned ethnobotany and medical anthropology in Nepal, especially with regard to interactions between local and scientific knowledge systems, and biological and socio-cultural landscapes. She died tragically on 23 September 2006.

Fei-Fei Li is an Assistant Professor in the Computer Science Department at Princeton University. She also holds courtesy appointments at the Neuroscience Institute at Princeton. She earned her Ph.D. from California Institute of Technology. Her main research area is computer and human vision, including statistical modelling and cognitive neuroscience. From 1999, she has spent many years studying Tibetan medicine with physicians at Lhasa Mentsikhang, including a clinical trial of Tibetan medicine for gastrointestinal disorders.

Margaret Lock is the Marjorie Bronfman Professor in Social Studies in Medicine, and is affiliated with the Department of Social Studies of Medicine and the Department of Anthropology at McGill University. She is a Fellow of the Royal Society of Canada, was awarded the Prix du Québec, domaine Sciences Humaines, in 1997, and in 2002 the Canada Council for the Arts Molson Prize. Lock's monographs include *East Asian Medicine in Urban Japan* (University of California Press, 1980), *Encounters with Aging: Mythologies of Menopause in Japan and North America* (UC Press, 1993) and *Twice Dead: Organ Transplants and the Reinvention of Death* (UC Press, 2002); her books have received numerous prizes. She has edited or co-edited ten other books and written over 160 scholarly articles. Her current research is concerned with post-genomic biology and its impact in the clinic and among families and the public at large.

Colin Millard first carried out research in medical anthropology in 1992 in Ladakh, the north-east Himalayan region of the Indian State of Jammu and Kashmir. Since that time he has maintained an interest in medical anthropology, particularly as it relates to Tibetan culture and medical practices in the South Asian region. In 2002 he completed his Ph.D. in the Department of Anthropology at

Edinburgh University, which focuses on learning processes in a Bonpo medicine school situated in the valley of Dhorpatan in the Baglung district of west Nepal. He is presently based in Edinburgh, where he is undertaking a research programme at the Tara Institute of Tibetan Medicine.

Laurent Pordié is an anthropologist, Director of the Department of Social Sciences at the French Institute of Pondicherry and Research Fellow at the Centre de Recherche 'Cultures, Santé, Sociétés' (CReCSS), Paul Cézanne University at Aix-Marseille. He is the General Co-editor of the academic book series 'Sous prétexte de médecines' (with A.-M. Moulin), with Editions aux Lieux d'Etre, Paris. His works and publications mainly concern the contemporary social dynamics of Tibetan medicine, and the anthropology of development, including the books *The Expression of Religion in Tibetan Medicine* (FIP, 2003) *Panser le monde, penser les médecines* (Karthala, 2005) and *Healing at the Periphery* (forthcoming with Duke University Press).

Geoffrey Samuel is a Professorial Fellow in the School of Religious and Theological Studies at Cardiff University. Since 1971, most of his research has focused on Tibetans, though he has also worked in South Asia and in Western societies. His specialist fields include the anthropology of Buddhist societies and of religion in South and South-East Asia, medical anthropology and the anthropological study of healing. At Cardiff, he is developing a series of research projects on mind–body processes in relation to healing, looking both at Tibetan medicine and yoga and at other Asian traditions, and also at the contemporary British usage of such techniques within the field of complementary and alternative medicine. He has produced a large number of publications, including the books *Mind, Body and Culture* (Cambridge University Press, 1990), *Civilized Shamans* (Smithsonian, 1993), *Healing Powers and Modernity* (Bergin & Garvey, 2001, with L. H. Connor), *The Daughters of Hariti* (Routledge, 2002, with Santi Rozario), *Tantric Revisionings* (Ashgate, 2005) and *The Origins of Yoga and Tantra* (Cambridge University Press, forthcoming).

Eliot Tokar practises Tibetan medicine in New York City, and is one of very few Westerners internationally to have received extensive textual and clinical training in this field by Tibet physicians such as Yeshi Dhonden and Trogawa Rinpoche. He was a nominee for the White House Commission on Complementary and Alternative Medicine Policy, and served as an adviser to the American Medical Students Association. He has lectured at institutions such as Washington University School of Medicine in St Louis, University of Pennsylvania School of Medicine and Princeton University. His publications concern the theory and practice of Tibetan medicine and the role of Tibetan medicine in the context of its current globalization.

Ivette Vargas received her Ph.D. in Indian and Tibetan Buddhism from Harvard University (2003) and is currently Assistant Professor of Asian Religions at Austin College, Texas. Her research interests concern the experiences of suffering and illness in Tibetan and Indian narrative and ritual literature, and the role of gender within these experiences; healing rituals; and the interface between religion and medicine. She has conducted research in Nepal, Tibet and Taiwan. She has published extensively on Tibetan and Indian Buddhist traditions.

Foreword

Margaret Lock

Rather than the eclipse by biomedicine of traditional practices that was prophesied in the second half of the twentieth century for the near future, medical pluralism flourishes in numerous geographical locations, and perhaps no more so than in Asia, with its long history of literate medical traditions. It is particularly appropriate that Tibetan medicine is the illustrative example for this volume because until recently, with a few notable exceptions, this particular tradition has been largely overlooked in publications about Asian medicine, to the detriment of our understanding of the complexity of the medical practices of the region as a whole.

In the influential 1976 volume *Asian Medical Systems: A Comparative Study*, the medical anthropologist Charles Leslie argued forcefully that medical systems cannot be fully understood outside the 'stream of history' and are subject to change as a result of both endogenous and exogenous forces. In part Leslie was reacting to certain scholars and observers of Asian medicine active at that time who can best be characterized as Orientalists, individuals who assumed that, although Asian medical systems may formerly have been systematically coherent and integrated, contemporary practices had become a pale reflection of the past – opportunistic, unsystematic, and no longer authentic.

This highly instructive volume on Tibetan medicine eradicates any lingering nostalgia for a purist past, and informs us in no uncertain terms, in part because the research is multi-sited, just how inappropriate was such an attitude. In reading these essays, we are catapulted into the postmodern, globalized era and exposed to the remarkable pastiche of contemporary Tibetan medical knowledge and practices that parenthetically make it abundantly clear that pluralism, innovation, conservatism, and competition were all inevitably at work, even when Tibetan medicine was confined largely to the Himalayan region. The extent of the spread of Tibetan medicine today will no doubt surprise some readers; this is in part due to the large numbers of Tibetans exiled from their homeland, and also due to the craving of many Westerners for what they believe Tibetan medicine has to offer. In this book, in addition to reading about practices in Tibet, Mongolia, Nepal, the Indian Himalayas, and mainland China, we learn about the forms that Tibetan medicine takes in London, New York, and the state of Massachusetts. In these latter sites it becomes integrated into the panoply of alternative medicines available everywhere today. Tibetan medicine can no longer be thought of as confined to the local, nor should it be described as traditional; while healers who reside in remote villages may self-consciously become the guardians of tradition, numerous others are active participants in the enormous transformations in the Himalayan region associated with modernity – these healers are deeply implicated with innovation, and may even think in terms of progress.

Making extensive use of historiography and ethnographic methods, the contributing authors ably contextualize Tibetan medical knowledge and practices with respect to politics, global and local, and specific social exigencies, emphasizing not only the perspectives of involved practitioners but also those of patients and clients, including a few of the numerous tourists who seek out this medicine. As Laurent Pordié notes in his introduction, Tibetan medical practices are today international in character, and a remarkable heterogeneity is undeniably evident, even though, wherever it is practiced, orientations common to virtually all forms of Tibetan medicine are apparent. These orientations provide the circumscribing framework for what Pordié characterizes as a newly emerged 'neo-traditional' Tibetan medicine.

Drama, hope, and tragedy unfold in these chapters with the recounting of the everyday reality of Tibetan medical practices. We read about a brain-drain, as eminent practitioners depart the villages for urban environments, leaving some villagers in effect without any form of medical care. Several of the chapters in this book dwell at length on the escalating encounter of Tibetan medicine with biomedicine. This frequently involves attempts to respond to demands by authorities or, at times, equally to practitioners' own inclinations, to standardize, secularize, and thus legitimate practices. This association with science, often involving a mimesis of aspects of scientific practice, can result in validation of the very tradition of Tibetan medicine as a science.

Tibetan medical practitioners have also had to confront the enormous challenges posed by commoditization and the neoliberal global market, including direct-to-consumer advertising on the internet and mass production of standardized medications. Ingenious practitioners engage in negotiations with drug companies and NGOs about intellectual property rights and the market price for herbal medications, while the most obvious effect of the market locally is the creation of a scarcity of medicinal plants, increased expenses for treatment, and reduced access to medical practitioners by poor people. Healers in more remote areas exhibit other forms of flexibility in searching out new ways of legitimizing their authority and power; in Northern India, for example, religion may be self-consciously integrated into medical practice for political ends. Elsewhere, in Tibet, the symbolic power associated with Tibetan medicine, derived in large part from its historical association with Buddhism, holds, even under extreme duress.

The allure of Tibetan medical knowledge that so many of us experienced in the 1970s when reading for the first time Rechung Rinpoche's *Tibetan Medicine* is still alive, and accounts in large part for the success of this particular form of Asian medicine in the world today. But the moment the reader's attention is drawn, as it so often is in this book, to the effects this neo-colonial appetite for Tibetan medications and medical practices has on people living in the Himalayas, the allure is abruptly dissipated to be replaced by unhappy reflection on the far-reaching impact of the neoliberal global economy.

This book is good to think with; it has theoretical and practical import, and will surely revitalize research into Asian medical systems as a whole, even as it makes abundantly clear that detailed ethnographic knowledge about the context and specificities of Tibetan medical knowledge and practices are essential if we are to grasp the particular place it has in the world today.

Acknowledgements

It was an afternoon in the summer of 2001 when Calum Blaikie encouraged me to bring together specialist researchers on the social dimension of Tibetan medicine to come up with a book on the subject. We felt that such a volume was missing, despite the exponential increase in Tibetan medical studies worldwide, and were excited by the possibility that a book of this kind could both present the current state of scholarship in the domain and provide avenues for fruitful work in the future. We were in Ladakh together with a team of researchers working on Tibetan medicine in the framework of a regional programme supported by the Research Unit, Nomad RSI. The aim of this programme was to explore the transformations of Tibetan medicine, focusing on the social and political dimensions of medical practice. It provided the foundations for various publication projects and engaged me in conceptualizing the present volume. The support that Florian Besch, Stephan Kloos, Vincent Brisard and Pascale Hancart-Petitet also gave me in the field at that time was instrumental in transforming this volume from a vision to a reality.

I wanted to compile a volume that would bring a comparative scope to contemporary studies of Tibetan medicine, based on multi-sited research, while keeping the focus on its social and political aspects. In this respect, a number of scholars in Tibetan medical studies were invited to contribute, some of whom were specifically requested to research and write on predefined topics and others who were already working on issues within the proposed framework. The project then took shape over the next five years and can perhaps best be considered as a collective work – a characteristic that has greatly enhanced its coherence and added to its heuristic potential. Without the agreement and efforts of the authors, this book would not have come into existence. I am humbled by their enthusiastic reception of the proposal and their patience, and I gratefully acknowledge them all.

The initial project was further supported by the Centre de Recherche 'Cultures, Santé et Sociétés' (CReCSS) at the Paul Cézanne University in Aix-Marseille. I would like to extend my gratitude to Alice Desclaux and to my fellow researchers at the Centre.

During the editing phase of this book, I have been heading the Department of Social Sciences at the French Institute of Pondicherry. I wish to offer my sincere thanks to the Institute for its funding, as well as to my colleagues and friends for feeding me regularly with their insights and providing a great working atmosphere.

I offer special thanks to the forty or so members of the 'Societies and Medicines in South Asia' programme, who have contributed a great deal to both broadening and deepening my perspectives on health and healing in South Asia.

Besides the French Institute of Pondicherry, extra material support has been granted by the Transversal Programme 'Democratic Transformations in Emerging Countries', coordinated by the IFAS in Johannesburg for the French Ministry of Foreign Affairs. I would also like to acknowledge the French Ministry of Research and Technology and the French Ministry of Foreign Affairs for the support they have provided over these years.

I also wish to thank the people at the Needham Research Institute (NRI), Cambridge, for their support, and especially the NRI Director Christopher Cullen, who has been positive about this project ever since he first received the proposal. Susan Benneth at NRI has also been very helpful and reactive, and I would like to thank her sincerely. By the same token, Stephanie Rogers and her assistants Hayley Norton and Leanne Hinves at Routledge have greatly facilitated the smooth progress of the manuscript and its transformation into the present book. I thank Taï Walker for his early editorial assistance with some of the texts, Ann King for her work on parts of the manuscript, and Helen Moss for her work in copy-editing. The comments provided by two anonymous reviewers have also been instrumental in shaping the present form of the book.

I will not attempt to cite here all of those who have been inspirational and supportive during this project, and I apologize to those who have been overlooked. Some colleagues, in India and elsewhere, have been especially supportive both practically and intellectually. Besides those already cited, I first offer my warm thanks to Jean Benoist, for the inspiration he has brought to my work. I am also grateful to Madhulika Banerjee, Rémi Bordes, Margaret Lock, Evelyne Miccolier, Anne-Marie Moulin, Jean-Pierre Muller, Harish Naraindas, Taeko Okaniwa, David Picherit, Geoffrey Samuel and V. Sujatha. My greatest acknowledgements go to Fernand Meyer, who guides me in the complex field of Tibetan medical studies despite my many weaknesses. He has brought tremendous support to the project and offered invaluable reviewing and advice throughout. I thank him for his strict rigour and his kindness – a rare blend that only great teachers have.

On a sadder note, I must express my deep regrets. Yeshi C. Lama, an author in this book, died in a tragic helicopter crash in Nepal on 23 September 2006. A colleague and friend to some of us in this volume, Yeshi was a young and incredibly active woman who was entirely dedicated to the establishment of people-sensitive environmental conservation programmes in her country. This book is dedicated to her memory.

It is not my intention however to finish on such a poignant note. I would rather prefer to celebrate what is too often left in the shadows of academic scholarship. I shall therefore offer, on behalf of my co-authors, heartfelt thanks and gratitude to our many friends, *amchi* and others, in the Himalayas and elsewhere, to whom we entirely owe our ethnographies.

Laurent Pordié
Pondicherry

Introduction

1 Tibetan medicine today

Neo-traditionalism as an analytical lens and a political tool

Laurent Pordié

Notwithstanding a marked increase in academic publications pertaining to the contemporary dynamics of Tibetan medicine in the past two decades, the light cast in this domain by the social sciences is still diffuse and the corresponding studies are scattered.[1] There is no specialized work that thoroughly examines this medicine in diverse regions for a given period and, a remarkable fact, Tibetan medicine has long remained absent from fundamental collective works and special issues of international journals dealing with Asian medicines (cf. Bates 1995; Leslie 1976; Leslie and Young 1992; Pfleiderer 1988).[2] The only comparative endeavour was the work by Connor and Samuel (2001), who included in their book three chapters on Tibetan medicine (by Adams, Janes and Samuel) concerned with the Tibet Autonomous Region (TAR) and exiled Tibetans in India (Dalhousie). This edited volume examines the articulation between the global and the local in various Asian societies in order to account for the way in which modernity is manifested or produced through medicine by means of negotiation, appropriation and transformation. This was the first time that Tibetan medicine appeared in a work on social sciences specializing in Asian therapies. However, studies in comparative anthropology were never extended to the whole of the Tibetan cultural area, even though the first works on Tibetan medicine go back to the end of the 1980s (e.g. Adams 1988, 1992; Kuhn 1988; Meyer 1986, 1987, 1993) and the number of studies subsequently saw an exponential increase.[3]

This volume therefore occupies a space left vacant both by the anthropology of Asian scholarly medicines and by Tibetan studies. It thus responds to an imperative need for the advancement of research on Tibetan medicine by setting forth in a comparative approach the attention currently given to it in the social sciences and by deepening the knowledge developed up until now. The authors brought together in this book offer a collective reflection on the social, political and identity dynamics of Tibetan medicine in Nepal, India and the People's Republic of China (Tibet Autonomous Region and urban China), in Mongolia and in the West. The comparative perspective presented here obviously exhausts neither the questions relating to Tibetan medicine nor the areas in which it is found. Nevertheless, the subjects broached and the variety of contexts studied provide a heuristic dimension that makes it possible to obtain a reference image on this theme, as well as to reformulate a number of questions central to 'traditional' medicine and to the social and political fields of health. This book answers three fundamental questions: What are the modalities and the issues involved in the social and therapeutic transformations of Tibetan medicine? How are national policies and health reforms connected to the processes of contemporary redefinition of this medicine? What interpretive grid can one propose so as to obtain a circumspect understanding of Tibetan medicine in the current global context?

The social, political and identity dynamics, as well as the changes related to practice and, to a lesser extent, epistemology are today affecting Tibetan medicine with an intensity that is unequalled in the modern period (Adams 2001a, 2002a, 2002b; Janes 1995, 2001; Meyer 1993). Tibetan medicine is inscribed in the national and international medical, political and economic fields of contemporary history. It is thus redefined in the course of complex social processes involving state-controlled policies, the logics of a global liberal economy and the renewed aspirations of practitioners.[4] Moreover, the development of Tibetan medicine for the market brings about a change in medical provision on the national level (Janes 1999; Samuel 2001) and an unprecedented expansion on the international level (Janes 2002; Meyer 1986). Tibetan medicine today has an international character: the places where it is practised, the patients and the nature of therapeutic discourse extend beyond the Tibetan cultural area and idioms.

The anthropological investigation of these phenomena not only accounts for the social construction of this centuries-old medicine, but also provides information on the societies in which Tibetan medicine is endemic or imported, on the national and international modes of dissemination and on the types of relations it maintains with other health systems and other forms of Tibetan medicine in different geographic areas and among different ethnic groups.[5] Tibetan medicine must be studied in its plurality: the various areas in which it is found, their history, contemporary health policies, and social, economic and political configurations have shaped this medicine.[6] These changes correspond to varied contexts and allow over time the rising of socially, and to some extent medically, different medicines. There are, in a certain way, Tibetan *medicines*.[7] The generic term 'Tibetan medicine' tends to give the impression of homogeneity to what in fact remains, anthropologically speaking, deeply heterogeneous. It also contributes to ethnicizing medicine and does not reflect the way in which practitioners and populations from various Himalayan and Central Asian regions qualify Tibetan medicine in their own languages. Sowa Rigpa (*gso ba rig pa*[8]), which means the 'Science of Healing', is the term used in the vernacular in all of these regions. While making use of Sowa Rigpa in English is linguistically more accurate and sociologically significant in specific contexts, it also constitutes a supplementary generic in a general introduction such as this. In foreign languages, most non-Tibetans, apart from Western practitioners, differentiate their medicine from 'Tibetan medicine' for reasons pertaining to medical and social identities: 'Amchi medicine' is common in North-West India, 'Himalayan medicine' in Nepal, 'traditional medicine' in Bhutan, 'traditional Mongolian medicine' in Mongolia, or again 'Buddhist medicine' is common elsewhere. These terms are constructions essentially directed towards external use. They actually best express the various forms of Sowa Rigpa and the plurality of 'Tibetan medicine'. These qualifications being made, I will use the term 'Tibetan medicine' in the remainder of the text to simplify the reading.

In this context, it is expedient to then raise the question of the relations that the diverse types of Tibetan medicine maintain among themselves – in a limited geographic area (rural/urban) and between geopolitical entities (Nepal/Ladakh or Tibet/Mongolia). In turn, this plurality is involved in the emergence of local modernities. It sheds light on singular situations that make it possible to revise and adapt theories relating to the modern world (Adams 2001a) and to better understand the manner in which populations fashion their period. It also informs on the contemporary 'politics of culture' (Alter 2005) pertaining to Tibetan medicine.

The various forms and expressions of Tibetan medicine reflect sometimes divergent interests, giving rise to and/or underscoring relations of power. They constitute a rich field for the study of legitimating modalities used by the practitioners and their institutions. The processes of social and medical legitimization are at the centre of contemporary changes in Tibetan medicine. Their varied and sometimes conflicting expressions are largely part of the social redefinition of the practice. As shown by Didier and Eric Fassin (1988), the study of the types of legitimacy makes it possible to understand the social manoeuvres implemented by healers in their quest for legitimization. We will see in numerous chapters of this book that the implicit goal of the practitioners is to consolidate their social status and, at times, to reinforce their social power. Practitioners may use to their advantage the norms and rules governing the systems, and the situations through which these norms and rules are manifested (Balandier 1974). This process corresponds to an attempt to maximize power in the limits of the existing social order. It also contributes to forging the actors' political identity, which is directly situated in the medical field.

For the requirements of analysis, I will consider this field, in Bourdieu's sense (1980), as an autonomous space of social life structured by power relations between social groups, individuals and institutions. Therefore, societal issues, as characterized by conflicts of legitimacy and identity, also play a role in the medical field. These societal issues allow new places and new expressions of power to appear. The quest for legitimization thus imposes the political redefinition of its basic principles and prompts reformulation of the very question of legitimacy (Fassin and Fassin 1988). In this context, the examination of medical legitimacy must be linked to a study of social legitimacy and the logics underlying it. This approach would therefore be incomplete without focusing attention on the way contemporary transformations of Tibetan medicine pertain to identity, and to the corresponding strategies employed on the individual, collective and institutional levels. As much as, if not more than, the legitimacy of Tibetan medicine and its practitioners, it is also their identity that is called into question. Practitioners attempt to acquire valorized social identities and to reconstruct the coherence of their relation to others in a context of accelerated and increased transformations of social and power relations (Tonda 2001). It is, of course, incorrect to view the changes that result from these contemporary phenomena as simply passive responses to a dominant agent or system (Landy 1974). They are active transformations brought into play by the actors themselves (practitioners, but also institutions and entrepreneurs). They broaden and reconstruct the field of Tibetan medicine, while adapting it to new contexts.

This book has a dual purpose. It offers a rereading of Tibetan medicine in the twenty-first century both by considering the contemporary reasons that have led to its diversity and by bringing out the common orientations of this medical system, considered here as a social institution. Several tendencies reflect the contemporary situation: 1) the recourse to external instances of legitimization (such as bio-medicine, 'science' or national policies), juxtaposed with traditional orders of legitimacy; 2) the political re-invention of tradition according to historical and/or ecological arguments: 3) the multiplication of activities belonging to therapists, more particularly to those having entered the complex milieu of 'development'; 4) the industrialization, commoditization and marketing of medicine; and 5) the transnational diffusion of Tibetan medicine and deterritorialization of practitioners and practices. These phenomena may exist independently of each other or indeed intermingle. Although these tendencies assume a particularly crystallized form in the urban medical institutions, it should be noted that they are no less indicative of a general orientation, to which their even partial penetration into rural areas testifies (Pordié forthcoming). This book takes this into account by shifting the analysis from the non-institutionalized milieu to the urban institutional environment in Asia, and then in the West.

These observations suggest a renewal of the 'grids of interpretation' that are applied to Tibetan medicine. In this respect, I will consider the categories that are classically applied to medicines by proposing a descriptive model, namely neo-traditionalism, which will serve to circumscribe the contemporary tendencies characterizing Tibetan medicine. It will contribute an additional perspective to the chapters that make up this volume. Finally, I will conclude this general introduction by briefly examining the book's structure.

Interlude: An amchi in the city

Impeccably dressed in crimson flannel trousers and a mustard yellow shirt, a Buddhist rosary clasped between the fingers of one hand and a passport replete with visas clutched in the other, the *amchi* from the mountains of the western Himalayas returns to his country after another visit to the United States of America, where for two months he had delivered his teachings on his centuries-old medical art. I meet up with him again at the airport in Delhi. After exchanging the usual courtesies and evoking briefly our earlier encounters, we share a taxi to the city centre.

As soon as we get out of the car, the *amchi* invites me to accompany him to the nearest cybercafé. He wants to check his e-mail immediately. He announces proudly that he is expecting an official invitation abroad. This man, who a few years earlier had marvelled at my laptop computer, is today a confirmed internet user. He even amiably makes fun of me when he notices my astonishment at the speed at which his messages appear on screen. 'You stayed too long in the mountains', he says, and bursts out laughing. My surprise is total as I observe how the broadband connection seems so familiar to him, an extension of his worn fingers. Had I too fallen into the trap of assumptions regarding the static, backward-looking and inert character of so-called traditional societies?

These societies are often represented like artefacts, museum pieces inspiring vague feelings of loss. Other images depict decadent societies corrupted by the race towards progress or economic growth. Is it possible to view traditional societies in their contemporary state in a balanced manner? How do we avoid romanticizing their supposed 'tradition' and lamenting their 'modernity', seeing in the former an ideal and in the latter an appalling danger? In any case, that is not where the problem lies; these questions are red herrings for the anthropologist. These are contemporary societies, some of which use or re-invent their traditions in an attempt to better define their role in today's world. Tibetan medicine may be understood in this way. It is because it is 'traditional' that this branch of medicine is so coveted by societies that believe they have lost contact with their origins and the mysteries that go with them. Tibetan medicine 'speaks' to the West. This medical language has however been reinterpreted there; it fills a void in both the Western medical and the popular imagination.

So, after all, why not the internet for everyone? This mountain dweller with long hair tied in a chignon, a Tibetan physician by trade, a Tantric practitioner returning from the Americas with an ultra-bright smile and brand new spectacles, who happily gazes at me without being distracted by the Ray-Ban label still stuck to his left lens: why shouldn't he communicate with all corners of the planet thanks to a high-speed electronic connection? Why should this man remain trapped in the mountains, an image from a postcard or tourist's photo album, when his role is also to provide remedies for illnesses afflicting people elsewhere? We will accept for now that this is one of the profiles that globalization must assume. This *amchi* cannot be dismissed as inauthentic.

While I am thinking about all the issues that this encounter raises for me, a jumble of thoughts as disorderly as the section above, the *amchi* shakes me by the arm, bringing me back to the present. It's done; he will soon make another trip across the Atlantic. He does not attempt to conceal his candid joy; the diffusion and worldwide popularity of his medicine are a windfall for him.

We set off for a fast food restaurant at Connaught Place, a spot frequented by the trendy youth of Delhi. The *amchi* chooses this place, thinking I will enjoy it. As my host, he wants to entertain me in style. I am convinced he would have preferred a plate of momos, but the choice of fast food symbolizes his social status, a status consolidated by his travels. The restaurant's infamous golden arches are emblems of the West. We are even offered a small red and yellow cuddly toy representing the mascot of the international chain, 'for our children'. For a moment, I consider using mine as a voodoo doll before refusing it. Quite manifestly, the *amchi* and I have different perspectives on this type of place. But it doesn't matter; we discuss our common projects and the problems the Indian *amchi* from the rural milieu confront when practising medicine under better material and social conditions and, above all, in perpetuating them. Generally speaking, Tibetan medicine in the remote Himalayas is facing great difficulties in the very areas where it is the primary form of health care and often the only medical provision. This situation has been the subject of diverse so-called development programmes targeting rural populations, but the impact of these programmes has been marginal. My friend, moreover, is very actively involved in a local association devoted to the development of his medicine. Despite that, health development is left in the hands of the overwhelming majority of rural *amchi*. This situation is not found exclusively in the Indian Himalayas, but may be found throughout areas of Tibetan cultural influence.

Paradoxically, while Tibetan medicine today is foundering in the rural regions where it has been established for centuries, it is experiencing an unprecedented prominence at the international level. Its world expansion camouflages the mediocrity of the situation in the rural milieu where it is considered to be most vital. Tibetan medicine is today a global phenomenon. It has become a division of the international industrial edifice of alternative medicines. The development of Tibetan medicine is today characterized by clinical research and pharmacology, pharmaceutical industrialization and mass production of medicines, the modernization of urban hospitals and, above all, the implementation of export policies. Whether it is a question of Chinese pharmaceutical policies in Tibet, of post-socialist reconstruction of the health system in Mongolia or of programmes involving several million euros implemented by the European Commission in Bhutan, the fate of Tibetan medicine seems to be doomed to the vagaries of international commerce. Of course, the rural Tibetan world only ever sees scant benefits from this form of 'development'.

This medicine is accordingly produced and reproduced as an international commodity and is generally consumed for its indigenous traditional virtues. It embodies moral (Buddhist) values, and a Tibetan view of the world that exerts a notable seductive power in Western societies. It represents a medical, ecological and social alternative, while the very logics that make this medicine accessible in the West depend upon an ideological and economic domination to which its sympathizers would object in principle. This situation is part of the construction of the reality of the Tibetan world and of its medicine. The often idealistic preconceptions that beset them both do not necessarily help them, because they refine the camouflage mentioned above.

The Indian *amchi* listens to me between two mouthfuls of vegetarian hamburger. He seems conscious of the expectations the New World has of him and adds: 'You know, Laurent, I tell them something of what they expect me to tell them. I adapt myself but without, for all that, losing the essence of my teachings . . . What they want to see is the image they have made of me before seeing me. I actually put them in front of a mirror. It is themselves that they see in me . . . I reflect the ideas they have about the world.' In this way a virtual image of Tibetan medicine is propagated.

What is there to say about this *amchi* who embodies therapeutic globalization and is one of its vehicles? He travels the world to speak of his own world, but his own world today shares an increasing number of traits with the World itself. He represents an emerging fringe among the *amchi*, well beyond archetypal descriptions. He belongs to the very influential minority who have achieved a certain degree of social success. These therapists are often regarded as examples by their fellow *amchi*: they convey certain values and ideologies that are disseminated in their community of practitioners. That is how this medical art is in part socially redefined. Tibetan medicine is subject to profound social and practical reconstructions that put to a severe test the classical categorizations that are applied to it.

Tibetan medical neo-traditionalism

The contemporary dynamics of Tibetan medicine seem to defy classical categorization (e.g. Dunn 1976; Kleinman 1980). However, does that justify the development of another descriptive category? Would the effort of conceptual unification from which it would follow be in vain? It may be that one simply observes therapeutic reconstructions promoted by actors who reinterpret and re-elaborate discourses and practices according to what is made available in a given socio-cultural whole. Yet, as we just observed, there are an increasing number of portraits of Himalayan healers that largely depart from standard descriptions. However, is there really something new that would justify the use of the prefix 'neo' in conjunction with a medicine that was up until now seen as 'traditional'? This chapter provides a few elements in response: neo-traditionalism could thus characterize a diversification of healers' activities and a multiplication of legitimating instances, their proximity to biomedicine on the practical, epistemological and symbolic planes, or the fact that they would be both subject to and participants in globalization (deterritorialization of actors and practices, modern transnationalization of knowledge) and that they would make systematic use of 'tradition' to legitimate new practices.

Although neo-traditionalism disseminates an image of Tibetan medicine, it is also a concept that makes it possible to develop comparative studies and to propose paths of research. Neo-traditionalism accounts for a modern socio-political phenomenon. That is to say, neo-traditionalism both *describes* the contemporary trends that characterize Tibetan medicine and *represents* Tibetan medicine (as a potential political tool for the healers and their institutions). Neo-traditionalism involves various domains of medicine (ideology, practice) and modulates the political and social behaviours of the actors. It thus participates in the social construction of Tibetan medicine. Neo-traditionalism not only elucidates, and contributes to, social transformation; it also is involved in gradual medical innovation. While the changes are just perceptible in the latter domain, we will see that neo-traditionalism fosters innovation.[9]

Let us make an initial comment. Even though it would sometimes be used in the literature the concept has never been fully developed in the study of health systems. For more than two decades, anthropologists have observed the emergence of 'new healers', 'syncretic' healers and 'neo-TM practitioners', the proportion of whom among all healers is today increasing in a remarkable manner. There are healers who use biomedical products, concepts or symbols to legitimate their practice and assert their identity (Bourdarias 1996; Gruénais 1991; Leslie 1992; McMillen 2004; Wolffers 1988), members of the biomedical profession who use so-called traditional practices (Barges 1996), health practices that emerge from drawing a parallel between, or from the integration of, non-biomedical therapies and treatments related to an alleged tradition (Ghasarian 2005), in which the notion of 'energy' can become central (Benoist 1996; Schmitz 2005). Today, these new healers cannot be ignored in the therapeutic field (Le Palec 1996). Gruénais (2002), for example, taking up again the chronological classification by Last (1986), sees among these new healers a 'third generation' of healers in Africa. The latter reconstruct their practice without necessarily having recourse to biomedicine, but they are nevertheless in direct competition with it on the social, geographic and economic planes.[10] The study of these new healers reveals many other types of combination, borrowing as much from the medical as from the social and political domains. The list is long.

Their emergence is generally understood to be a product of cognitive, practical, social or political developments inscribed in the continuity of a medicine or of a given medical field. The essays collected in the recent book *Asian Medicine and Globalization* (Alter 2005) open up a fruitful avenue, examining the relationship between medicine and the national and transnational politics of culture, at the level of both the production of medical theory and the modern transnational flow of knowledge. These healers may also be viewed as showing new syncretic models that have become gradually independent of the systems from which they arose (e.g. Ernst 2002). Syncretism has moreover been understood by some authors as the continuation of a tradition in itself for a particular medical system. However, these *bricolages* of practices – hybrid therapeutic knowledge – and the renewed identities of these 'new healers' have not until now involved new descriptive categorizations in medical anthropology.

In the case of Tibetan medicine, this situation indicates a very clear caesura between diverse types of practitioners within one and the same system. This caesura is straightforward, and the reconfiguration of the therapeutic field (on local and global levels) that is engendered is profound. Modern institutionalization, the globalization of medicine, the appropriations of medical paradigms or the change in legitimacy thus account for the transformation of Tibetan medicine, characterized by rapid and fundamental changes (acceleration of social transformations, new directions). They have thus given rise to a new category of practitioners of Tibetan medicine, whom I propose to call 'neo-traditional'.

It is important to make clear that in what follows the term 'neo-traditional' will mainly serve to qualify these new practitioners of Tibetan medicine and to distinguish them from their counterparts. 'Neo-traditionalism' will be used to describe and circumscribe the social phenomenon – and its political ramifications – in which these new healers participate. In our case, neo-traditionalism is distinct from what Croizier calls 'pure traditionalism', a traditionalism that rejects what comes from Western science and medicine (Croizier 1976: 344). However, neo-traditionalism shares similarities with some forms of traditionalism involved in medical revivalism, such as promoting and making use of tradition while engaging in modernity, but it is not restricted to it. We will see that neo-traditionalism revisits and opens up traditionalism; it is rooted in and legitimized by tradition but it welcomes and provokes change and innovation. Its scale goes from the most localized areas to the wider global arena.

Change, identity and new practitioners

There is a strong identity dimension in the emergence of neo-traditionalism. A fringe of the medical elite today masters the art of expressing Tibetan medicine in terms of identity, not only among the Tibetans dramatically affected by China, but also in Mongolia, Ladakh or upper Nepal. However, Tibetan medicine's neo-traditional practitioners are not individuals with a weak legitimacy in their community. On the contrary, they generally come from legitimated milieux – by tradition (family, lineage) or institutionalization – and benefit from a high recognition. The situation consequently differs quite significantly from African medicine in which the 'new healers' seem to have suffered individually from a lack of legitimacy (Gruénais 2002; Tonda 2001).[11] Fassin observes in this regard that the therapists who have the least traditional legitimacy attempt to gain new forms of legitimacy (rational-legal) by positioning themselves on new terrains and by playing according to new rules (1994: 351).[12] For this reason, some Africanists use the adjective 'neo-traditional' in quite a pejorative way. Neo-traditionalism easily signifies imposture (cf. de Rosny 1996), thus condemning traditional practices to a certain inertia.

This is not the dominant tonality of neo-traditionalism in Tibetan medicine. These men and women are genuine therapeutic figures of modern times. In addition, while the identity strategies are borne by particular individuals – who thereby unquestionably consolidate their social status – these strategies also stem from institutions.

The identity to which I refer always ultimately has repercussions on the identity of the medicine. The identity claims concern the status of medicine as a social and medical institution, as well as the status of the whole community of practitioners or, in the case of the exiled Tibetans in particular, of the nation.

The transformation that neo-traditionalism both accounts for and engenders has a bearing on the *categories*. Tibetan medicine is both 'traditional' (in Tibet, Ladakh, Bhutan) and alternative (in Europe, the USA). The schematic descriptions to which systemic analyses give rise no longer allow that this medicine be explained as a *traditional* or *local system*.[13] The therapeutic field not only becomes blurred and more complex on the world scale, but also on the local scale. Although practised exclusively by the inhabitants of the regions of Tibetan culture, it is no longer exclusively theirs. A schism of classical diagnostic categories could be added when this medicine is delivered through the internet. Neo-traditionalism also involves a historical dimension. The actual situation exhibits unique characteristics in the development of Tibetan medicine since its genesis. The rapidity with which the changes occur, the magnitude of the geographic diffusion of medicine and the role that it obtains in the international health scenario are major characteristics.[14] The next caesura is social. The knowledge and ambitions of neo-traditional practitioners, who are generally boosted by an urban institutional environment, reinforce the subordination of their fellow practitioners, who are usually located in the rural areas. The existing congruence between social power and the forms of knowledge acquisition (institutionalization) thus appears very clearly among neo-traditional practitioners. Their aspirations go far beyond the (Tibetan) medical field. Neo-traditionalism today accounts for a very pronounced demarcation between healers. This divide pertains not only to medical erudition or techniques, or even to social status, but more generally to the *space of possibilities* that opens up to neo-traditional healers, inside or outside of their medical field, their regions of origin and their societies. However, the coexistence of classical, village-based healers and their neo-traditional homologues generally does not pose problems.[15] On the contrary, although they tend to be hierarchically ordered, each type of practitioner legitimizes the other: while most village-based healers become in a way guarantors of tradition (a central legitimating instance for the neo-traditional healers), their neo-traditional fellows embody a valued form of social success and are more directly equated with the exigencies of modern society. The contemporary success of the latter benefits the image of Tibetan medicine and its practitioners as a whole. As suggested, the change also potentially concerns, to a lesser extent, medical epistemology. Through exploring the space that is offered to them, the neo-traditional healers may be innovative and creative in the therapeutic field. As we will see below, they attempt to build 'epistemological bridges and shortcuts', without necessarily being disturbed by the incoherence therein.

Characteristics of neo-traditionalism

I do not suggest that there are currently uniform categories of practitioners of Tibetan medicine, or even that the neo-traditional practitioners would be homogeneous. However, neo-traditionalism in Tibetan medicine characterizes a new type of elite that has arisen in a new socio-political and economic environment. These therapists are practitioners who are generally institutionalized (associations, medical centres, government structures) in urban areas or located near urban centres and the social and political life of towns. They belong to a relatively well-educated fringe and often have a good command of the English language. Belonging to nationalities issuing mainly from the Himalayan chain, a tiny minority also comes from the West. These practitioners are regularly present on the political medical scene on the regional and/or global level. Although this is in itself nothing new for the Tibetan medical elite, apart from its global perspective, the political role of these neo-traditional practitioners is significant. As we understand it, neo-traditionalism grants a better political representation to Tibetan medicine. This characteristic does not suffice to define neo-traditionalism,[16] but explains it to a large extent.

A fundamental characteristic of neo-traditionalism concerns the *appropriation* of ideologies and epistemologies, the use of modern rhetoric and practices that are, at least initially, foreign to Tibetan medicine. The clearest example is that of biomedical science (concepts, apparatus, discourses). One could cite the use of the sphygmomanometer or of the ultrasound scan along with the traditional urine analysis, the emergence of biomedical concepts (immunity translated in humoral terms), the renaming of diseases according to biomedical terminology, the practice of clinical trials and so on.[17] Banerjee, for instance, used the term 'neo-traditionalism' in relation to biomedical science to refer to the emergence of ideological movements involving Ayurvedic medicine at the time of colonial modernity in India (2004: 89). The 'traditionalists', wanting to preserve the purity of the tradition as it is, confronted the 'neo-traditionalists', for whom the only way to preserve tradition was to make it conform to the modern orders of legitimacy, in particular reflecting biomedical authority.

Science is a tool used by neo-traditional Tibetan medical practitioners for 'confirming' the validity of Tibetan medicine as a science in itself.[18] These practitioners may also intend to show that the theories and findings of biomedical science were somehow anticipated in Tibetan medicine. In other words, they reverse the legitimizing principle mentioned above: indigenous medicine is then understood as validating modern science.[19] Generally speaking, the rapprochements with biomedicine and, in particular, the establishment of scientific proof, when it is the case, lend Tibetan medicine a presence superior in the global scenario. The normative dimension of science also tends to reduce differences between medical systems. In short, we witness a process of withdrawal from the *medical culture* that consequently allows *medicine*, as a category, to appear more clearly. This process, by making Tibetan medicine more universal, favours all the more its commercial development on both national and international levels (Pordié 2005).

However, the principle of appropriation does not happen only with respect to biomedical science and ideology. Some individuals trained in Tibetan medicine do not hesitate to integrate theoretical or practical elements from other types of non-biomedical therapies. There are Tibetan doctors who practise Chinese acupuncture or offer reiki and 'singing bowls' healing sessions together with their medicine, and Western practitioners of Tibetan medicine who combine in the same manner various alternative approaches to healing with their own. Conversely, other practitioners, including biomedical personnel, may integrate what they consider to be Tibetan medicine (or 'Tibetan medical philosophy') into their practice as an attempt to bring new, alternative approaches to health care.[20] This trend gives a new tinge to Tibetan medicine and facilitates its entrance to the 'mystic-esoteric nebula' (Champion 1994) of the New Age milieu in the West (see Vargas, Chapter 9).[21] These medical practices embody ideologies that attempt in particular to evade the individualism and formidable materiality of industrial societies. While their status was once located at the cultural periphery of Western societies, these healing practices have today become increasingly closer to the centre. They convey a morality of being and well-being. This morality is based on holistic, energy-based, even transcendental, and generally pro-environmentalist, medical discourses.

The appropriation of environmentalist narratives and precisely the idea of nature as aesthetics central to medicine also constitute a main feature of Tibetan medical neo-traditionalism. The idea that people living in distant places from Western powers and Western cultural norms are closer to nature has particularly marked out the Orientalist discourses (Clarke 1997). As far as Himalayan Buddhists are concerned, their religion is commonly perceived as compatible with conservation and environmentalist agendas.[22] Buddhists are generally thought to be inherently ecologists (Huber 1997). Such discourses are today adopted by the neo-traditional practitioners of Tibetan medicine and translated into medical language. The integration of ideas concerned with the benefits of medicine as 'natural medicine' devoid of secondary effects and near to the 'natural' functioning of the body reflects this tendency. 'Environmental awareness' is a modern production, the appropriation of which in the medical field of traditional societies is facilitated if it is established on a basis that is meaningful for local actors. In this respect, the five elements theory in Tibetan medicine and the resulting similarity between microcosm and macrocosm allow a closer connection of the medical discourse to certain holistic ideologies that are prevalent among ecology movements. In Ladakh, the omnipresent mountains, where the basic essentials of plants and minerals are found, are the archetype 'of nature valued as good and pure' (Dollfus and Labbal 2003: 94), which also greatly facilitates the shifting of nature to the medical sphere. Beyond the merging of traditional conceptions and relatively recent concepts, these discourses are elaborated in counterpoint to the structural and therapeutic 'violence' of biomedicine, both in the East and the West.[23] They favour natural treatments, the 'taking into account of the individual in his totality', and underscore the importance of the relation between patient and therapist in the healing process. The Tibetan medical discourse turns towards the patient and tends to redefine his relationship to healing as well as to the body/bodies.[24] It is directed at the behaviours of users and is manifested through Buddhist ethics and the related modes of relation to others and to the environment.

The ecology of the theoretical medical foundations mentioned above therefore also results from a principle of accentuation – and/or distortion – of existing characteristics of Tibetan medicine. The same is true for external and manual therapies pertaining to re-invented traditions in the East,[25] to Tibetan treatments with minerals and crystals in the West, and to the practical reinterpretation of massage (*bsku mnye*) as described in the classic texts. This kind of *selective accentuation* is very typical of neo-traditionalism. In this light, neo-traditionalism also reappraises the relation between medicine and religion. The growing market of Tibetan medicine in the West and for Westerners is largely based on a practice that accentuates very adroitly the presence of religious foundations. Some authors have thus emphasized the display of symbolic religious objects (i.e. *thang kha*) and the contemplative mood or the quasi-monastic atmosphere that is to be found in the clinics in this context (Janes 2002; Samuel 2001).[26]

The media are also instrumental in diffusing partial, approximate or distorted images of Tibetan medicine, along lines which unwittingly reflect neo-traditionalist features. The media propagate neo-traditionalism and make it more real than the real thing. 'Tibetan medical spirituality', 'Tibetan crystal therapy', the efficacy of 'natural' medicines for certain ailments, and the inherent ecological ethics of medicine and its practitioners are some recurrent themes alternatively or simultaneously put to the fore, so as to meet the desires and fantasies of both the users and the market.

However, we should bear in mind that the emphasis of a presumed spiritual dimension in Tibetan medicine may also be combined with the de-contextualization of the practice from its religious foundations (through science). The 'scientific tradition' and the 'religious tradition' can be used by practitioners of Tibetan medicine according to context as instances of legitimization and identity (Pordié 2003). They make acceptable, respectively, the withdrawal and the underscoring of religion. Thus, neo-traditionalism, by borrowing from multiple orders of legitimacy, makes it possible to reconcile ostensibly contradictory characteristics (scientific medicine/spiritual medicine). The pharmaceutical industry typically combines these aspects. The search for new products derived from Tibetan medicine is scientific (clinical trials, screening of isolatable active principles). Marketing and packaging then combine this modern scientific character (legitimating tradition at the same time) with the myth of Shangri-La and the whole esoteric dimension that goes with it. In the West, Mainland China or Tibet itself, this kind of strategy favours selling to consumers who want to take with their medicines a portion of Tibet itself.[27]

Indeed, neo-traditionalism is found in the pharmaceutical milieu, which revisits the tradition through new galenic methods and sometimes modifies the ancestral formulae, or creates 'new ancestral formulae', so as to facilitate market penetration. The legitimating order of these new products is precisely the 'medical tradition' to which they supposedly belong. The 'remedies' can therefore also have a neo-traditional character.[28] The same holds for the reformulation of the contents of contemporary institutional training, which discards in some instances modules involving the preparation of medicines, and incorporates elsewhere rudiments of biomedicine (Garrett 2005; and, in this volume, Adams and Li, Chapter 5; Janes and Hilliard, Chapter 2; Millard, Chapter 8).

Thus, neo-traditional Tibetan medicine is partially or largely a reconstructed medical practice. These combinations lead to new discourses, knowledge and practices, the legitimacy of which, for its part, rests explicitly on the therapeutic tradition, whether real or invented. Neo-traditionalism is based on tradition as much as it allows the tradition to be legitimated. It is also for this reason that neo-traditionalism, which arises from and accounts for a multiple schism in Tibetan medicine and which largely borrows elements foreign to 'tradition', stands in a relationship of continuity with the latter.

The next order of central characteristics of neo-traditionalism extends these principles. It is a matter of *multiplication and diversification* of the medical practitioners' activities.[29] The physicians of today must be, undeniably, more so than in the past, technicians and specialized bureaucrats (health care, development, research). They diversify their activities and redefine their social role. They are involved in the defence of intellectual property rights relating to medicinal plants (Pordié, Chapter 6, this volume); they become environmentalists and intervene in the framework of conservation (Aumeeruddy-Thomas and Lama, Chapter 7, this volume). They depart from the field of medical technique to act as developers (Craig, Chapter 3, this volume). This extension of the domain of classical (therapeutic) activity to that of development – in which conservation, indigenous rights, and health care fall – ensures that healers gain or consolidate their social status. As for those in responsible positions in associations or specific programmes, development facilitates entry into a fringe of the urban intellectual elite. Although these are also conditions to enter 'development' (higher education, social network and status), they are originally circumscribed within one particular field, here Tibetan medicine. The particularity of development is that it confers recognition on a larger scale, beyond the (social and technical) boundaries delimiting the original field. The multiplication of activities of neo-traditional healers shows the capacity of (individual) subjects to be recognized as social actors.

As the case of development indicates, neo-traditionalism accentuates the larger social networks (Castells 1996), rather than the very group of origin, as the main structural concept. This appears all the more clearly in its following characteristic: the *transnationalization* and the physical or virtual (internet) *deterritorialization* of Tibetan medicine (institutions, practices and practitioners).[30] The most reputed practitioners traverse the world to give lectures and seminars, even at elite universities; clinics of Tibetan medicine are established in various European countries and in America; the origin and the places where Tibetan physicians practise no longer reflect the 'ethnographic Tibet' (see the chapters in this volume by Millard, Vargas and Tokar – Chapters 8, 9 and 10); medicines are dispensed subsequent to virtual consultation. By moving around geographically, Tibetan medicine changes status. Once an indigenous medicine, it becomes an alternative medicine. Such aspects have been underscored by Micollier (2004), through a study of the international diffusion of the religious form of Chinese *qi gong*. This author shows how this diffusion relies, on the one hand, on the representation on the internet of *qi gong* schools and masters and, on the other, on the establishment of social networks.[31] Micollier describes the process of transnationalization as a circular phenomenon of 'deterritorialization' and of 're-territorialization' that is also relevant in the case of Tibetan medicine. First, the practice is transformed according to 'contextualities' and follows an intrinsic logic of global practices and local significations. Second, this international diffusion grants the practice social status from which it benefits back home (ibid.). Indeed, Tibetan medicine takes various shapes and meanings according to locations and conjectures, and its international popularity confers on it a new order of legitimacy in numerous countries where it is endemic or very ancient. Alter moreover shows in the case of Asian medicines how 'transnationalisms, in highlighting links or possible links, either destabilize medicine as a category or complicate its structure, function and meaning' (2005: 16).

The neo-traditional healers contribute not only to the diffusion of medicine (as a total and unfragmented entity) but also, and perhaps mainly, to the diffusion of some key and selected concepts, to behaviours, to imaginative worlds concerned by a particular medical tradition. Hence, while it is true that the market for Tibetan medicine dramatically increased during the past decade, it is not only medicine per se which is marketed but also a way of life that goes with it. This way of life then becomes another commodity to consume and sell (Lau 2000).

I mentioned earlier the new international scope acquired by Tibetan medicine (diffusion, therapeutic validation, international clientele), and the way this 'universalization' strengthens the very category of medicine, but it must be said that it does not, for all that, completely replace the culture that a given 'medicine' embodies. On the contrary, it also diffuses fragments of culture, such as a certain *Lebensphilosophie*.[32] As already noted, the combination of science and Tibetan culture not only is favourable to the introduction and success of Tibetan medicine in the international market of alternative medicines, but furthermore gives substance and magnitude to identity claims. This linkage is adroitly mastered by neo-traditional practitioners (Pordié, Chapter 6, this volume). Neo-traditionalism contains the necessary elements to foster regionalist and nationalist claims. Thus, a nationalist tonality readily coexists with the universalist ideal in the new forms of Tibetan medicine.

Towards a descriptive and political category?

What I propose in this text gives a representative idea, without, however, claiming to be comprehensive. The analysis is confined to Tibetan medicine and must not be extrapolated without adjustments or revisions except, perhaps, for Asian scholarly medicine – and that too only with extreme prudence. Not all terms characterizing neo-traditionalism have been exhausted, and neo-traditionalism is only one possible way for interpreting the contemporary tendencies in Tibetan medicine. However, although it does not involve all locations and forms of Tibetan medicine, the penetration of therapeutic neo-traditionalism as a social fact becomes increasingly prominent. It must also be said that, however significant neo-traditionalism may be for the anthropologist, it does not always imply dramatic changes in the practice (and, even less so, theory) of Tibetan medicine. The degree to which medicine is transformed or affected may vary from one context to the other. Furthermore, the neo-traditionalist features I described do not mean that neo-traditional Tibetan medicine is a diluted form of a more authentic Tibetan medicine. Therapeutic neo-traditionalism is indicative of the course and development of Tibetan medicine, as much as it reveals the social transformations surrounding medical practice. The fields in which neo-traditionalism is manifested contain the medical system but are not limited to it. This descriptive model can be of help in understanding Tibetan medicine today.

Neo-traditional practitioners are the best placed to respond to the actual challenges of their medical system, being located precisely at the interface of the societies of Tibetan culture and the worlds that encompass them. They are able to make connections between and actuate contradictory and/or distant sectors. A few fundamental characteristics have been included in this chapter: individual, collective and institutional inflection of neo-traditionalism; multiplication of practitioners' activities; complete or partial appropriation of modern ideologies and rhetoric (environmentalism, development), and of medical practices and, to a lesser extent, epistemologies (biomedicine and 'alternative medicines'); selective accentuation of existing characteristics, such as the reorganization of religion around medicine; transnationalization and deterritorialization of practices and practitioners; and development of information and communication technologies.[33]

Neo-traditional practitioners and institutions thus mobilize diverse orders of legitimacy, borrowing as much from the ideologies of modernity as from science or from the ancestral ethic and moral foundations of the medical practice. The types of legitimacy are also multiple according to the levels with which they are concerned and on which they are based, ranging from the local to the global. Neo-traditionalism both induces the actors to find new modes of legitimization and highlights them. However, neo-traditional practitioners systematically use tradition in their quest for legitimization and refuse to break with it. Conversely, they in return are instrumental in legitimating it. The tradition to which they refer can be geographically and temporally distant, localized or universalized, real or invented. Types of legitimacy meet, but today they always include references to a certain 'tradition'. This, and the fact that the neo-traditional healers practise, above all, Tibetan medicine and are generally grounded in their communities of origin, is the reason why neo-traditionalism is perceived as a continuous process in the evolution of the system.[34]

The neo-traditional actors construct and reconstruct their medicine, not with the aim of radically changing it or in order to create a new therapy, or even simply to improve it, but so as to meet political and economic, individual and collective objectives. Neo-traditionalism is therefore intimately enmeshed with issues pertaining to the social and medical identities of both the practitioners and their medicine. It gives rise to strategies of identity that materialize in the mixing of domains that are mutually exclusive in terms of classical socio-epistemological orthodoxies (Tonda 2001). Neo-traditionalism helps to mitigate a certain deficit of social and medical legitimacy of the medicine-as-institution, which does not, as noted above, refer to a lack of individual legitimacy within the community of practitioners. Furthermore, the identity dimension which is involved in the rise of neo-traditionalism also consolidates the latter: every register of medicine brought into play by such healers subsequently becomes a pole of identity for the whole community. Neo-traditionalism fashions a space of collective representation, which is also a relational space that reassures the practitioners and gives them new points of reference in contexts where Tibetan medicine is challenged.

Neo-traditionalism also renders Tibetan medicine compatible with other cultures and other worlds, without for all that renouncing its anchorage in its identity, culture and history. In this way, it possesses a certain political dexterity in gaining access to new geographical and identity territories. The role of the media and of new information technologies is here very central and relays neo-traditionalism. Neo-traditionalism forms a new category for the classification of medicine that makes it possible to circumscribe certain attributes of so-called 'postcolonial' sciences. Therapeutic neo-traditionalism goes beyond boundaries and reappraises orthodoxies.

Neo-traditionalism is both a descriptive tool for analysis and a socio-political phenomenon contributing to the global development of Tibetan medicine, as it combines economic growth, legitimization of tradition, cultural preservation and relative localization of power. It represents a modern type of relationship of authority and legitimization. Neo-traditionalism is not content to challenge and transform political behaviours; it also affects the social structures of Tibetan medicine. It modulates the loci where power is expressed and gives rise to new power relations. Neo-traditional practitioners indeed constitute an influential and decisive elite. They are veritable men and women of power.

We may therefore ask if the Tibetan medical neo-traditionalism of today does not foreshadow the Tibetan *traditional* medicine of tomorrow.

The book in a nutshell

The preceding sections have gone through the book by contextualizing or developing some of the texts composing it. It is therefore now time to briefly present the sequence and specific content.

The first part of this volume explores the modern institutionalization of Tibetan medicine in Mongolia, Nepal, the Tibet Autonomous Region, and Mainland China, with a special emphasis on legitimization and identity. Institutionalization comprises here the logics of both governmental structures and contemporary associations of healers. It is a process that produces the neo-traditional elite. The chapters forming this part show how institutionalized Tibetan medicine leads to a modification of the types of legitimization, and how these new legitimization modalities create new relationships between practitioners on the one hand and medicine and the state on the other. The role of individuals in the construction of their future within their institutions is also explored in these chapters and, by the same token, in the construction of the future of their institutions. Craig R. Janes and Casey Hilliard use a comparative approach to show how the historical events in Mongolia and Tibet in the context of late-twentieth-century capitalist development and post-socialist state processes have produced distinct local medical traditions and thus different identities. As for medicine in Mongolia, about which very little has been known up until now, these authors show how this re-invented tradition is today particularly intended for the global market. This comparative view highlights the degree to which global-level forces – economic and ideological – as transformed by state constructions of science and national identity affect the training, practice and accessibility of Tibetan and Mongolian medicines on the local level. The question of identity is central in the chapter by Sienna R. Craig. She studies the professionalization of the Nepali *amchi* through the ethnography of a practitioners' association. The effort of construction and explanation the *amchi* undertake regarding their professional identity reveals the weakness of their position in the nation-state. This author thus shows how practitioners in Nepal are reshaping their collective identity as healers, as Nepali citizens and as practitioners of a Tibetan healing system. Chen Hua concludes this part by describing the nature and modalities of the diffusion of Tibetan medicine in various regions of the People's Republic of China. This chapter does not constitute a theoretical reflection on Tibetan medicine but should be taken as a representative documentation of Tibetan medicine, to which this volume provides further problematization and political nuance.[35] This contribution contains, however, precise and detailed factual materials that were not readily accessible until now, partly because they rely on literature in the Chinese language.

Part II explores the politics of knowledge in the Tibetan world. Vincanne Adams and Fei-Fei Li study the significance and practical realities of 'integrative medicine' in the context of Lhasa's Mentsikhang (*sman rtsis khang*) efforts to survive in the climate of creeping biomedicalization. The authors are interested in the areas in which medical theories, practical knowledge and epistemologies conflict,[36] as well as in the domains in which the political and economic imperatives of biomedical modernity tend to dramatically affect the practice of Tibetan medicine. Based on a perspective that is first historical and then epistemological, the authors examine the meaning, practice and consequences of medical integration in the case of diagnosis, therapeutic treatment and the interpretation of results. While integration can appear in a quite naïve way to be a valid means of medical synergy (cf. Lee 2001), in reality, the encounter between biomedicine and Tibetan medicine generally takes place to the detriment of the latter. The encounter is systematically expressed in a normative framework in which the scientific markers are intended to delimit the realm of possible actions. The singularity claimed by Tibetan medicine is first advanced, to then be gradually swallowed up and diluted in clinical practice. In this context, the idea of *medical disintegration* appears to be more appropriate.[37] In Tibet, 'the effort to integrate in Lhasa's Mentsikhang most often means adopting biomedical standards and authority and eliminating perceptions that Tibetan medicine is capable of advancing on its own, by its own rules or standards' (Adams and Li, Chapter 5). Although biomedical epistemology is in no way wholly accepted by the practitioners of Tibetan medicine, and generally not considered as an absolute truth to which the relative truth of Tibetan medicine must be subordinated, biomedicine fulfils its normative function. The complex and non-egalitarian nature of medical integration thus devalues Tibetan medicine. This chapter indicates the precariousness of the Tibetan medical identity in contemporary Tibet, as well as the new forms through which it reveals itself when confronted with biomedicine. The chapter that I wrote also investigates the encounter between Tibetan medicine and biomedicine, and the way biomedical power is locally domesticated in the context of bioprospecting. This study is concerned with bio-pirates, imaginary pharmaceutical industries and the (at times virtual) theft of medical knowledge in India. In this country, a series of measures bearing on the utilization, protection and preservation of phytogenetic resources and related knowledge have been established. Intellectual property rights regimes are one such measure. This national movement has repercussions throughout the land, including Ladakh, a region of the north-west Himalayas. However, although the local protagonists agree to follow the national policy, they redefine its meaning and purposes to serve their interests on the levels of their community and of national society. This chapter is therefore concerned with questions of social, ethnic and medical identities, which are expressed through 'hijacking' a relatively new subject in the field of medicine in Ladakh: intellectual property rights. This situation must not be understood as a product of modernity but as a conjectural element favourable to the introduction of Tibetan medicine to modernity, which has in turn the power to transform modernity. In both Craig's chapter and my chapter, the *amchi* hold off the force of external and dominant powers – medicine, state, religion – over their own world. They endeavour in these contexts to consolidate their community and/or individual power, to affirm their ethnicity and their medical identity. In these cases, indigenous medicine is an effective means of expressing medical and social identities in societies dominated by other health care systems and in which the non-Hindu minorities are largely marginalized. These *amchi*, in Dolpo or in Ladakh, must however combine a particular identity in their country, Buddhist but Nepali or Indian, with a medicine known and recognized as Tibetan. The actuation of a Tibetan medical identity, of minority ethnic and religious identities in Nepal or in India, and a national identity in each of these cases, characterizes these therapists. To conclude this part, Aumeeruddy-Thomas and Lama explore the manner in which Tibetan physicians in a region of upper Nepal have entered, at a particular point in global conservation history, into certain forms of partnership with local and foreign conservationists. They examine how the process of forming these partnerships has created new social dynamics. Such an encounter between different worldviews, knowledge systems and practices carries various epistemological and social implications. In this context, the authors study the reciprocal redefinitions of practices and representations between the *amchi* and the team of an environmental conservation project. While this approach is essential to elaborate, community-based conservation programmes (Law and Salick 2007), Aumeeruddy-Thomas and Lama also show how the idea of 'local knowledge' is reconstructed in the process, and examine the consequences of this reconstruction in the practice of conservation and the future of Tibetan medicine.

This encounter between global politics and local practices ushers in Part III of this book, where we deal with the relations between the West and Tibetan medicine.

The chapter by Colin Millard provides a reflection on four domains in which Tibetan medicine must adapt itself in the United Kingdom: the legal domain, the socio-economic and political environment, 'medical ideology' and clinical practice. Millard provides a detailed analysis of what persists in Tibetan medicine, or is reinforced, and what is transformed, or disappears. This chapter revises the idea of monolithic 'traditional' Tibetan medicine by offering a framework for comparison with the practice of medicine in a particular context in Nepal. It shows not only the perspicacity of the actors in defining a new form of political efficacy for Tibetan medicine, but also the plasticity and the tolerance of Tibetan medical paradigms (Meyer 1987; Pordié 2007). Such tolerance is largely explored in the West, as Ivette Vargas shows, by reviewing the transformation of Tibetan medicine in the American state of Massachusetts. The medicine becomes energy-based, overlaps with the nebulous domain of Tibetan spiritualism and is reconstructed through additions of therapeutic practices. This chapter approaches in particular the scene of alternative therapies (and therapists) at Harvard University, where heterodoxy appears to prevail. This situation accounts for the composite tendency in North America in terms of 'alternative medicines'. Tibetan medicine becomes there a 'holistic medicine', particularly calling to mind the discourses of the millenarian movements. This part concludes with a chapter written 'from the inside' by a Western practitioner of Tibetan medicine. Eliot Tokar firmly takes sides. He rejects the current approaches to the integration of Tibetan medicine into the modern medical industrial complex, which subjects this branch of medicine to certain corrosive vagaries of globalization, especially in the form of bio-piracy and the hegemony of biomedicine. Based on his own Tibetan medical practice in New York City, the author enquires in particular about the rapprochements between Tibetan medicine and the industry of complementary and alternative medicines (orchestrating especially the ballet of dietary supplements and nutriceuticals). Tokar shares his opinion on the social, moral and medical significance of the transformation of Tibetan medicine in the context of American normative public health policies. In this context, this chapter shows the manner in which the author/practitioner views and constructs his neo-traditional practice, so as to evolve a medicine that is, as far as its legitimization is concerned, traditional. Most significantly, he further shows how his clinical setting advances the translation of Tibetan medical concepts and terminology in a way that both is intended to be faithful to its theory and makes it accessible and useful to the broad spectrum of patients living in New York City. This section offers a fundamental perspective on 'Tibetan-medicine-as-a-medical-alternative' and on the profound social modifications of which it is a reflection.

This book thus opens up several research paths. It marks out trails that we may follow to the end, but which quite distinctly clear prospective avenues for the researcher, the student or the informed layman. The encounter of social sciences and Tibetan medicine set forth in this book hopes to contribute in a constructive manner to studies on Asian medicine. Tibetan medicine has never before been the subject of such a broad collective reflection, even though today it plays a role that is far from being socially and sociologically insignificant on local and international levels. Moreover, Tibetan medicine has been undergoing for more than a decade a development that is as remarkable as it is ambivalent. One witnesses today the entrance of this medicine into a major new period in its history. Its popularity, the magnitude of its diffusion and its international dynamism indicate a very clear change of scale and a no less considerable change of course. The golden century that Tibetan medicine experienced from the second half of the seventeenth century (Meyer 1997) appears set to repeat itself at the beginning of the twenty-first century. But it remains to be seen if the gold in question should still be understood metaphorically, or if the literal sense will prevail at the risk of Tibetan *medicine* itself.

Notes

1 Despite their fundamental interest for our research, I intentionally omit works on history, philology and medical theory that do not directly concern the subject of this book (e.g. Avedon *et al.* 1998; Finckh 1980, 1985, 1994; Garrett 2006; Gyasto 2004; Meyer 1981, 1987, 1990, 1992a, 1992b, 1995; Parfionovitch *et al.* 1992; Rechung 1973).

2 I will forgo in this introduction a detailed review of these important works on Asian medicines, in particular what they have provided in terms of epistemological understanding. The interested reader may consult the texts by Connor (2001) and by Lock and Nichter (2002).

3 We note nevertheless the existence of collective publications on Tibetan medicine that ensued as a result of conferences and in which a number of social science articles appeared. These are the proceedings of the International Symposium on Tibetan Medicine organized in 1996 in Germany (Aschoff and Rösing 1997) and the proceedings of the International Academic Conference on Tibetan Medicine, which took place in Lhasa in 2000 (CMAM 2000). However, these two volumes were inadequately disseminated, and their comparative dimension in social sciences is absent. The recent publication of the proceedings of a seminar on Tibetan medicine (Sources, Concepts and Current Practices) organized in 2006 in Metz by the French Society for Ethnopharmacology (Fleurentin and Nicolas 2006) also comprises papers that do broach social issues, but their essential relevance for current research lies in the ethno-botanical factual data presented therein. While it was not designed with the exclusive aim of exploring the contemporary social dimensions of Tibetan medicine, I shall also mention the Special Issue of the *Tibet Journal* (Boesi and Cardi 2006), which brings an interesting contribution to Tibetan medical scholarship (history, anthropology, ethno-botany and medical theory). More directly related to this volume is the forthcoming publication of the proceedings of the Panel on Tibetan Medicine held during the Tenth Seminar of the International Association for Tibetan Studies, Oxford (Schrempf 2007), which contributes a range of comparative material that partially mitigates the shortcoming mentioned above.

4 The usual Tibetan word for a practitioner of Tibetan medicine, which occurs in both colloquial contexts and the classical texts, is *sman pa*. Practitioners may also be called *am chi* or *em chi* (*amchi*). This is a Mongolian loan word, which is widely used in Himalayan areas for traditional physicians. The term *lha rje* also qualifies the practitioners and/or their families in some regions. Bhutan is a unique case where the practitioners are called *drung tsho*, although this term may also designate elsewhere in the Himalayas a family in which healers are or have been present. Increasingly in Asia and in the West, practitioners are called doctors and may adopt the title 'Doctor'. This is a potentially controversial matter insofar as in the West the title 'Doctor' used in the medical context takes on a legal connotation. Where this is the case, the authors in this

book have used the term *amchi* or the title Doctor, which corresponds to the common usage in their field of research.

5 Tibetan medicine is found among communities scattered from west to east along the Himalayan chain, in India (Ladakh, Himachal Pradesh, Sikkim and Arunachal Pradesh), in Nepal (Mustang, Dolpo and the Mount Everest region), in the People's Republic of China (Tibet Autonomous Region, Yunnan, Sichuan, Qinghai and inner Mongolia) and in Bhutan, as well as in Mongolia and in Buryatia. It is also practised in urban China as far as Hong Kong and Beijing, and is exported with some success to the West.

6 While the geographical origin of Tibetan medicine is Tibet, I do not imply that some original and unique form of 'Tibetan medicine' had existed at some point in history. The early various schools and lineages have led to more or less significant diversity. Intra-local variations and heterogeneity of knowledge and practice also characterize Tibetan medicine.

7 In the same way as there exist diverse forms of biomedicine (cf. Berg and Mol 1998; Lock 1980).

8 A note regarding transcription in this volume: the terms are transliterated in accordance with the system devised by Turrell Wylie (1959) for the Tibetan language. Phonetic transcriptions are generally given in the case studies and refer to the local pronunciation of Tibetan and/or Tibetan dialects, which vary greatly across the Himalayas (the physician of Tibetan medicine, for example, transliterates as *sman pa*, and is pronounced as *menpa* in Tibetan or *smanpa* in Ladakhi). They are followed by the transliteration in brackets. One exception concerns the name of the Tibetan College of Medicine and Astro-computation (*sman rstis khang*), which, following the common usage, is written Mentsikhang for the Lhasa-based original institution, and Men-Tsee-Khang for the reinstituted college in Dharamsala, India. Transliteration alone will be given for Tibetan terms when the region is not specified.

9 On the subject of innovation in pre-modern Chinese medicine, see the excellent volume edited by Hsu (2001). In our case, however, medical innovation does not happen systematically through the 'interplay of convention and controversy', for, as we will see, controversy does not characterize Tibetan medical neo-traditionalism as such.

10 Gruénais calls the third generation '*néo-tradipraticiens*' – using the neologism '*tradipraticiens*' created by the Organization of African Unity (OAU) and later diffused by the World Health Organization (WHO) in French-speaking countries – and divides it into six classes (Gruénais 2002: 225–229).

11 There exist, however, cases where the neo-healers have a traditional legitimacy in Africa, but they seem to belong to a recent and emerging fringe.

12 Parallel to this, the development of therapeutic neo-traditionalism has greatly benefited from the poor image of biomedicine in Africa in the context of an inadequate health system (Dozon 1995).

13 I refer to the works by Kleinman (1980) and Dunn (1976) which, notwithstanding their high heuristic value, no longer reflect the contemporary situations of numerous health practices.

14 Although the phenomenon is today at the height of expansion (Janes 2002), it nevertheless dates back more than twenty years. Meyer (1986) has already analysed the reasons for the diffusion of Tibetan medicine in the West, and Leslie observed in 1980 that Asian medicines were an integral part of the globalized world. See also Leslie (1989).

15 When dissension occurs, it is more likely to happen between neo-traditional practitioners in the form of jealousy of displays of wealth, foreign travel and so on.

16 For instance, the Ayurvedic revivalist movement during the last century in India was deeply political. Brass spoke of this movement in terms of 'traditionalistic revivalism' (1972).

17 In this volume, Adams and Li provide a detailed ethnography of 'integrative' processes pertaining to Tibetan medicine. On clinical trials, see Adams (2002a) and Adams *et al.* (2005).

18 Throughout the Tibetan world, Tibetan medicine claims to be a 'science' (*rig gnas*) on its own terms, that is, a traditional domain of knowledge that is logical, valid and proved. While the practitioners distinguish the science of healing (*gso ba rig pa*) from 'modern' science (*tshan rig*), this distinction accounts for a certain art of equilibrium and ambiguity between what constitutes science and knowledge. Vincanne Adams has moreover explored the ambiguous relations that science maintains with the sacred, in the case of the Tibet Autonomous Region, in a very interesting work on the semantic uses of science by physicians and on related discursive strategies (Adams 2001b). See also Adams (2002b). Audrey Prost has explored the meaning and practices of Tibetan translation of science among exiled Tibetans, the aim of which is not to promote secular culture (such as in the TAR) but to stimulate dialogue between Buddhism and Western science (Prost 2006).

19 This type of discourse is still quite embryonic in the case of Tibetan medicine and only appears among the most inspired practitioners, whereas it is much more widespread in the case of Ayurveda (cf. Cohen 1995).

20 Salient examples are found in nursing (cf. Begley 1994) and childbirth practices (cf. Hubbell Maiden and Farwell 1997), for which Tibetan medicine becomes a model or a tool to improve existing practices.

21 New Age is a loose and vast category that would need to be precisely defined. This being so, in our particular case this term refers to a common understanding attributed to syncretic and holistic practices, sometimes connected with new forms of religiosity and combining different medical systems, the paradigms of which are at times very different. The production of this type of new therapy continues very actively today. On the subject of New Age therapies, see English-Lueck (1990), Ghasarian (2005) and Reddy (2004).

22 See, for example, the article 'Buddha and Mother Earth' by Robert Thurman (1997), published in a volume which underscores and interprets the relationship between Buddhist thought and the environment.

23 On the violence of science, see Nandy (1988). On the social re-transcription of the dialectic relation between the chemical violence of biomedicine and the natural, inoffensive character of traditional medicines, see Zimmermann on Ayurveda (1992) and Tan (1999) in the case of indigenous medicines in the Philippines.

24 Other Asian medical systems show similar patterns. See, for example, the article by Bode (2002) on the moral dimension of the concept of nature conveyed by Ayurvedic and Unani industrial pharmaceutical products in India.

25 Janes and Hilliard (Chapter 2 in this volume) show the existence of various re-invented forms of Tibetan medicine in Mongolia, some of which are very clearly based on external therapeutic practices.

26 However, a point should be made regarding this subject. An analysis of clinics intended for tourists in the region of Ladakh would lead to the same conclusions. Nevertheless, it would be exactly the same for all village 'clinics' (which are generally rooms in someone's house), or for government offices devoted to *amchi* medicine. Both are furnished with religious photographs, statues, *thang kha*, incense and so on. The perception of the atmosphere depends above all on the observer. I am not sure that a Ladakhi would find a clinic for tourists very different from any other (except, perhaps, for higher and fixed rates). And a tourist who experiences this 'spiritual atmosphere' feels this sentiment in any clinic, all the more, let us note, when the clinic is run by an *amchi*-monk. Moreover, some tourists in Ladakh are also heard to say, regarding clinics to which they were preferentially directed (explicit announcements in English or English-speaking *amchi*), that they were disappointed by the short time accorded to them by the *amchi* or by the lack of esotericism in his or her discourse.

27 Tibet, after having been described as a cruel and barbarous place, today has a highly valued image in Western societies. See on this subject Lopez (1998) and Brauen (2004). Tibetan treatments, such as the precious pills, are also valued in China because they

embody the esoteric knowledge of the 'mysterious Land of the Snow'. The cohort of clinical researchers investigating the therapeutic potential of Tibetan medicine in China would also, by their presence and enthusiasm alone, confer some paradoxical form of scientific legitimacy on this medicine.

28 The 'Tibetan' drug Padma 28(r) produced in Switzerland is an example. The same applies to the manufacture of day creams and anti-wrinkle and nourishing creams by the Dharamsala Men-Tsee-Khang, which therefore revisits 'tradition', upon which one expressly bases oneself to legitimate these products. Elsewhere in India, the range of health care products of the Himalaya company flaunts an 'Ayurvedic concept' (Ayurvedic Proprietary Medicine) for protective sunscreen lotions, toothpaste, gentle wash gels or lip balms. Cohen moreover mentions the 'neo-chyawanprashes' to underscore the recommoditization of Ayurvedic 'tonics' (chyawanprash) and their new uses (1995: 326).

29 It is interesting to note that, while the healers multiply their activities outside the field of medicine, their medical practice may become highly specialized in institutional settings. Some practitioners are today full-time pharmacists; others belong to specific medical yards and specialities. They may be relieved of anything that is non-therapeutic, such as taking money, packing medicines, keeping records and so on.

30 It should also be remembered that the drastic conjuncture of Tibet at the time of the Chinese invasion in the 1950s contributed to the international diffusion of Tibetan medicine. The exiled Tibetan communities have been very dynamic and enterprising in this respect, benefiting furthermore from the positive image Tibet has in the West.

31 Elsewhere, Kuczynski shows the role of international networks in the delocalization of the practices of African marabouts (2002).

32 For a detailed study in the case of Ayurveda, see the work by Zimmermann (1995).

33 Medical tourism was not considered in this section. Although it exists, it still remains very marginal in Tibetan medicine, but its actual development allows one to foresee a rosy future for it. On the subject of medical tourism in Ayurveda and its role in the recasting of certain social and medical aspects of the practice, see Langford (2002).

34 The marginal case of Western Tibetan medical practitioners raises another problem regarding the understanding of continuity or discontinuity in medical practice. I will not consider this here.

35 As this chapter shows, the Chinese government did not play the devastating role in respect of Tibetan medicine which has been commonly attributed to it. However, Tibetan medicine was severely oppressed and undermined during the Cultural Revolution owing to its affinity to religion and because it represented a clear expression of Tibetan culture, but the ambivalence stems from the fact that government policies have also supported Tibetan medicine by integrating it in socialist modernity (e.g. local recourse, complementarity with biomedicine, supposed affinity to Chinese civilization). The Chinese government has largely contributed to the transformation of Tibetan medicine according to this selective principle. See on this issue the article by Janes (1995), and the chapters in this volume by Adams and Li (Chapter 5) and Janes and Hilliard (Chapter 2).

36 On conflicting biomedical and Tibetan medical epistemologies see the article by Samuel (2006).

37 The case of Bhutan could be an exception, embodying a peculiar model of 'development', if we accept McKay and Wangchuk (2005). The Bhutanese National Health Care System integrates 'traditional medicine' (Sowa Rigpa) and biomedicine in the state health services, 'offering patients the choice of systems under one roof' (ibid.: 208). According to these authors, although biomedicine is hegemonic in certain domains, biomedical physicians' attitudes to traditional medicine are generally tolerant, and 'the two medical systems have positive interactions and personal links that determine patterns of referral' (p. 216). The very fact that the state supports traditional medicine also seems to confer social legitimacy on the latter (p. 215). Despite the fact that one would have wished a thicker ethnographic description to support the authors' assertions, no

definition is given, however, as to what 'integration' precisely means in this context, besides implying the ubiquitous presence of one system next to the other in the same medical structures.

References

Adams, V. (1988). Modes of Production and Medicine: An Examination of the Theory in Light of Sherpa Medical Traditionalism, *Social Science and Medicine* 27(5): 505–513.

Adams, V. (1992). The Production of Self and Body in Sherpa-Tibetan Society. In M. Nichter (ed.), *Anthropological Approaches to the Study of Ethnomedicine*, Amsterdam: Gordon and Breach Publishers.

Adams, V. (2001a). Particularizing Modernity: Tibetan Medical Theorizing of Women's Health in Lhasa, Tibet. In Linda H. Connor and Geoffrey Samuel (eds), *Healing Powers and Modernity. Traditional Medicine, Shamanism and Science in Asian Societies*, Westport, CT: Bergin & Harvey.

Adams, V. (2001b). The Sacred in the Scientific: Ambiguous Practices of Science in Tibetan Medicine, *Cultural Anthropology* 16(4): 542–575.

Adams, V. (2002a). Randomized Controlled Crime: Postcolonial Sciences in Alternative Medicine Research, *Social Studies of Science* 3, 32(5): 659–690.

Adams, V. (2002b). Establishing Proof: Translating 'Science' and the State in Tibetan Medicine. In M. Nichter and M. Lock (eds), *New Horizons in Medical Anthropology: Essays in Honour of Charles Leslie*, London and New York: Routledge.

Adams, V., Miller, S., Craig, S., Nyima, Sonam, Droyong, Lhakpen and Varner, M. (2005). The Challenge of Cross-Cultural Clinical Trials Research: Case Report from the Tibetan Autonomous Region, People's Republic of China, *Medical Anthropology Quarterly* 19(3): 267–289.

Alter, J. (ed.) (2005). *Asian Medicine and Globalization*, Philadelphia: University of Pennsylvania Press.

Aschoff, J. C. and Rösing, I. (eds) (1997). *Tibetan Medicine: 'East Meets West – West Meets East'*, Ulm: Fabri Verlag.

Avedon, J., Meyer, F., Bolsokhoyeva, N. D., Gerasimova, K. M. and Bradley, T. S. (eds) (1998). *The Buddhist Art of Healing: Tibetan Paintings Rediscovered*. New York: Rizzoli.

Balandier, G. (1974). *Anthropo-logiques*, Paris: Presses Universitaires de France.

Banerjee, M. (2004). Local Knowledge for World Market: Globalising Ayurveda, *Economic and Political Weekly* XXXIX(1), 3–9 January: 89–93.

Barges, A. (1996). Entre conformismes et changements: le monde de la lèpre au Mali. In J. Benoist (ed.), *Soigner au pluriel: Essais sur le pluralisme médical*, Paris: Karthala.

Bates, D. (1995). *Knowledge and the Scholarly Medical Traditions*, Cambridge: Cambridge University Press.

Begley, S. S. (1994). Tibetan Buddhist Medicine: A Transcultural Nursing Experience, *Journal of Holistic Nursing* 12(3): 323–342.

Benoist, J. (1996). Carrefours de cultes et de soins à l'île Maurice. In J. Benoist (ed.), *Soigner au pluriel: Essais sur le pluralisme médical*, Paris: Karthala.

Berg, M. and Mol, A. (eds) (1998). *Differences in Medicine: Unravelling Practices, Techniques and Bodies*, Durham, NC and London: Duke University Press.

Bode, M. (2002). Indian Indigenous Pharmaceuticals: Tradition, Modernity and Nature. In W. Ernst (ed.), *Plural Medicine, Tradition and Modernity, 1800–2000*, London and New York: Routledge.

Boesi, A., Cardi, F. and guest eds (2006). *Tibet Journal* (Special Issue on Tibetan Medicine), XXX(4), Summer 2005 and XXXI(1), Spring 2006.

Bourdarias, F. (1996). Bamako: les guérisseurs du 'bout du goudron', *Journal du Sida*, numéro spécial Afrique 86–87: 49–52.

Bourdieu, P. (1980). *Questions de sociologie*, Paris: Minuit.

Brass, P. R. (1972). The Politics of Ayurvedic Education: A Case Study of Revivalism and Modernisation in India. In S. H. Rudolph and L. I. Rudolph (eds), *Education and Politics in India: Studies in Organization, Society and Policy*, Cambridge, MA: Harvard University Press.

Brauen, M. (2004). *Dreamworld Tibet, Western Illusions*, Trumbull, CT: Weatherhill.

Castells, M. (1996). *The Rise of the Network Society*, Oxford: Blackwell.

Champion, F. (1994). La 'nébuleuse mystique-ésotérique': une décomposition du religieux entre humanisme revisité, magique, psychologique. In J.-B. Martin and F. Lapalantine (eds), *Le défi magique: Esotérisme, occultisme, spiritisme*, Lyon: Presses Universitaires de Lyon.

Clarke, J. J. (1997). *Oriental Enlightenment: The Encounter between Asian and Western Thought*, London: Routledge.

CMAM (2000). *Anthology of 2000 International Academic Conference on Tibetan Medicine*, Beijing: Chinese Medical Association of Minorities (CMAM).

Cohen, L. (1995). The Epistemological Carnival: Meditations on Disciplinary Intentionality and Ayurveda. In D. Bates (ed.), *Knowledge and the Scholarly Medical Traditions*, Cambridge: Cambridge University Press.

Connor, L. H. (2001). Healing Powers in Contemporary Asia. In L. Connor and G. Samuel (eds), *Healing Powers and Modernity: Traditional Medicine, Shamanism, and Science in Asian Societies*, Westport, CT: Bergin & Harvey.

Connor, L. H. and Samuel, G. (eds) (2001). *Healing Powers and Modernity: Traditional Medicine, Shamanism, and Science in Asian Societies*, Westport, CT: Bergin & Harvey.

Croizier, R. C. (1976). The Ideology of Medical Revivalism in Modern China. In C. Leslie (ed.), *Asian Medical Systems: A Comparative Study*, Berkeley: University of California Press.

Dollfus, P. and Labbal, V. (2003). Les composantes du paysage ladakhi. In J. Smadja (ed.), *Histoire et devenir des paysage en Himalaya: Représentations des milieux et gestion des ressources au Népal et au Ladakh*, Paris: Editions du CNRS.

Dozon, J.-P. (1995). Quelques réflexions sur les médecines traditionnelles et le sida en Afrique. In J. Benoist and A. Desclaux (eds), *Sida et Anthropologie: Bilan et Perspectives*, Paris: Karthala.

Dunn, L. F. (1976). Traditional Asian Medicine and Cosmopolitan Medicine as Adaptative Systems. In C. Leslie (ed.), *Asian Medical Systems: A Comparative Study*, Berkeley: University of California Press.

English-Lueck, J. A. (1990). *Health in the New Age: A Study in California Holistic Practices*, Albuquerque: University of New Mexico Press.

Ernst, W. (ed.) (2002). *Plural Medicine, Tradition and Modernity, 1800–2000*, London and New York: Routledge.

Fassin, D. (1994). Penser les médecines d'ailleurs: La reconfiguration du champ thérapeutique dans les sociétés africaines et latino-américaines. In P. Aïach et D. Fassin (eds), *Les métiers de la santé: Enjeux de pouvoir et quête de légitimité*, Paris: Anthropos.

Fassin, D. and Fassin, E. (1988). De la quête de légitimité à la question de légitimation: les thérapeutiques 'traditionnelles' au Sénégal, *Cahiers d'Etudes Africaines* 110, XXVIII-2: 207–231.

Finckh, E. (1980). Tibetan Medicine: Theory and Practice. In M. Aris and Aung Sang Suu Kyi (eds), *Tibetan Studies in Honor of Hugh Richardson*, Warminster: Aris and Phillips.

Finckh, E. (1985). *Grundlagen tibetischer Heilkunde*, Uelzen: Medizinisch Literarische Verlagsgesellschaft.

Finckh, E. (1994). Behavior: An Important Part of Tibetan Medicine. In P. Kvaerne (ed.), *Tibetan Studies*, Vol. 1, Oslo: Institute for Comparative Research in Human Culture.

Fleurentin, J. and Nicolas, J.-P. (eds) (2006). *La médecine tibétaine: Sources, concepts et pratique actuelle. Actes de la Journée du 8 avril 2006 à Metz (France)*, Metz: Société Française d'Ethnopharmacologie et Institut Européen d'Ecologie.

Garrett, F. (2005). Hybrid Methodologies in the Lhasa Mentsikhang: A Summary of Resources for Teaching about Tibetan Medicine, *Tibet Journal* XXX(4)–XXXI(1): 55–64.

Garrett, F. (2006). Buddhism and the Historicizing of Medicine in Thirteenth-Century Tibet, *Asian Medicine* 2(2): 204–224.

Ghasarian, C. (2005). Réflexions sur les rapports entre le corps, la conscience et l'esprit dans les représentations et pratiques néo-shamaniques. In O. Schmitz (ed.), *Les médecines en parallèle: Multiplicité des recours au soin en Occident*, Paris: Karthala.

Gruénais, M.-E. (1991). Vers une nouvelle médecine traditionnelle: Exemple du Congo, *La revue du praticien* 141: 1483–1490.

Gruénais, M.-E. (2002). La professionalisation des 'néo-tradipraticiens' d'Afrique centrale, *Santé Publique et Sciences Sociales* 8/9, Juin: 217–239.

Gyatso, J. (2004). The Authority of Empiricism and the Empiricism of Authority: Medicine and Buddhism in Tibet on the Eve of Modernity, *Comparative Studies of South Asia, Africa and the Middle East* 24(2): 83–96.

Hsu, E. (ed.) (2001). *Innovation in Chinese Medicine*, Cambridge: Cambridge University Press.

Hubbell Maiden, A. and Farwell, E. (1997). *The Tibetan Art of Parenting: From before Conception to Early Childhood*, Somerville, MA: Wisdom Publications.

Huber, T. (1997). Green Tibetans: A Brief Social History. In F. J. Korom (ed.), *Tibetan Culture in the Diaspora: Proceedings of the Seventh Seminar of the International Association for Tibetan Studies (PIATS), Graz, June 18–24, 1995*, Österreichischen Akademie der Wissenschaften, Philosophisch-historische Klasse, Denkschriften, 262, Vol. 4, Vienna: Verlag der Österreichischen Akademie der Wissenschaften.

Janes, C. R. (1995). The Transformations of Tibetan Medicine, *Medical Anthropology Quarterly*, 9(1): 6–39.

Janes, C. R. (1999). The Health Transition, Global Modernity and the Crisis of Traditional Medicine: The Tibetan Case, *Social Science and Medicine* 48: 1803–1820.

Janes, C. R. (2001). Tibetan Medicine at the Crossroads: Radical Modernity and the Social Organization of Traditional Medicine in the Tibet Autonomous Region, China. In L. Connor and G. Samuel (eds), *Healing Powers and Modernity: Traditional Medicine, Shamanism, and Science in Asian Societies*, Westport, CT: Bergin & Harvey.

Janes, C. R. (2002). Buddhism, Science, and Market: The Globalisation of Tibetan Medicine, *Anthropology and Medicine* 9(3): 267–289.

Kleinman, A. (1980). *Patients and Healers in the Context of Culture*, Berkeley: University of California Press.

Kuczynski, L. (2002). *Les marabouts africains à Paris*, Paris: Editions du CNRS.

Kuhn, A. (1988), *Heiler und ihre Patienten auf dem Dach der Welt: Ladakh aus ethnomedizinischer Sicht*, Frankfurt am Main: Peter Lang.

Landy, D. (1974). Role Adaptation: Traditional Curers under the Impact of Western Medicine, *American Ethnologist* 1(1): 104–127.

Langford, J. (2002). *Fluent Bodies: Ayurvedic Remedies for Post-Colonial Imbalance*, Durham, NC and London: Duke University Press.

Last, M. (1986). The Professionalisation of African Medicine: Ambiguities and Definitions. In M. Last and G. L. Chavundunka (eds), *The Professionalisation of African Medicine*, Manchester: Manchester University Press.

Lau, K. J. (2000). *New Age Capitalism: Making Money East of Eden*, Philadelphia: University of Pennsylvania Press.

Law, W. and Salick, J. (2007). Comparing Conservation Priorities for Useful Plants among Botanists and Tibetan Doctors, *Biodiversity Conservation* 16: 1747–1759.

Le Palec, A. (1996). Mali: Les nouveaux guérisseurs urbains en quête d'identité, *Journal du sida*, numéro spécial Afrique 86–87: 45–48.

Lee, R. V. (2001). Doing Good Badly, *Ladakh Studies* 16, December: 26–28.

Leslie, C. (ed.) (1976). *Asian Medical Systems: A Comparative Study*, Berkeley: University of California Press.

Leslie, C. (1980). Medical Pluralism in World Perspective. In C. Leslie (ed.), Medical Pluralism, *Social Sciences and Medicine* (Special Issue) 14B(4): 190–196.

Leslie, C. (1989). Indigenous Pharmaceuticals, the Capitalist World System, and Civilization, *Kroeber Anthropological Society Papers* 69–70: 23–31.

Leslie, C. (1992). Interpretations of Illness: Syncretism in Modern Ayurveda. In C. Leslie and A. Young (eds), *Paths to Asian Medical Knowledge*, Berkeley: University of California Press.

Leslie, C. and Young, A. (eds) (1992). *Paths to Asian Medical Knowledge*, Berkeley: University of California Press.

Lock, M. (1980). *East Asian Medicine in Urban Japan: Varieties of Medical Experience*, Berkeley: University of California Press.

Lock, M. and Nichter, M. (2002). Introduction: From Documenting Medical Pluralism to Critical Interpretations of Globalized Health Knowledge, Policies and Practices. In M. Nichter and M. Lock (eds), *New Horizons in Medical Anthropology: Essays in Honour of Charles Leslie*, London and New York: Routledge.

Lopez, D. (1998). *Prisoners of Shangri-La: Tibetan Buddhism and the West*, Chicago, IL: University of Chicago Press.

McKay, A. and Wangchuk, D. (2005). Traditional Medicine in Bhutan, *Asian Medicine* 1(1): 204–218.

McMillen, H. (2004). The Adapting Healer: Pioneering through Shifting Epidemiological and Sociocultural Landscapes, *Social Science and Medicine* 59: 889–902.

Meyer, F. (1981 [2002]). *Gso-Ba-Rig-Pa, Le système médical tibétain*, Paris: Editions du CNRS.

Meyer, F. (1986). Orient–Occident: un dialogue singulier. In Autres médecines, autres moeurs, *Autrement* 85, 124–133, Paris: Editions Autrement.

Meyer, F. (1987). Essai d'analyse schématique d'un système médical: La médecine savante du Tibet. In Anne Retel-Laurentin (ed.), *Etiologie et perception de la maladie*, Paris, L'Harmattan.

Meyer, F. (1990). Introduction à l'étude d'une série de peintures médicales créées à Lhasa au XVIIe siècle. In *Tibet: Civilisation et société*, Paris: Editions de la Maison des Sciences de l'Homme/Fondation Singer-Polignac.

Meyer, F. (1992a). Introduction: The Medical Paintings of Tibet. In Y. Parfionovitch, F. Meyer and G. Dorje (eds), *Tibetan Medical Paintings: Illustrations to the Blue Beryl Treatise of Sangye Gyamtso (1653–1705)*, New York: Harry N. Abrams.

Meyer, F. (1992b). Histoire et historiographie de la médecine en Asie, *Médecine et Hygiène*, 50(1936), Juin: 1681–1685.

Meyer, F. (1993). La médecine tibétaine: tradition ancienne et nouveaux enjeux. In Olivier Moulin (ed.), *Tibet, l'envers du décor*, Genève: Olizane.

Meyer, F. (1995). Theory and Practice of Tibetan Medicine. In J. V. Alphen and A. Aris (eds), *Oriental Medicine: An Illustrated Guide to the Asian Arts of Healing*, London: Serindia Publications (republished by Shambhala, Boston, MA, 1997).

Meyer, F. (1997). Le siècle d'or de la médecine tibétaine. In F. Pommaret (ed.), *Lhasa, Lieu du divin: la capitale des Dalaï-Lama*, Genève: Olizane.

Micollier, E. (2004). Le qigong chinois: enjeux économiques et transnationalisation des réseaux, pratiques et croyances, *Journal des Anthropologues* 98–99: 107–146.

Nandy, A. (ed.) (1988). *Science, Hegemony and Violence: A Requiem for Modernity*, Tokyo and Delhi: United Nations University and Oxford University Press.

Parfionovitch, Y., Meyer, F. and Dorje, G. (eds) (1992). *Tibetan Medical Paintings: Illustrations to the Blue Beryl Treatise of Sangye Gyamtso (1653–1705)*, 2 vols, New York: Harry N. Abrams.

Pfleiderer, B. (ed.) (1988). Permanence and Change in Asian Health Care Traditions, *Social Science and Medicine* 12(5): 411–567.

Pordié, L. (2003). *The Expression of Religion in Tibetan Medicine: Ideal Conceptions, Contemporary Practices and Political Use*, Pondy Papers in Social Sciences 29, Pondicherry: FIP.

Pordié, L. (2005). Emergence et avatars du marché de l'évaluation thérapeutique des autres médecines. In L. Pordié (ed.), *Panser le monde, penser les médecines: Traditions médicales et développement sanitaire*, Paris: Karthala.

Pordié, L. (2007). Téléscopages religieux en médecine tibétaine: Ethnographie d'un praticien musulman, *Puruṣārtha* 27, Paris: Editions de l'EHESS (forthcoming).

Pordié, L. (forthcoming). *Healing at the Periphery: Ethnographies of Tibetan Medicine in India*, Durham and London: Duke University Press.

Prost, A. (2006). Gained in Translation: Tibetan Science between Dharamsala and Lhasa. In T. Herman (ed.), *Translating Others: Translations and Translation Theories East and West*, Manchester: St Jerome Press.

Rechung, R. (1973). *Tibetan Medicine*, Berkeley: University of California Press.

Reddy, S. (2004). The Politics and Poetic of 'Magazine Medicine': New Age Ayurveda in the Print Media. In R. D. Johnstan (ed.), *The Politics of Healing: Histories of Alternative Medicines in Twentieth-Century North America*, New York and London: Routledge.

Rosny, E. de (1996). *La nuit, les yeux ouverts*, Paris: Seuil.

Samuel, G. (2001). Tibetan Medicine in Contemporary India: Theory and Practice. In Linda H. Connor and G. Samuel (eds), *Healing Powers and Modernity: Traditional Medicine, Shamanism, and Science in Asian Societies*, Westport, CT: Bergin & Garvey.

Samuel, G. (2006). Tibetan Medicine and Biomedicine: Epistemological Conflicts, Practical Solutions, *Asian Medicine* 2(1): 71–84.

Schmitz, O. (2005). Des fleurs pour soigner les affects: L'usage des remèdes du Dr. Bach par les guérisseurs syncrétiques. In L. Pordié (ed.), *Panser le monde, penser les médecines*, Paris: Karthala.

Schrempf, M. (ed.) (2007). *Soundings in Tibetan Medicine: Anthropological and Historical Perspectives. Proceedings of the 10th Seminar of the International Association for Tibetan Studies (PIATS)*, Oxford, 6–12 September 2003, Leiden: Brill Publishers.

Tan, L. M. (1999). *Good Medicine: Pharmaceuticals and the Construction of Power and Knowledge in the Philippines*, Amsterdam: Het Spinhuis.

Thurman, R. (1997). Buddha and Mother Earth. In J. Martin (ed.), *Ecological Responsibility: A Dialogue with Buddhism*, New York: Tibet House.

Tonda, J. (2001). Le syndrome du prophète, *Cahiers d'Études africaines,* 161 (http://etudes africaines.revues.org/document69.html).

Wolffers, I. (1988). Traditional Practitioners and Western Pharmaceuticals in Sri Lanka. In J. Van der Geest and S. Whyte (eds), *The Context of Medicines in Developing Countries*, Boston, MA and London: Kluwer Academic Publishers.

Wylie, T. (1959). A Standard System of Tibetan Transcription, *Harvard Journal of Asiatic Studies* 22: 261–267.

Zimmermann, F. (1992). Gentle Purge: The Flower Power of Ayurveda. In C. Leslie and A. Young (eds), *Paths to Asian Medical Knowledge*, Berkeley: University of California Press.

Zimmermann, F. (1995). *Généalogie des médecines douces: De l'Inde à l'occident*, Paris: Presses Universitaires de France.

Part I
Modern institutionalization

2 Inventing tradition

Tibetan medicine in the post-socialist contexts of China and Mongolia

Craig R. Janes and Casey Hilliard

By the mid-1980s Tibetan physicians in China had largely shaken off the effects of the Cultural Revolution and had turned their energies to restoring the institutions of Tibetan medicine – the hospitals, clinics, and medicine factories – to their formerly integral position in Tibetan society. Bolstered by support from the Tibet Autonomous Region's Ministry of Health and aided by a more liberal attitude toward Tibetan cultural traditions by Beijing, senior physicians began the work of reintegrating Tibetan medicine into the public health and primary medical services provided to Tibetans living throughout south and southwestern China. Hospitals were built; a medical college was established; the older and experienced physicians who had been sent during the Cultural Revolution into the countryside to work as peasants and herders were found and brought to Lhasa to supervise clinics and medical curricula; and a new generation of Tibetan physicians entered training. By the mid-1990s, Tibetan medical practitioners were fully integrated into the primary health care system down to the county level. Yet the hard-won successes of Tibetan physicians, propelled by the economic and social liberalization of the preceding two decades, opened Tibetan medicine up to international trade, foreign influence, global health reform initiatives, and the potentially transformative force of the Western imagination. These new and essentially global pressures represent a significant challenge to Tibetan medicine's role in the primary health care system, and are a threat to its ability – intellectually and organizationally – to meet the health needs of Tibetans, particularly the rural and urban poor.

To the north, Tibetan medicine was subject to another, yet to some degree similar, series of transformations at the hands of socialist reformers. Established in Mongolia through centuries of contact and scholarly exchange, Tibetan medicine became the dominant professional system of healing during the time of the Qing hegemony. Until the early part of the twentieth century it is evident that the principal theoretical precepts of Mongolian and Tibetan medicine – what Unschuld (1985) terms the "paradigmatic core" – were closely shared by Tibetan and Mongolian physicians, supported by the overarching intellectual framework of the Gelugpa tradition of Tibetan Buddhism to which most subscribed. This Tibetan-Mongolian medicine, practiced largely by Buddhist monks, dominated Mongolian healing systems until the Mongolian socialist revolution of 1924. For the next seven decades, Mongolians embraced a Soviet-style socialist reform program which championed technological modernization along largely Western lines. Soviet-style biomedicine became the only legitimate medical system, and all other competitors were legally restricted. As a consequence of the Stalinist purges of the 1930s in which thousands of monks were killed and their monasteries looted and destroyed, Mongolian medicine largely disappeared from the scene. In 1990, after severing its ties with the Soviets and embracing a pro-market, Western-style "democracy," Mongolia sought to revitalize its native institutions. Mongolian medicine, though by 1990 having precious few knowledgeable practitioners and thus possessing little of an active intellectual tradition, was nevertheless reborn with the full backing of the state. By the end of the 1990s, Mongolian medicine was offered as a separate curriculum in the national medical university, two private traditional medical colleges had opened, and several public and private hospitals and clinics were established. As with medicine in Tibet, Mongolian medicine is now practiced in a context in which state interests and global health policy largely determine its content and availability. In both – now post-socialist – contexts, indigenous medicine is entangled with, and thereby constrained by, state-level concerns over national and/or ethnic identity, global economics, and international health development agendas which champion "traditional" medicine as cost-effective and push market approaches to health care distribution.

In this chapter we undertake a comparison of the recent socialist and post-socialist histories of indigenous medicine in Tibet and Mongolia. Our concern here is not to explore how social and political histories may have acted on the core intellectual tradition once, and arguably still, common to Mongolian and Tibetan medicine, but rather to analyze the processes by which identifiable state and global-level forces have shaped the organization, practice, distribution, and, ultimately, accessibility of the tradition to Mongolians and Tibetans. The comparative approach that we employ here will identify several common threads in the development of these "modern" indigenous medical systems. It will also reveal significant differences. Taken together, these cast light on the processes that link global discourses, state interests, and local therapeutic politics. Our argument here will focus on three such processes: 1) the degree to which programs or "projects" of socialist modernity determined the long-term development of these indigenous medical traditions; 2) the importance of problematizing identity, i.e. what it means to be Tibetan or Mongolian in socialist/post-socialist contexts, in order to reveal how indigenous medical systems operate, or are allowed to operate; and 3) the degree to which the many dimensions of globalization – cultural, economic, and political – affect the social organization of indigenous medicines at the level of the community.

We draw on data collected between 1988 and 1994 in the central prefectures of Lhasa, Tsethang, and Shigatse in the Tibet Autonomous Region, China, and between 2000 and 2002 in urban Ulaanbaatar and the rural northwestern province of Huvsgol in Mongolia. In both settings, methods included interviews with physicians, patients, and policy-makers. In Mongolia we conducted a structured survey of community members living in urban and rural environments designed to elicit experiences with and perceptions of access to health care – both cosmopolitan and "traditional." One of the authors (Janes) has published extensively on the modern history and globalization of medicine in Tibet; this information will be provided here in highly summarized form. Greater emphasis will therefore be placed on presenting the Mongolian materials in the greatest detail. Readers interested in a longer discussion of the modern history and social organization of Tibetan medicine in China and South Asia should consult the works of Janes (1995, 1999a, 1999b, 2001, 2002), Adams (2001a, 2001b, 2002), and the many excellent works in this volume.

A critical ethnography of Tibetan-Mongolian medicines

Our comparative approach draws on a framework established initially by Unschuld (1975) and developed in medical anthropology by Crandon-Malamud (1991). In this framework, the "content" of a medical system, termed its "primary resources," is distinguished from its organizational, political, and economic effects, termed "secondary resources." Primary resources refer to the activities or content of healing per se: theories of etiology, both specific and general; nosology; the *materia medica*; and therapeutic techniques more generally. In providing, or pursuing access to, these primary resources, patients and healers may realize other benefits. From the perspective of healers, control of primary resources brings with it social and economic rewards, including influence, legitimacy, prestige, authority, and power. From the perspective of patients, health care decisions often reference the gritty details of life – illness and suffering – and it is important to recognize that most such decisions are motivated largely by such pragmatic concerns. However, it is also the case, as Crandon-Malamud (1991) has eloquently argued, that a health care decision may assert a particular social and/or ethnic identity vis-à-vis others – dominant or subordinate, modern or "traditional." Primary resources are not isolated from secondary ones. Patient demands, healers' pursuits of influence, prestige, and economic benefits, and state attempts to control and/or transform healing practices have a certain impact on the epistemology, theory, and knowledge in the indigenous system. Unschuld (1985), for example, documents how temporally specific social and political events, exigencies, and ideologies led to the development of historically contingent Chinese medicines. Although in Unschuld's reading the paradigmatic core of the tradition did not change much – e.g. the etiologic centrality of the system of correspondences – the application of core ideas to understanding socially and environmentally specific patterns of cause and effect did. Unschuld's focus is identifying and explaining the relationship of this shifting "surface" or "soft" covering of the paradigmatic core tradition to events in wider Chinese society.

We find the distinction between primary and secondary resources, and between the core elements of medical traditions – in this case based on that blend of Ayurvedic humoral theory, Buddhist epistemology, and the pragmatic therapeutic rationalism that makes up the root texts, or *Gyü-Shi* (*Rgyud bzhi*), of Tibetan medicine, and the application of these ideas within rapidly changing social and political contexts – to be a particularly useful device for understanding the parallel courses taken by Tibetan and Mongolian medicine through the twentieth century.

Thus, as the various interested parties, acting out of contextually specific interests, and within particular constraints, exploit the primary resources of a medical tradition, it is put into motion – made social – leading to many effects, only one of which is strictly, or even, the amelioration of symptoms and suffering. One effect, certainly, especially under the political-economic terms of post-socialist transformation, is a reformulation of the content of a tradition. In this way, primary and secondary medical resources clearly interact; this interaction is in turn largely determined by factors operating at the level of the nation-state and, increasingly, within global systems of economic, political, and cultural exchange.

Our argument is "critical" in the sense that we see transformative power flowing from groups who have vested interests (direct or indirect) with respect to the organization and development of traditional medicine. This power, we argue, is principally political-economic in origin, e.g. associated with interests in the global trade of "herbal" pharmaceuticals, or nation-building, but is experienced at local levels through the deployment of those ideological and symbolic devices that attempt to create particular identities, bodies, and modernities.

Globally, such discourses with regard to science, medicine, and tradition develop within the major Western-dominated intergovernmental institutions, e.g. the development banks, the World Health Organization, and, increasingly, international non-governmental organizations. These discourses have a powerful influence at national levels, where lenders, development experts, and resident expatriates work to bring national practices in line with global ideologies. As Escobar (1995) argues, those in power globally set the rules of the game at the local level:

> who can speak, from what points of view, with what authority, and according to what criteria of expertise; it sets the rules that must be followed for this or that problem, theory, or object to emerge and be named, analyzed, and eventually transformed into a policy or a plan.
>
> (Escobar 1995: 41)

These discourses are operationalized through the processes of labeling, monitoring, institutionalization, bureaucratization, and professionalization. As we shall argue, in Tibet and Mongolia neoliberal policies of health reform – rationalization, privatization, and cost-efficiency – have had a pronounced effect on the primary and secondary resources offered by indigenous medical systems.

States are not passive players in determining health policy, but stand very much in between global interests and local action. Governments, as Starr (1982) pointed out, have a clear interest in being identified with the distribution of desirable social services; this interest provides both an incentive and a logic to intervene. Insurance schemes which recognize traditional medicine, state sanction of professionalization, and celebration of "native genius" may all flow from such political interests. On the other hand, political exigency, for example concern over unchecked expressions of ethnic identity, or the potentially politically destabilizing demands of a restive population, may require that states interfere in the content of services offered so that they do not offer potent challenges to the status quo. Above all, states self-consciously interact with global ideologies of modernity, particularly those which emanate from the North and West. The products of such interactions in the case of medicine are ideas, translated into policy, about processes of healing vis-à-vis Western science.

Not to be neglected, of course, is the fact that communities of individuals and practitioners may offer various kinds of resistance to programs, changes, or mandates from above. Our critical approach, cognizant of the many potential loci of power, asserts that social change, in this case transformations to indigenous Tibetan-origin medicines, is a product of conflicts occurring at many levels, from the community and clinic to the nation-state and global health development agencies. These conflicts in part explain how the relationships between primary and secondary resources shift, and how these shifts in turn determine the historically contingent character of indigenous medicine.

Lastly, we believe it is important to acknowledge at the outset that our interests in understanding the transformations of indigenous medical systems are guided by principles of equity and social justice. We believe that, for a host of reasons that have been described elsewhere (Janes 1999a), the availability of a diverse array of therapeutic resources is a good thing. Our exploration of how medical traditions have become entangled in a web of global discourses is motivated by trying to understand how and why so many Tibetans and Mongolians have access to a rather impoverished array of health services, and what the experiences of these two peoples, each with a different history but both sharing the legacy of post-socialist social and economic transformation, might tell us about how globalization affects one important feature of local social life.

Mongolian medicine

In 2002, Mongolia had eleven public Mongolian medical hospitals, thirty-five public outpatient clinics (mostly associated with district and provincial hospitals), sixty-five private clinics, and three state-licensed colleges of Mongolian medicine (Bold and Ambaga 2002).[1] In addition to the clinics and colleges were five government-regulated traditional medicine manufacturing companies. In 2002 these companies produced over 270 types of Mongolian medicines with raw materials (herbs, minerals, and animal products) primarily collected in the Mongolian countryside. A number of the manufactured drugs were patented and licensed for sale in several Eastern European countries. Remarkably, this active, integrated, and developed traditional medical culture is mostly a recent phenomenon. It is an artifact of post-socialist nation-building and externally imposed health reform efforts which began just over a decade ago.

As we shall argue, Mongolian medicine as it is taught and practiced today is an eclectic mix of beliefs and therapies. From the perspective of its current practitioners, the traditional medicine of today is the product of an unbroken lineage of a rich nomadic and Buddhist tradition dating back at least to the thirteenth century. Despite such claims, however, its foundations are recent. Seventy years of political repression and Soviet-style modernization effectively disrupted Mongolia's ties to the Tibetan medical and Buddhist traditions of the past. Mongolian medicine is a creative reconstruction of that past, a project that is grounded in the social, political, and economic exigencies of the present. Its current character is a reflection of the global and national discourses that have shaped and reshaped the face of Mongolia over the past century, and particularly the past decade.

For six centuries Tibetan medicine was the only formal medical system in Mongolia. Introduced to Mongolia in the thirteenth century along with Buddhism, Tibetan medicine was quickly adopted and assimilated by the nomadic population. By the seventeenth century, a uniquely Mongolian Tibetan medical system was found throughout the country. Colleges for the formal training of medical practitioners were established, and Mongolian scholars began to gain impressive reputations as healers throughout central Asia. Tibetan medicine was a thriving tradition in Mongolia. By the early 1920s, however, Mongolia's struggle for independence from China effectively severed its ties to the Tibetan scholarly tradition.

A loosely organized feudal state at the turn of the twentieth century, Mongolia was in Marxist theoretical terms among the least likely candidates for a socialist revolution. In 1924, however, it became the first socialist state in Asia, and the world's second socialist state after the Soviet Union. This dramatic change in political philosophy and social organization was not at the outset the consequence of Mongolia's deep-seated commitment to revolutionary values but a desperate political attempt to escape hated Chinese hegemony and secure international recognition of their independence and sovereignty (Baabar 1999). The parallels between the efforts of the Mongolians and of the Tibetans to establish states independent of China are striking (e.g. Goldstein 1989). Unlike Tibet, Mongolia was ultimately successful in its attempts to assert independence, although this success was achieved at the expense of Soviet domination.

Given Mongolia's largely rural, pastoral economy, and the entrenched social and political power of the religious elite (40 percent of the male population were reported to have been monks [Baabar 1999]), initial political and economic reforms promulgated by Mongolia's new socialist government were quite moderate. Religious tolerance was the policy of the government, and indigenous medicine was not only tolerated but actively supported. Indeed, as was then the case in Tibet as a consequence of social and political reforms promulgated by the thirteenth Dalai Lama (Janes 1995; Goldstein 1989), concern over the health needs of a vast, underserved rural population led to active support of Tibetan-Mongolian medical training and practice. This support came to an abrupt end with the Stalinist purges of the 1930s and 1940s, when superstitious, religious, feudalist, and traditional medical practices became direct targets of government control and subject to organized, and horrific, violence.

The Great Purges, begun in 1937 and designed to cleanse Mongolia of its feudalist leanings, stand out as the harshest examples of the repressive Soviet era. Over the course of seven years, the government executed over 30,000 Mongolian men, mostly monks, and displaced many others. The terror campaign devastated the traditional culture of Mongolia. Writes the Mongolian historian Baabar (1999: 355),

"Through the Great Purges, Stalin eliminated the heirs of 2000 years of Mongolian aristocratic tradition, whose civilization, historic continuity, oral literary traditions, rules of conduct, customs, and habits had been passed on from generation to generation." The religious institutions that had served to integrate the dispersed Mongolian population were dismantled. The medical system that had served the Mongolian population for centuries was on the verge of extinction.

In the years that followed, a massive, Soviet-style socialist program of modernization was undertaken. This program, linked to a commitment to technological development along Western lines, had dramatic social and economic effects. Mongolia moved rapidly from a feudal state based on loosely organized nomadic groups to an industrial state embracing "high modernist" (cf. Scott 1998) efforts to establish communal agricultural enterprises, rationalize public education, promote science and technology, and introduce Soviet-Western biomedicine to all sectors of the population. Tibetan medical practice was rejected as a remnant of the feudal past. Mongolia established a fully modern and technological health care system based on the Russian model.[2] For the next seventy years, Mongolia embraced a Soviet-style socialism which, by advancing a competitive orientation to Western scientific and industrial development, radically transformed traditional Mongolian society. In juxtaposition to its old nemesis of China to the south, Mongolia was not only an utterly transformed state, but ideologically it embraced uncritically the benefits of Western-style industrial and technological development (Baabar 1999).

The invention of Mongolian medicine

By the late 1980s, as was occurring throughout Soviet Central Asia, the socialist government had begun to falter. In 1990 Mongolia's socialist party[3] led a peaceful transition to an elected, parliamentary-style pro-market government. By this time, owing to the socialist repression of the previous seventy years, there was no longer an intact traditional medical system. Thus, in 1990 when efforts to develop Mongolian medicine were begun, the process was less one of revival than one of 'invention' (Hobsbawm and Ranger 1983).

The political and economic transition of the early 1990s precipitated a national crisis of character. For seventy years Mongolians had embraced a European-oriented Soviet identity and had thoroughly renounced those Buddhist traditions that were associated with the "undeveloped" and feudal institutions of traditional Mongolia. Yet the sharp turn in orientation away from the Soviet Union left the Mongolian state bereft of an unambiguous national identity – was it Asian or Western, and how would this identity influence its relationship with its economically powerful neighbors? Soviet society was crumbling at the time, the thousands of Russian expatriates who had established residences in Mongolia began to leave in large numbers, and the pent-up resentment of Russia burst forth in a wholesale rejection of Russian cultural hegemony. Mongolia began a nationalist revival, which both embraced and eulogized its traditional nomadic culture and the dominant historical role once played by Mongolia throughout Asia (Bulag 1998).

This nationalist revival was rapid and far-reaching. Chinggis Khan was reclaimed as the Mongolian national hero, the traditional Mongolian script was reintroduced, mass production of the traditional costume, the *deel*, was begun, shamanism was rediscovered (especially for the benefit of increasing numbers of Western tourists), and Buddhism was re-designated as the state religion (Kotkin and Ellman 1999; Ole and Ole 1996). The vast rural countryside, once associated with backwardness and untoward conservatism, was portrayed increasingly as the wellspring of a nearly lost, authentic, Mongolian culture. The movement redefined Mongolia's distinctiveness, its bounded significance in a global world, while at the same time building a cultural identity that enhanced its competitive value on the global marketplace (Yoshino 1998; Hae-Joang 1998). As part of this renewed tradition and market-oriented national identity, Mongolia embraced, redefined, and encouraged the development of Mongolian medicine.

The political-economic transition, although it opened the door for the discovery of and experimentation with a new cultural identity, also dealt a severe blow to the economic and social stability of the country. The withdrawal of Soviet aid (35 percent of Mongolia's GDP) and the neoliberal economic reforms that accompanied Mongolia's democratic transition affected all sectors of the Mongolian infrastructure (Pomfret 2000). The economy collapsed, the highly rationalized, Soviet-style health care system largely disintegrated, and urban areas grew rapidly owing to the decollectivization of the rural areas, poorly implemented privatization schemes, and a run of bad weather that displaced many herders. With the assistance of international financial aid, Mongolia has showed some signs of economic recovery. Mongolia has become, in many ways, the post-socialist "poster-country" for international aid, attracting substantial interest, and investment, from many quarters. However, social inequality is cited by many Mongolians to be a continued threat to the integration of their communities; the GINI index (an index of income inequality), for example, rose by nearly 20 percent in the five-year period between 1995 and 1998 (Government of Mongolia 1999).

Mongolian medicine's modern development was in many ways spurred on by the initial economic crisis that crippled the nation. Highly dependent on Soviet aid, drugs, and equipment, Mongolia's health care system experienced an overwhelming challenge to its ability to address the needs of the population. As a result, for the first few years of the 1990s life expectancy declined, infant and maternal mortality rose, and the general health status of the nation suffered. In response to this situation, several physicians reported being motivated to learn about alternatives to biomedicine in order to better serve patients. The experience of one physician, now a teacher of acupuncture to students in the main public college of traditional medicine, is typical. Dr Delgermaa received a degree in biomedicine from a Russian medical college in 1991. She completed her internship and residency in Mongolia during the period when biomedicine was "in shambles" owing to the economic transition. "There were no medicines and doctors had difficulty helping their patients. This led me to my interest in traditional medicine." Delgermaa consulted with her Russian professors, and eventually enrolled in a traditional medicine program in Korea, specializing in acupuncture. She has become one of the leading intellects in Mongolian medicine.

Like Delgermaa, and lacking access to any formal training in traditional medicine in Mongolia, a number of physicians traveled to other Asian countries (China, Tibet, and Korea primarily) for training, and began a dialogue with the few physicians who had studied traditional medicine in secret. Through these efforts, these early physicians played a significant role in the reconstruction of Mongolian medicine. It is notable that the development of Mongolian medicine was shaped, in large part, by the interest of a number of biomedically trained physicians.

As we shall discuss in greater detail below, this experience, coupled with the oversight of the Ministry of Health, itself dominated by Russian-trained physicians, shaped both the content and the institutional role created for Mongolian medicine. The result was the development of an "adjunct" or complementary tradition, which initially at least was somewhat of a pan-Asian medicine, borrowing liberally and eclectically from other Asian medical systems. More recently, however, with the establishment of stronger ties to Tibetan institutions in exile, and with greater attention given to study of the Mongolian medical texts, many of which are written in Tibetan, there has been a greater effort to historicize Mongolian medicine and thus to construct a more culturally "authentic" tradition. These efforts are particularly evident in the main private medical college of Manba Datsan (discussed in more detail below), which is run by a Buddhist monk trained in India.

We observed the practice of Mongolian medicine in the main public in- and outpatient clinics in Ulaanbaatar. These clinics provide the main practical training opportunities for the vast majority of Mongolian medical physicians and thus represent the dominant mode of traditional healing nationwide. Outpatient diagnostic practices are similar to what has been reported for Tibetan medicine in China and India (Janes 1995; Samuel 2001). Pulse diagnosis is the principal technique used and, combined with an interview of the patient, suggests an initial diagnosis. Inpatient diagnostic practices are more complex, involving urine diagnosis (urine is not stirred or whipped as in Tibet, simply observed and smelled) and a battery of biomedical tests as well. The treatment regimen offered to patients is in some ways distinctive from that which Janes has observed in China (1995, 2002) and which Samuel (2001) has described in India. It involves a mix of herbal medications, regular massage, mud baths, medicinal baths, Chinese-style acupuncture, heat and light therapy, blood-letting, and cupping.

In addition to the standardized and diverse traditional medicine practiced at the public clinic, the nationalist movement has encouraged the revival of the Buddhist healing traditions. During the socialist period monasteries, which had once been, as in Tibet, key social, political, and economic institutions in local communities, were either destroyed or abandoned. Buddhist rituals, where they were still performed at all, were done in secret. Most religious activity was restricted to the domestic sphere. By 1987 there was only one operating monastery in the entire country (Sanders 1987). However, the declaration of Buddhism as the state religion in 1990 encouraged proactive efforts to resurrect the tradition, and monasteries were rebuilt throughout the country. As part of this initiative the "Monastery of Medicine to Help People" (*Busdad Tuslahui Anagaah Uhaani Khiid*), a monastery in Ulaanbaatar destroyed in 1937, was restored as Manba Datsan[4] (to which we refer above), and a Mongolian medical practice closely associated with its Buddhist foundations has been developed. The government-backed center contains an outpatient clinic, hospital, traditional medical college, and active monastery.

Religious healing is an integral part of this medical practice. Chanting and ritual often accompany other features of patient care. For instance, Manba Datsan houses a monastery with monks trained to perform special rituals for the restoration of physical, emotional, and mental harmony. Also, the prayers, ceremonies, blessings, meditations, and healing rituals at the monastery are specially focused on repelling misfortune and sickness. Patients treated at Buddhist private traditional medical clinics may be provided advice to organize and participate in longer rituals, which are performed by specially trained monks for a set fee. This Buddhist Mongolian medicine is licensed, regulated, and supported by the government. Its overtly religious foundations are embraced as part of the Mongolian national identity, and the medicine has been supported for this reason.

The traditional medical system practiced throughout Mongolia today is thus an eclectic mix of theories and practices. Drawing from ancient Mongolian medical texts, historical texts, contemporary Tibetan medicine, new "research" designed to assess the biomedical relevance of traditional theories and medicaments, and training received in other Asian countries, scholars of Mongolian medicine have built a system that is designed for and shaped by the social, scientific, and thoroughly modern exigencies of the present historical moment. Its current reality is less a reflection of the past than it is the product of rational efforts, spurred on by the democratic transition in 1990, to create a marketable, efficient, and complementary medical system that resonates with global discourses on the value of traditional medicines, efforts at Mongolian nation-building, and the imposition of neoliberal reforms to the human services sector. Mongolian medicine is today celebrated as an important part of Mongolian heritage. Its "natural" medicines, grown on Mongolian soil, are considered best suited for the Mongolian bodies, and its practitioners and users laud its effectiveness.

Training in Mongolian medicine

The Mongolian government early on made an effort to systematize training in Mongolian medicine, establishing a School of Mongolian Traditional Medicine within the National Medical University of Mongolia in 1990. It is clear from the beginning that, despite the celebration of "native genius" inherent to government decisions to legitimize traditional medicine, and its strategically symbolic importance to nation-building, Mongolian medicine was in practical terms seen as a resource complementary, and thus secondary, to biomedicine. Training in Mongolian medicine was developed as a layer of elective coursework on top of a core curriculum of basic biomedicine. Students deciding to specialize in Mongolian medicine complement this biomedical core curriculum with courses in the Tibetan language, Tibetan medical theory, and Mongolian additions to/modifications of that basic theory. Students of Mongolian medicine are, for example, expected to study and memorize selected portions of the core texts – *Gyü-Shi* (*Rgyud bzhi*) – of Tibetan medicine, and are expected to master basic medical terminology in three languages – Tibetan, Russian, and Mongolian.[5]

Parallel training in biomedicine and traditional medicine continues through the fourth year of instruction. At this point internship and residency training is completed in Mongolian medicine. Altogether the length of training is six years; students are awarded dual baccalaureate degrees in family medicine and Mongolian medicine. As of 2002 there were 251 graduates from the traditional medical program and approximately 1,000 biomedical physicians who had received three to twelve months of postgraduate training at the School. The School has trained the vast majority of Mongolian medical practitioners in Mongolia.

Graduates from the program are licensed as both biomedical and traditional medical practitioners. Reflecting health care reforms designed to promote primary health care, based on the European "family doctor" model, the graduates of this program are considered the ideal primary care physicians equipped with "holistic skills" to address a full range of patient needs. The traditional medical training is considered a useful asset for the biomedical doctor. As of 2002, however, few Mongolian medical doctors have been hired to work as family doctors; most choose to work in hospitals and clinics which specialize in traditional medicine. Also, many have left the country to establish lucrative practices in Europe. Generally speaking, it is far more attractive economically to work in private settings than in the quasi-public family doctor clinics which form the core of Mongolia's primary health care system.

Aside from the main public training program and hospital, there are two other colleges of Mongolian medicine. Both are private and represent a slightly different form of Mongolian medicine than that which is taught and practiced in the School of Mongolian Traditional Medicine at the National Medical University. The two colleges, Monos[6] and Otoch Manramba Institute at Manba Datsan, offer five-year programs and award graduates a baccalaureate degree in traditional medicine with the professional title of "physician of traditional medicine." The colleges have been reviewed and granted formal accreditation by the Mongolian government. Unlike the graduates of the National Medical University, graduates of these institutions are only permitted to practice traditional medicine. Nearly all have gone into private practice.

The Otoch Manramba Institute at Manba Datsan was established in 1991. To date there have been 100 graduates from the program who now practice as private physicians, teachers, and researchers. Eight of the twenty-five teachers at the college are Otoch Manramba graduates and the rest are biomedical doctors, scientists, and religious figures with advanced degrees in Buddhist philosophy (many earned in Tibetan monastic colleges in India). The curriculum is 70 percent traditional medical topics, 25 percent Western medical subjects, and 5 percent "general knowledge."

Graduates describe the biomedical curriculum as limited to the interpretation of biomedical diagnostic tests, which, as in the case of the public university, are required in order to rule out an acute biomedical disease prior to treatment. The study of traditional medical theory is emphasized, mastery of literary Tibetan is required, and all four books of the *Gyü-Shi* (*Rgyud bzhi*) are memorized.[7]

The Institute is housed within an active monastery. The prayers, ceremonies, blessings, meditations, and healing rituals at the monastery are specially focused on repelling misfortune and sickness. The monks are trained in rituals intended to restore physical, emotional, and mental harmony. Thus, the medical training at this college is closely associated with Buddhist religion and spiritual healing. A number of the Institute's graduates are monks.

In practice, the medicine taught at Otoch Manramba is characteristic of the traditional medical practice closely associated with Mongolia's revival of Buddhism and, as a consequence, it is in some ways distinct from that taught in the biomedically dominated Mongolian traditional medicine program at the National Medical University (described above). For example, biomedical diagnostic tests are absent from the Otoch graduates' practice. The traditional diagnostic techniques, pulse diagnosis, interrogation, and examination are similar in method, but the Otoch physicians do not use biomedical instruments. They look at X-rays, ultrasounds, and lab results if brought by the patient and comfortably refer patients for testing, but sphygmomanometers, stethoscopes, and ECGs are noticeably absent from examination rooms.

An additional distinction in practice is the use of treatments. Unlike the liberal use of diverse, external therapies by the School of Mongolian Traditional Medicine's graduates, Otoch traditional physicians rely primarily on herbal medications. The students are trained in massage, moxibustion, acupuncture, cupping, and blood-letting, but the treatments are rarely employed in the outpatient setting. In addition to their reliance on herbal medications, Otoch practitioners employ Buddhist rituals in their healing practice. Thus, religious healing is an integral part of their medical practice. The director of Manba Datsan is famous for his special secret mantras for infertility and prevention of miscarriage. He said the success of his mantras was "guaranteed" and noted that he had traveled to London and Japan to help infertile couples.

Mongolian medicine in the Mongolian health sector

Subsequent to the political-economic transition, and recognizing that significant resources were tied up in expensive curative, tertiary services, the Mongolian government, in consultation with (some would say at the behest of) international donors and policy-makers, tentatively adopted a primary health care strategy as the centerpiece of health care reform. Universal access by all citizens to primary health care was legislated as early as 1990, and some services, mainly care to women and children, were to be provided free of charge. A national health insurance system was legislated in 1994, and has been consistently revised since then to regulate costs and expenses, and to address problems of access by, and exclusion of, so-called "vulnerable" subpopulations.

Little substantive reform was accomplished until the Asian Development Bank (ADB) entered the picture in the latter half of the 1990s. It has to date provided loans in the amount of approximately US$24 million in support of a "Health Sector Development Programme" (HSDP). Although there are many formal goals of ADB-sponsored health reform, the core themes can be reduced to two: a) the shifting of health care costs, and activities, from public to private sectors, accomplished through the application of compulsory insurance, co-payments, and user fees; and b) the establishment of a system of family doctors, providing full and equal access by urban and provincial center populations to basic primary health care services, and acting as gatekeepers to secondary and tertiary care facilities.

The cornerstone of ADB-funded primary care development in Ulaanbaatar and the provincial centers is the "family group practice" (FGP). Within each practice, several doctors, ideally (but not always) trained in primary care, provide services to a defined population of patients. Family doctors are paid on a capitation basis, adjusted by population risk and socioeconomic factors. The capitation scheme is designed both to recognize different health needs in a community and to give incentives to the family doctors to provide quality service to needy groups (Hindle *et al.* 1999).

Family doctors are prohibited from selling drugs or otherwise collecting user fees. They are obligated to provide services to all those registered in their communities. They are charged with referring patients, if deemed necessary, to higher-level treatment or diagnostic work-ups in district or specialty hospitals. Funding for establishing the FGPs came originally from the ADB's first health sector development program grant. It has now been partly shifted to local government and, in 2003, funding was beginning to flow into the system from the national health insurance fund.

As has been described, doctors trained in Mongolian medicine at the National Medical University are also licensed to practice as family doctors. It is clear from our interviews with medical college and ADB staffs that there is great hope that cadres of family doctors, with some knowledge of traditional medicine, will become important, if not central, to the delivery of primary health care. One of the ADB representatives has suggested that the idea behind the FGP model is that family doctors will be fully able to offer "holistic medicine" to all citizens, regardless of their ability to pay. Traditional medicine, according to one of the professors in the School of Mongolian Traditional Medicine, is "ideally suited" to provide such care, insofar as it relies on therapies and medicines that are easily and cheaply available. A WHO report on the Mongolian health sector very much embraced this efficiency argument (WHO 1999):

There is potential for wider application of traditional medicine practices of proven value in Mongolia. For example, acupuncture as an effective, inexpensive and readily transportable modality could be used to improve the delivery of health care service in Mongolia, considering the shortage of essential drugs available for the treatment of common diseases.

(Section 6, p. 19)

Although it is early in its development, the family group practice model has yet to achieve its goal of providing holistic care on an equitable basis, particularly in poor communities (Janes *et al.* 2006). Restricted access to basic drug supplies and diagnostic tests, problematic and highly bureaucratic funding arrangements, and thus financial limitations of doctors' abilities to offer anything but a referral service to patients, who may not be able to afford the services to which they are referred, has resulted in, as one of us has argued, a system of attenuated and thus ineffective primary care (Janes *et al.* 2006). Given these significant structural constraints and financial disincentives, traditional medicine has thus been largely kept out of the family group practice system. To date physicians with Mongolian medical training work primarily in specialized traditional medical hospitals or private clinics, and even the few traditionally trained family doctors practicing primary care are disinclined to offer traditional medicine. For example, we interviewed a family physician who received training in Mongolian medicine and uses her skills each summer when she travels to Poland, earning in a few weeks what she earns in a year as a family doctor, but offers it only rarely to her low-income patients in Ulaanbaatar.

Further weakening efforts to integrate Mongolian medicine into the primary care delivery system is the lack of interest or faith in traditional medicine exhibited by patients from the poorest segments of Mongolian society, the intended beneficiaries of traditional medical services. During the course of our research in Mongolia, we completed a survey of rural and urban residents who live in low-income communities. We interviewed members of sixty-one households who lived in the squatter-type "ger settlements"[8] on the outskirts of Ulaanbaatar, and members of thirty households in rural Huvsgol province in northwestern Mongolia. These households were selected randomly, using a multi-stage, cluster sampling technique. These households are thus representative of the parts of the country, and the communities, from which they were drawn. We asked about access to, use of, and opinions about various health resources, and collected narrative histories of illness events that had occurred in the month prior, and year prior, to the interview. Traditional medicine, which included self-treatment with collected herbs (domestic medicine), was used in approximately 16 percent of illness incidents reported in the preceding year (35 out of a total of 219 incidents). However, when we asked about patterns of resort to health care providers, for all illness incidents reported formal traditional medicine was used as a first resort in just 2 percent of cases, second resort in about 5 percent of cases. We also asked individuals to discuss their opinions of traditional medicine. Most individuals claimed to be ignorant of traditional medicine and, of these, the majority expressed an equivocal or negative opinion, claiming to have greater faith in biomedicine. Clearly, for this population of Mongolians, and for the health problems they experienced, traditional medicine is not valued as a health care resource, and this opinion translated into very low rates of use.

The picture that emerges from our study of patients, community members, and hospital staffs is that Mongolian medicine is largely an urban health care resource offered to relatively affluent patients in private hospitals and clinics. Within such settings, Mongolia's national health insurance system provides reimbursement for inpatient care with Mongolian medicine. While health insurance is available to all Mongolian citizens, substantial co-payments and user fees restrict access. From the perspective of practitioners, though, insurance reimbursements, when combined with these patient fees, make the practice of Mongolian medicine particularly lucrative. Mongolian medical hospitals and clinics are now the fastest-growing sector in the new private medical market. As Table 2.1 shows, the number of traditional medical clinics and hospitals equals the number of non-specialized private biomedical clinics.

This integration of Mongolian medical practitioners into the biomedical health care system as specialists rather than primary care physicians is based on a division of labor encouraged by the pervasive belief that traditional medicine is best suited for treating illnesses that biomedicine does not satisfactorily treat. Doctors and patients argue that traditional medicine is effective for treating the cause of the illness and restoring health, whereas biomedicine is effective at relieving acute disorders and in treating trauma and other emergent conditions. It is also suggested that biomedicine's alleviation of symptoms does not heal the "root causes" of disease, turning it, therefore, into a chronic, periodically recrudescent condition. Therefore, traditional medicine with its focus on the roots of disease is considered the necessary complement to biomedical treatment. In this way, a rational system of medical care has been defined that employs biomedicine for the relief of acute symptoms and traditional medicine for the cure of the illness's root causes. Of course, the distinction between "chronic" and "acute" is characteristic of many, if not most, pluralistic medical systems. In Mongolia, however, the distinction is explicitly coded in health policy and insurance reimbursement mechanisms and, as such, takes on a character which appears to distinguish it from other Asian

Table 2.1 Private health care institutions in Mongolia in 2001

Type of service or institution	Number in all Mongolia	Number in Ulaanbaatar
Private hospitals with beds	75	45
Private pharmacies	320	184
Drug wholesale agencies	42	42
Dental clinics	148	83
Gynecological clinics		
(abortions and STI treatments)	60	43
Traditional medicine clinics	59	45

Source: Government of Mongolia, Ministry of Health and Social Welfare

contexts. Of greatest interest is the degree to which the distinction derives principally from a biomedical frame of reference, which then dominates diagnostic and therapeutic decision-making even though these may be exclusively "traditional." An example will illustrate how this distinction works in practice.

Patients seeking admission to the main public Mongolian medical hospital in Ulaanbaatar are typically referred by a primary care physician or by a practitioner working in a district hospital facility. The demand for admission to the hospital is very great, especially during the winter, and the waiting list for a bed may be as long as three months.[9] Prior to admission the patient undergoes a biomedical screening which is intended to rule out any potentially serious conditions. Only those patients who have certifiably chronic but stable and non-serious diseases will be considered for admission. Patients with acute conditions, or serious chronic diseases such as cancer, will be referred instead to a biomedical facility. Subsequent to admission, the patient undergoes a complete diagnostic work-up. Patients are given two diagnoses. The first, and required for insurance reimbursement, is the biomedical diagnosis. This diagnosis is often based on a combination of history, previous laboratory tests, and biomedical tests given at the time of admission. There are a number of biomedical specialists who work in the hospital; their job is to assist with making an accurate biomedical diagnosis; this becomes the primary diagnosis, and is written in Russian, or a combination of Russian and Mongolian, on the patient's chart. Traditional diagnoses are then determined on the basis of history, pulse-taking, and traditional urinalysis (smell, appearance, color). A traditional diagnosis is then given and written in Tibetan on the patient's chart. According to physicians, the treatment plan, which may include herbal medications, massage, medicinal baths, acupuncture, blood-letting, and cupping, is entirely in keeping with the logic of, and any subsequent refinements to, the traditional diagnosis. Our observations of and interview with patients in this hospital suggest that biomedicine – either institutionally or in terms of its primacy as the cognitive model which guides the primary diagnostic effort – is a gatekeeper of access to Mongolian medicine in the public sector. Patients are referred by biomedical practitioners, and upon admission are evaluated to insure that they do not have an acute or serious (read: "treatable") condition. Only after the basic steps of biomedical diagnosis have been satisfactorily completed is a patient able to take advantage of the facilities. As one young physician remarked, traditional medicine is in many cases the "last" resort after all other measures have been exhausted or found to be ineffective.

This same young physician admitted that the dominance of biomedical thinking, both in terms of her own training and in terms of admission to the public inpatient hospital, affects the way she thinks about Mongolian medicine. She noted that, for the first part of her training, she learned almost nothing but biomedicine, and thus concentrated on what she termed "scientific" understandings of the body. This, she noted, is the study of "real" and "material" things. The terminology of Mongolian medicine, when it was introduced, was much more difficult to comprehend. It is quite abstract, and lacks the "materiality" of "scientific" medicine. It was very difficult for her at the beginning to truly comprehend traditional theories of the body, and they definitely took a back seat to her training in biomedicine. It is for this reason, she said, that she relies primarily on biomedicine when she approaches a patient (although she did note that she is new to the practice of medicine and that some of her teachers don't do this at all). The primary history, diagnosis, lab tests, and so forth are all rooted in biomedicine. Only when bio-medical techniques are "exhausted" does she turn to traditional techniques, except in cases where she has learned from experience that traditional medicine really works – she mentioned cerebral palsy and rehabilitative medicine – where Mongolian medicine would be the treatment of first resort.

This faith in the tangible, material aspects of biomedicine manifests itself in the considerable anxiety among practitioners of Mongolian medicine over the potential harm of a 'wrong' diagnosis using traditional medical techniques. Patients and doctors both suggested that one of the only disadvantages to traditional medicine was the greater risk for misdiagnosis and, hence, mistreatment. This reflected the belief that the pulse exam was a subjective and possibly unreliable way of assessing the health of the whole body, while biomedical tests were objective and valid. If done properly, by an experienced physician, the pulse-taking was considered an accurate means of diagnosing the body, though the potential for error was believed to be greater. Given this level of uncertainty and anxiety, biomedical diagnostic tests were used to support traditional medical assessments and validate the success of traditional treatments, for example a reduction of blood pressure or shrinkage of an ovarian cyst.

The shape and content of training in and practice of Mongolian medicine clearly demonstrate the conflict between the desire to instantiate an important feature of Mongolian history and culture, on one hand, and the requirement that care be fully "modern" in the sense that biomedical theory and knowledge provide the primary logic for diagnosis and therapy. The result of this conflict has been the development of a system which at the surface level is "traditional," with ample symbolic connections to religion and spirituality. On another level – the level of practice – traditional medical practitioners are expected to adhere to the basic formulation that traditional medicine is complementary and secondary to biomedicine. In the private hospitals and clinics, while this feature of modern practice may not be as evident as in the public clinics, the requirements imposed by health insurance, by licensing, and by accreditation insure that the boundaries of the complementary role remain fixed. The important question, and one which we cannot at this point answer, is whether and to what extent the complementary role to which Mongolian medicine is now restricted has had an impact on the theoretical basis – such that it exists – of the tradition. There is some evidence to suggest that, as a consequence of placing Mongolian medicine in a close and direct relationship with biomedicine, traditional practitioners are engaged in a project of reconciling traditional theory with what they know of biomedical theory. In a recent text describing the fundamentals of Mongolian medicine, Bold and Ambaga (2002) devote an entire chapter to a "New era for scientific research into traditional medicine." In it they argue that the abstract notions of the humors are in effect metaphors for the "three basic states of membrane structure."

Of equal importance and as a consequence of the more significant of neoliberal transformations to the Mongolian health system – privatization and gate-keeping by primary care physicians – access to Mongolian medicine is restricted largely to individuals who can draw on the resources required to gain admission to one of the public or private hospitals or who can pay for consultation and medicines in one of the many private clinics. Despite global discourse on the role of traditional medicine in providing cheap and efficient therapy in the context of holistic primary care, it is principally available to the urban elite. Economic rewards, locally, and abroad, particularly in Eastern Europe, where Mongolian physicians have found opportunities for lucrative practice and drug sales, attract traditional doctors into the private sector. Local and global demand is driven by those whose desire for alternatives to biomedicine is matched by their access to social and economic resources. This is not to suggest, however, that there is necessarily a great, unmet demand for traditional medicine among the urban and rural poor. Mongolian medicine, as we have discussed, has been created out of a project of nation-building and, as such, is largely an intellectual product of the same classes to which it now primarily offers its services. Individuals in poor communities – urban and rural – know relatively little about Mongolian medicine, often evince equivocal attitudes about it, and therefore use it relatively little.

Indeed, one reading would suggest that the creation of traditional medicine in Mongolia is in many ways an exercise of political elites who have embraced neoliberal reform while at the same time deploying powerful symbols of Mongolian identity in order to contend with the demons of the socialist past. Although the invention of Mongolian medicine may have begun as an overtly political, and thereby cynical, act, its creation has captivated the imagination, both local and global. Its eminent marketability has enormous appeal in an economic context of liberal markets and the growing global trade in herbal medicines. Traditional medicine, a showcase element of an imagined Mongolian identity, also bears the global imprimatur of market efficiency. And what could be more attractive to the modern liberal state than this?

The transformations of Tibetan medicine

The modern history of Tibetan medicine in China differs from that of Mongolian medicine primarily in the degree and intensity of efforts by the state to destroy it. Whereas in Mongolia three generations of violent oppression effectively extinguished the tradition, in China two factors insured the continuity of the indigenous medical system. First, as a result of efforts by the thirteenth Dalai Lama to "modernize" Tibet in the early twentieth century, a non-monastic tradition of Tibetan medicine was established. This non-monastic tradition, based in Lhasa at the first Mentsikhang[10] by virtue of its independence from the great monasteries and lack of any explicit ties to the feudal past, survived the early years of Chinese political control and socialist reform. The first director of the Mentsikhang, an accomplished student of the great twentieth-century physician Khyenrab Norbu, became an influential Tibetan member of the Chinese Communist Party, and used this position and influence to protect the main elements of training and practice. In many ways, he is principally responsible for the contemporary structure and character of Tibetan medicine in China. Tibetan medicine was early on defined as a secular institution, separated from the politically and ideologically problematic religious sector, and associated with the principles of social justice that formed the core of Chinese revolutionary discourse. Second, the government in Beijing has never pursued a coherent or consistent policy in the Tibet Autonomous Region with regard either to traditional medicine or to Tibetan cultural institutions more generally. Attitudes toward traditional medicine in Tibet were in large part like attitudes toward traditional Chinese medicine – these were a potentially valuable resource, illustrative of native genius, and thus inseparable from those elements of Chinese civilization that were, in Maoist thinking, to be blended with the uniquely Chinese socialist project of modernization. Tibetan medicine was identified as one of the "family" of Chinese medicines. On the other hand, Tibetan medicine was associated with Tibetan ethnic expression, a problem that has plagued Chinese attempts to integrate the region more thoroughly with the interior, predominately Han, state. It is fair to say that, given these countervailing interests, the attitude of the government toward Tibetan medicine was, and continues to be, ambivalent.

The Cultural Revolution in Tibet, as throughout China, had serious consequences for scholarly institutions, but it was relatively short-lived, and damage done during the period was repairable. Tibetan medicine was thus poised for rapid development when the Mao government fell and Deng Xiao-Ping initiated liberal macroeconomic and political reforms. Tibetan medicine was rapidly expanded into the sparsely populated rural regions where it was intended to become an important component of primary health care.

As in Mongolia, these efforts at rationalization had a certain impact on the content and practice of the tradition. Tibetan medicine was set into conversation with biomedicine and science (as these are represented in China), and the training of medical practitioners was incorporated into the standard undergraduate university curriculum. Through training, and limitations on practice, the state is able to control the secondary and, to a great extent, the primary resources of Tibetan medicine. Janes (2002) has summarized these efforts at control as follows: First, the state controls the content of education in traditional medicine. Although these days faculties are given significant latitude in discussing the philosophical underpinnings of Tibetan medical theory, both they and their students interact with this knowledge in a context where religion, because of its association with Tibetan independence sentiments, is a touchy subject. Scholars and students are careful to frame their discussions in such a way that their explicitly religious connotations are downplayed or articulated in "scientific" terms (Adams 2001b). Second, the line that distinguishes the sacred from the scientific is drawn carefully in the context of an educational system that early on sets students in conversation with biomedicine, science, and political theory. Scholars and practitioners must resolve disparities between the theoretical elements of Tibetan medicine and biomedicine in a context where anything other than scientific discourse is problematic. As with Mongolian medical scholars, the effort is to demonstrate correspondences between traditional and modern medical theory. Third, the social organization of Tibetan medical practice seriously limits the degree to which medical theory and the traditional logic of treatment can be thoroughly applied. For example, the theory of humors suggests that each individual possesses a particular "character." This character predisposes the individual to particular diseases and, therefore, must be taken into consideration in determining treatment. Disease is thus individual- and context-specific, and care must be taken in determining a particular diagnosis and treatment regimen. In the setting of the busy clinic, where, as one of us has discussed (Janes 2002), physicians may take just a few minutes for treatment, the individualized approach is abandoned in favor of a more standardized model of diagnosis and treatment.

The consequences of such state-led practices of rationalization are summarized as follows:

> Tibetan medicine is becoming fully modern in its social structure and cultural content. . . it is becoming disembedded from local contexts of practice and reconstituted as part of a centralized system of technical accomplishment and professional expertise, which in turn is expected to conform to the pervasive and powerful cultural standards of rational science and biomedicine . . . [W]hen ethnomedicines are sanctioned and supported by the state the resulting pluralism is orchestrated by institutions and structures built out of the culture of biomedicine and, therefore, entails a transformation of medical care and training so that it is consistent with the epistemological, symbolic, and sociologic attributes of biomedicine . . . The modernization of ethnomedicines in such a fashion is represented by shifts in epistemology and practice that favor a standardized and radically materialistic perspective on the body, an objectification and thus desocialization (decontextualization) of disease, and transformations in the social relations of healing that put emphasis on professionalism, contribute to asymmetries of power in healing encounters, and objectify/reify the patient.
>
> (Janes 1995: 24–25)

By the early 1990s, global discourses around reform, "efficiency," and, somewhat later, "competition" and "decentralization" invaded and displaced the state's discourse on the rational deployment of indigenous medical institutions. By the early 1990s, the clinics, hospitals, and medicine factories of Tibetan medicine saw their state-appropriated budgets slashed by as much as 50 percent. Throughout the region, Tibetan hospitals began competing with one another, not in Tibet so much, but in Beijing, Shanghai, Xian, and Chengdu, as they strove to open for-profit clinics catering to both Chinese and non-Chinese. Representatives of the different regional hospitals traveled abroad to negotiate deals with purveyors of Asian medicine in Paris, Geneva, Munich, and New York.

By 2002, Tibetan medicines had become a hot commodity in the global pharmaceutical marketplace. In one report aired on Chinese national television in early 2001, it was reported that "Tibetan traditional medicines are getting more and more popular both at home and abroad. The *China Business Times* is reporting that the Tibetan herbal medicine industry has an annual output value of over US$2.5 billion." In a follow-up article that appeared in the *People's Daily* the next day, it was concluded that, "in order to fully develop Tibetan medicine, several local governments are looking for foreign investment" (*People's Daily*, January 15, 2001). In December of 2001, China's Xinhua news agency reported that "wild herbal medicines are poised to become big profit makers." Under the terms of entry into the World Trade Organization, replications of foreign patented medicines – something China's large pharmaceutical industry has been dependent on – would be forbidden. As a consequence, "the domestic medicine sector is now actively readjusting its operating strategies, relying on traditional medicine techniques to participate in future competition" (Xinhua News Agency, December 10, 2001).

Preparing Tibetan and other indigenous medicines in China for the global market-place has had predictable consequences on their local practice and availability. In Janes's study of rural health in the summer of 1992 (Janes 1999a, 2002), he found that relatively few rural clinics had sufficient personnel or medications to provide even basic care to local farmers and herders. The best and most experienced doctors had been called to service profit-generating enterprises in Lhasa and beyond. The most desirable medications rarely made it out of Lhasa, unless for transport to Chengdu, Shanghai, Beijing, or Paris. Young, inexperienced doctors, lacking the skills needed to identify and manufacture their own medicines, were left in the expanses of Tibet beyond the capital and major towns, and were unable to provide the kind of care available to urban-dwellers. With the collapse of rural health insurance schemes and the move toward privatization of the health sector, rural biomedicine was largely in the same state. Increasingly in China, access to all medicines, including traditional medicines, is largely a privilege of the urban elite (Hsiao 1995; Hsiao and Liu 1996).

Conclusions

The institutions of indigenous medicine in Mongolia and the Tibet Autonomous Region are both products of socialist modernity. Although the forms that state interest took are quite distinct, and proceeded along different ideological and political lines, the outcomes, in terms of the local structure of primary and secondary resources, share many features. In Mongolia the project of Soviet-socialist modernity was to quash Mongolian traditional identity and, most particularly, those elements associated with the feudalism of the past. Unlike Tibetan medicine, which had to some extent been shielded from feudalist associations, Mongolian medicine, learned and practiced in the context of the monastery, was the object of violent repression. Yet when Mongolian medicine "emerged" in the 1990s subsequent to the collapse of the socialist state, ostensibly to showcase a recovery and cele-bration of a historically rooted yet modern Mongolian identity, its content and the structure of its practice were defined, at least in the initial years, by the high modernist sensibilities that were particularly characteristic of the Soviet enterprise in Central Asia (Scott 1998). Mongolian medicine was invented as a tradition, but subject to the widespread and thoroughly modernist belief that it should be an "adjunct" or complement to biomedicine, a treatment of "last resort." It is possible that Mongolian medicine may over time escape this particularly confining role in the health system, particularly if privatization and economic liberalization weaken the control of the Ministry of Health over its content and practice.

In Tibet, the modernist project was far more moderate than it was in Mongolia: Mao had, especially after the failed Great Leap and his disenchantment with the Russians, little interest in the heavy-handed and Western-oriented approach of the Soviet Union. Yet, as in Mongolia, the relationship between indigenous medicine and identity was a problem, though of a different order, and Tibetan medicine has been forced to maintain a clear boundary between what it calls Tibetan medical "science" and the "sacred" philosophical and soteriological underpinnings of the tradition that are clearly Buddhist and thus, to China, ideologically and politically problematic (Adams 2001b). State control of the medical curriculum, the rationalizing consequences of the modern bureaucracy and, more recently, the impact of health reform have produced in Tibet a standardized, secular tradition.

Thus, in both Tibet and Mongolia, larger state agendas have produced a carefully orchestrated pluralism in which the role played by traditional medical institutions is carefully defined, particularly in juxtaposition to biomedicine. State interests have revolved around two principal motives: concern over the relationship between medicine and identity – championed in one context and feared in the other – and controlled deployment of a valuable health care resource along lines established by the dominant intellectual and political position of science and acceptance of global standards of modernity. Regardless of its political and ideological starting point, orchestrated pluralism has had the same effect in both settings: a desocializing of traditional medicine and a preparation of indigenous therapies and medicines for the global marketplace. On the global scene, these indigenous medicines take on a very different character, and meaning, than they do locally, engaging, in particular, the Western imagination about the wisdom of the East.

Appadurai (1996) argues that imagination, as a social practice which has "broken out of" the past and entered the "logic" of ordinary life, has become a central feature of globalization. The idea that imagination is somehow a newly emergent cultural phenomenon of the global age is probably overstated. Imagination would seem to be central to the representational processes through which groups define and address an array of social problems and from which various discourses, both local and global, are produced. What is a qualitative break from the past is the degree to which imagination as a local social practice is affected by the desires of those at great social, cultural, and geographic distance. Imagination provides people with a new vocabulary for thinking about suffering and its causes and consequences, and thus plays an important role in local medical practices (Janes 1999b). The technicians of development interact with state officials in imagining a health sector and the interventions to it that will create good health at low cost. As well, Western desires for alternative modes of healing, whether empowered by fantasy (e.g. Janes 2002) or the terrifying costs of the health transition in rapidly aging societies (Janes

1999a), engage with global capital in the exploitation, and thus transformation, of local medical traditions. Indigenous medicines in Tibet and Mongolia are enmeshed in, and transformed by, these thoroughly global processes of imagination and the practices that they entail.

Janes (2002) has argued that Tibetan medicine is unique in the degree to which it has become both globalized as Asian medicine and entangled in the complex political and ethical discourse that surrounds the Tibet question. This fact produces several distinct lines of transnational discourse. In the context of global human rights dialogues, Tibetan medicine, like Tibet itself, is construed as subject to ruinous suppression and reorganization at the hands of the Chinese, impairing its authenticity and requiring, if possible, repair and salvage. Given that there is a substantial Tibetan community that lives outside Tibet, one which engages fully in keeping this image of a suffering Tibet on the global human rights agenda, a genuine alternative is always available – an authentic counterpoint to an inauthentic Chinese fabrication (Lopez 1998).

Not unrelated, but in a telling which celebrates its "native genius," Tibetan medicine is center stage among exported Asian medicines, where the transnational deployment of a set of understandings about Buddhist spiritualism pervades its theory and practice (Janes 1999b, 2002; Samuel 2001). As a feature of Tibetan culture, particularly a threatened one, long the subject of Western interest, Tibetan medicine may evoke a longing for imagined things that have been or will soon be "lost" through the processes of modernity (Appadurai 1996; Foucault 1978; Giddens 1990; Lopez 1998). Threatened by the Chinese, Tibet-as-Shangri-La emerges as a threatened source of exceptional, disappearing medical knowledge for maintaining physical and spiritual health. Although Mongolian medicine has not been the object of the same kind and level of Western fascination, the fact that it is an Asian-Tibetan medicine, one which advertises its distinctiveness and which has now fully embraced its Buddhist roots, may promise to attract similar trans-national curiosity. These ideas likely resonate with the changing health needs of the aging populations in the resource-rich Western states of North America and Europe (Janes 1999a).

In Mongolia, a different kind of imagination has been brought to bear on the development of indigenous medicine – the imagination of a health sector as a distinct social world, and the subsequent construction of tools and apparatuses for intervening in that world (e.g. Escobar 1995). As in most countries in the grip of neoliberal health reform, the bearers of this imagined world are the technicians of globalization – a loosely affiliated and cosmopolitan mix of economists, financiers, physicians, health administrators, and public health practitioners – who together link the global possibility of health reform, as it is imagined in the halls of the development banks and other intergovernmental institutions, to local institutional realities. Central to this imagining is the idea that the privatization of some aspects of the health sector is the only avenue to providing "efficient" and "high-quality" health care at low cost.

Privatization stimulates paradigmatic shifts in health policy and a structural reorganization of health care institutions. Under pressures to privatize, the health care "system" is pulled apart at the seams. Traditions, specialties, therapists, and styles of care are set in competition with one another, diversity is encouraged, and market mechanisms are left to order the relationships between kinds and levels of services. In the context of political decentralization, the consequence is an anarchic fragmentation of services (Janes *et al.* 2006).

Conceptually, this fragmentation of the health care system is accomplished through a series of representational dividing tactics, informed principally by neoclassical economic thought (Laurell and Arellano 1996; Paalman *et al.* 1998). A logic of "public" versus "private" goods is invoked to rationalize privatization, with empirically weak arguments marshaled to argue that some kinds of health care are "private goods" insofar as they are drawn from a theoretically limited supply (and thus cannot be consumed by others), and benefit only the person who consumes them. Because these logics are intellectually compelling, resonate with a long intellectual tradition in public health which has tended to downplay the population-level biological efficacy of clinical health care (e.g. McKeown 1976), and, perhaps most importantly, coalesce with a general "economizing" of society that has accompanied the global penetration of capitalist political economy, they have come to dominate global health policy. In our view, these economizing discourses may free the social organization of therapeutic pluralism from the heavy hand of science (however construed).

In conclusion, these brief examples, drawn from two Asian sites, demonstrate that the development of traditional medicine is entangled in several national and transnational social, cultural, and economic processes. On the state and local level, socialist, and post-socialist, projects to rationalize medical systems in the context of managing national identities transform the practices and theories of traditional medicine. On the transnational level the cultural dimensions of globalization, to which Appadurai (1996) fixes the term "imagination," entail social practices by which local medicines are transformed. Asian medical traditions instantiate Western desires for a holistic or spiritual medicine that in the West has been "lost" to modernity, but may be recovered from an Eastern Shangri-La. In both Tibet and Mongolia the medical systems that we have described have been subject to practices produced out of the discourses of health development – where health care is seen in increasingly economic terms, segmented into types in relation to cost-utility, and valued in regard to its status as public or private goods. In the case of the latter two processes especially, these transnational products of imagination constitute both the rationale and the means to prepare medicines for the global marketplace. In such a way, the potential for the delocalization, if not wholesale appropriation, of local traditions is great. While the local never completely surrenders to the global, in the case of both Tibet and Mongolia there are significant pressures on the local level to reorganize and restructure the primary and secondary medical resources that form Tibetan medicine.

From the perspective of equity and social justice, our research suggests further that access to traditional medicine is increasingly a product of social privilege. In both Mongolia and Tibet, the political economy of health reform, coupled with global demands for the products of these medical traditions, has led to a hierarchical structuring of therapeutic pluralism. For those in the newly emerging, and now sizeable, lower classes, access to health care, any health care, is a problem. To invert a critical observation made by Paul Farmer (1999), whether or not traditional medicine is poor medicine, it is increasingly *not* for poor people.

Notes

1 The three colleges are the School of Mongolian Traditional Medicine at the National Medical University, Otoch Manramba Institute at Manba Datsan, and Manos College. Manos College was not observed. It is a private institution with a five-year program, and its graduates receive a bachelor's degree in traditional medicine.
2 The Russian system of health care emphasized inpatient services, the building of hospitals and clinics, and a reliance on biomedical diagnostic and therapeutic technology. Though rationally distributed and accessible throughout the country, given the reliance on hospital care and a lack of development of a public health system, health care in Mongolia was considered inefficient and expensive by the time of the economic transition of the 1990s.
3 The Mongolian People's Revolutionary Party, or MPRP, which, except for a period in the late 1990s during which a coalition government held power, has dominated national politics throughout the post-transition period.
4 Manba Datsan is the Mongolian transliteration of the Tibetan term for "medical college" (either *sman pa grwa-tshang* or *sman pa grva tshang*). This was the name given to the Tibetan medical schools found throughout Mongolia in the seventeenth to nineteenth centuries.
5 Russian is now giving way to English as the preferred language of scientific instruction.
6 This college was not observed and no graduates from this college were interviewed. It is relatively new and presumably similar to Otoch Manramba Institute.
7 It is unusual in Tibetan medical training for students to memorize all four of the texts; the third text, the Men-ngag Gyü, is in Tibet and India not memorized. It is the longest and most complex of the treatises, and is devoted to a detailed consideration of disease categories, causes, and particular treatments. It is the text subject to the greatest elaboration through commentary, and potential modification in light of "modern" conditions (Samuel 2001). Writes Samuel (2001: 261), "It would be interesting to know how far 'studying the Men-ngag Gyü' at the [colleges today] in fact means studying comparable material on disease categories that has been rewritten in light of present-day needs."
8 The "ger" is the traditional nomadic tent used by Mongolian herders. Known as a "yurt" in the West, this structure is relatively inexpensive and has the advantage of being easily moved. Many newcomers to Ulaanbaatar establish residence in one of the outlying districts of the city, setting up their gers wherever there is available land. These "ger districts" form the most socioeconomically deprived communities in Mongolia today.
9 Individuals may pay fees to move up on the waiting list; more affluent patients thus experience shorter waiting times.
10 The Mentsikhang (Tibetan: *sman rtsis khang*) or, literally, institute of medicine and astrology was established in Lhasa in 1916. It remains the intellectual center of Tibetan medicine in the Tibet Autonomous Region today.

References

Adams, V. (2001a). The Sacred in the Scientific: Ambiguous Practices of Science in Tibetan Medicine, *Cultural Anthropology* 16: 542–575.
Adams, V. (2001b). Particularizing Modernity: Tibetan Medical Theorizing of Women's Health in Lhasa, Tibet. In Linda Connor and Geoffrey Samuel (eds.), *Healing Powers*

and Modernity: Traditional Medicine, Shamanism, and Science in Asian Societies, Westport, CT: Bergin & Garvey.

Adams, V. (2002). Establishing Proof: Translating "Science" and the State in Tibetan Medicine. In M. Nichter and M. Lock (eds.), *New Horizons on Medical Anthropology: Essays in Honor of Charles Leslie*, pp. 200–220, New York: Routledge.

Appadurai, A. (1996). *Modernity at Large: Cultural Dimensions of Globalization*, Minneapolis: University of Minnesota Press.

Baabar, B. (1999). *History of Mongolia*, trans. D. Suhjargalmaa, S. Burenbayar, H. Hulan, and N. Tuya, Cambridge: Mongolia and Inner Asia Studies Unit, University of Cambridge.

Bold, S. and Ambaga, M. (2002). *History and Fundamentals of Mongolian Traditional Medicine*. Ulaanbaatar, Mongolia: S. Bold.

Bulag, U. (1998). *Nationalism and Hybridity in Mongolia*. Oxford: Clarendon Press.

Crandon-Malamud, L. (1991). *From the Fat of our Souls: Social Change, Political Process, and Medical Pluralism in Bolivia*, Berkeley: University of California Press.

Escobar, A. (1995). *Encountering Development*, Princeton, NJ: Princeton University Press.

Farmer, P. (1999). *Infections and Inequalities*. Berkeley: University of California Press.

Foucault, M. (1978). *The History of Sexuality*, Vol. 1, New York: Vintage Books.

Giddens, A. (1990). *Modernity and Self-Identity: Self and Society in the Late Modern Age*, Stanford, CA: Stanford University Press.

Goldstein, M. C. (1989). *A History of Modern Tibet, 1913–1951: The Demise of the Lamaist State*, Berkeley: University of California Press.

Government of Mongolia (1999). *Mongolian Statistical Yearbook 1999*, Ulaanbaatar, Mongolia: National Statistics Office.

Hae-Joang, C. (1998). Constructing and Deconstructing Koreanness. In Dru Gladney (ed.), *Making Majorities: Constituting the Nation in Japan, Korea, China, Malaysia, Fiji, Turkey, and the United States*, Stanford, CA: Stanford University Press.

Hindle, D., O'Rourke, M., Batsuury, R. and Bunijav, O. (1999). Privatising General Practice in Mongolia: A Trial of Needs-Adjusted Capitation, *Australian Health Review* 22(3): 27–43.

Hobsbawm, E. and Ranger, T. (1983). *The Invention of Tradition*, Cambridge: Cambridge University Press.

Hsiao, W. C. L. (1995). The Chinese Health Care System: Lessons for Other Nations, *Social Science and Medicine* 41: 1047–1054.

Hsiao, W. C. L. and Liu, Y. (1996). Economic Reform and Health: Lessons from China, *New England Journal of Medicine* 335(6): 430–432.

Janes, C. R. (1995). The Transformations of Tibetan Medicine, *Medical Anthropology Quarterly* 9: 6–39.

Janes, C. R. (1999a). The Health Transition and the Crisis of Traditional Medicine: The Case of Tibet, *Social Science and Medicine* 48: 1803–1820.

Janes, C. R. (1999b). Imagined Lives, Suffering and the Work of Culture: The Embodied Discourses of Conflict in Modern Tibet, *Medical Anthropology Quarterly* 13: 391–412.

Janes, C. R. (2001). Tibetan Medicine at the Crossroads: Radical Modernity and the Social Organization of Traditional Medicine in the Tibet Autonomous Region, China. In L. Connor and G. Samuel (eds.), *Healing Powers and Modernity: Traditional Medicine, Shamanism, and Science in Asian Societies*, Westport, CT: Bergin & Garvey.

Janes, C. R. (2002). Buddhism, Science, and Market: The Globalisation of Tibetan Medicine, *Anthropology and Medicine* 9(3): 267–289.

Janes, C. R., Chuluundorj, O., Hilliard, C. E., Janchiv, K., and Rak, K. (2006) Poor Medicine for Poor People? Assessing the Impact of Neoliberal Reform on Health Care Equity in a Post-Socialist Context. *Global Public Health* 1: 1–22.

Kotkin, S. and Ellman, B. (1999). *Mongolia in the Twentieth Century: Landlocked Cosmopolitan*, New York: M. E. Sharpe.

Laurell, A. C. and Arellano, O. L. (1996). Market Commodities and Poor Relief: The World Bank Proposal for Health, *International Journal of Health Services* 26: 1–18.

Lopez, D. S. (1998). *Prisoners of Shangri-La: Tibetan Buddhism and the West*, Chicago, IL: University of Chicago Press.

McKeown, T. (1976). *The Role of Medicine: Dream, Mirage, or Nemesis?*, Princeton, NJ: Princeton University Press.

Ole, B. and Ole, O. (1996). *Mongolia in Transition: Old Patterns and New Challenges*, London: Curzon.

Paalman, M., Bekedam, H., Hawken, L. and Nyheim, D. (1998). A Critical Review of Priority Setting in the Health Sector: The Methodology of the 1993 World Development Report, *Health Policy and Planning* 13: 13–25.

Pomfret, R. (2000). Transition and Democracy in Mongolia, *Europe–Asia Studies* 52: 49–58.

Samuel, G. (2001). Tibetan Medicine in Contemporary India: Theory and Practice. In Linda Connor and Geoffrey Samuel (eds.), *Healing Powers and Modernity: Traditional Medicine, Shamanism, and Science in Asian Societies*, Westport, CT: Bergin & Garvey.

Sanders, A. (1987). *Mongolian Politics, Economy, and Society*, London: Frances Pinter Publishers.

Scott, J. C. (1998). *Seeing like a State*, New Haven, CT: Yale University Press.

Starr, P. (1982). *The Social Transformation of American Medicine*, New York: Basic Books.

Unschuld, P. (1975). Medico-Cultural Conflicts in Asian Settings: An Explanatory Theory, *Social Science and Medicine* 9: 303–312.

Unschuld, P. (1985). *Medicine in China: A History of Ideas*, Berkeley, CA: University of California Press.

World Health Organization (1999). *Mongolia Health Sector Review*, June, Ulaanbaatar, Mongolia: WHO-Mongolia and the Mongolia Ministry of Health and Social Welfare.

Yoshino, K. (1998). Culturalism, Racialism, and Internationalism in the Discourse of Japanese Identity. In Dru Gladney (ed.), *Making Majorities: Constituting the Nation in Japan, Korea, China, Malaysia, Fiji, Turkey, and the United States*, Stanford, CA: Stanford University Press.

3 Place and professionalization

Navigating *amchi* identity in Nepal

Sienna R. Craig

Soma Namgyal sat outside his clinic in Mustang, Nepal, thumbing his prayer beads. A monk in his seventies, Soma Namgyal is also a Tibetan medicine practitioner (*amchi*[1]) of renown. In his youth, Soma Namgyal studied with senior *amchi* from Chagpori, before this institute of Tibetan medicine, founded in the seventeenth century, was destroyed in the aftermath of the Chinese occupation of Lhasa in 1959.

"I don't know what to make of things these days," he said.

> For years, we were unimportant to the Nepali government. Where is Mustang to them? Not much more than a backward place in the mountains. Now, since democracy came to Nepal, *rongba* [lowland, Hindu Nepalis] and foreigners talk about our medicine. Younger *amchi* say we need development to preserve our *amchi* tradition. But I've seen development. It's nothing more than moving to Kathmandu, buying a motorcycle, eating more rice than *tsampa*.[2]

"But what about the work some *amchi* are doing?" I asked. "Forming an organization, making connections to Dharamsala, Lhasa, and the Nepali government, publishing newsletters, having workshops?"

"I don't know," said the old *amchi*. "I joined the organization. I've been to meetings. But I'm too old. The best I can do is treat people until I die. What will happen? That is for the younger generation to decide."

In this chapter, I explore the circumstances under which *amchi* from Nepal are shifting the forms and, to a certain extent, the meaning of their medical practices: from vocation to profession, from master-apprentice instruction to more formalized, institutional learning, from medicines produced and prescribed by the same healer to the use of ready-made pills and powders. I argue that the professionalization of *amchi* in Nepal is occurring in partial and fragmented ways, despite the organizing principle of the Kathmandu-based Himalayan Amchi Association (HAA) and its state and non-governmental interlocutors; yet the impacts of professionalization are deeply felt and debated by the *amchi* with whom I work. This process of professionalization calls into question taken-for-granted distinctions between "tradition" and "modernity" as they relate to systems of healing, and provides further illumination to what is meant by the phrase "medical pluralism." The dynamics about which I write further complicate distinctions between professional affiliation and cultural identity, and relate to the boundaries – ideological and geographic, ethnic and linguistic – that partition modern Nepal. The story of *amchi* practice in Nepal today also reveals healing as a social process, enacted and embedded in the politics of the day. Practitioners of Tibetan medicine who are also citizens of Nepal navigate between individual and collective sensibilities and between forms of knowledge as well as between *at least* three nations, namely Nepal, exile-Tibet, and Tibetan areas of China.

In what follows, I ask how, why, and to what extent *amchi* from Nepal are seeking legitimacy and support from the Nepali state, non-governmental conservation and development organizations, and institutions of Tibetan medicine in India, China, and beyond. How does the fact that *amchi* from Nepal exist as historically marginalized citizens of the world's only Hindu polity[3] play against their identification as cultural, if not political, Tibetans? Finally, how does this collective positioning of *amchi* from Nepal vis-à-vis state-level and international agendas relate to individual renown, locality, and distinct ways of knowing and practicing Sowa Rigpa (*gso ba rig pa*), the "science of healing"? To address these questions, I focus on events surrounding the Second Annual National Conference of Amchi, held on January 4–6, 2002. The conference was organized by the HAA, a Nepali non-governmental organization (NGO) founded in 1998, whose more than 120 members hail from the high-mountain regions of Nepal, bordering the Tibet Autonomous Region (TAR) of China.

This chapter is divided into four sections. First, I sketch the founding of the HAA, as well as its current activities and future goals. I address issues of ethnicity, nationalism, and identity to frame encounters between *amchi* and the Nepali nation-state. I describe the official narrative the HAA produces about the history and current state of *amchi* medicine in Nepal. I sketch a few key biographies of the individual actors in the HAA, as they relate to the organization as a whole. I also touch on the ways that foreign models of organization – from large institutions of Tibetan medicine in India and China to international conservation and development programs – have influenced the sensibilities and goals of *amchi* from Nepal, and how this influence plays out in the internal politics of the HAA. Second, I examine the creation of HAA identity cards, the production of Amchi Profile Data sheets, and the inaugural session of the conference. Here, I aim to describe and analyze the varied, and at times conflicting, strategic essentialisms which contour *amchi* professionalization in Nepal. Third, I focus on the creation of a certificate that was given to each novice *amchi* who completed a month-long refresher training course, which occurred after the conference. This episode illustrates how the HAA and its individual members negotiate the politics of language and culture in Nepal, and explores the benefits and limitations of standardizing medical knowledge and practice through certification. I conclude by weaving the specifics of *amchi* practice in Nepal back into the more general tropes of "tradition" and "modernity." I offer a view toward how these concepts are deployed, as well as how they coexist, in the lives and work of Tibetan medicine practitioners in Nepal today. As such, this study of *amchi* professionalization is also an inquiry into different modes of knowledge transmission.[4]

Ethnography provides an entrée into many of the issues that both HAA members and I identify as pertinent aspects of professionalization, albeit with different philosophical and theoretical emphases. In the abstract, negotiation of the forms and structures of *amchi* practice exemplify a classic postcolonial paradox: how to simultaneously defend and transform "tradition"? Practically, this includes internal and external pressures to conserve medicinal plants, standardize medicines and medical practice, incorporate biomedicine into treatment regimes, and alter the forms and structures of *amchi* education. Partially through the efforts of the HAA, "*amchi*" is beginning to connote a fixed professional marker in Nepal, and yet it also continues to serve as a more fluid identity, emerging at the confluence of religious, political, and historical consciousness, played out distinctly across local cultural geographies. As such, these professionalizing processes signify new and conflicting agendas about what it means to be an *amchi* in Nepal today: discourses and practices that point toward larger anthropological questions about efficacy, medical pluralism, and the dynamics of being a "traditional medical practitioner" in a "modern" world.

The Himalayan Amchi Association: "Tibetanness" and the Nepali nation-state

The *amchi* with whom I work are speakers of Tibetan dialects who live in or retain ties to villages located in the fourteen districts that form Nepal's northern border with the Tibet Autonomous Region, China. They are also practitioners of Tibetan Buddhism and Bön. These *amchi* and their fellow villagers are often labeled by the rather awkward term "Tibetanid" or, in Nepali vernacular, by the derogatory term "*bhote*" (Höfer 1979; Ramble 1993). Ramble (1997) describes what he calls "Tibetan pride of place" against the notion that Nepal's high-mountain populations can be considered an ethnic group. It is perhaps more accurate, he argues, to understand identity as a local and relational phenomenon, tied to cults of mountains, village protector deities, and other place gods.[5] We must remember that many of the borderland regions of Nepal, in which today's *amchi* live and work, were once part of the network of vassal states and principalities that formed historical Tibet (cf. Jackson 1984; Snellgrove 1961). Although these border regions have been a part of the nation-state of Nepal since the eighteenth century, most of these areas have remained peripheral to the state. My own fieldwork in these Nepali borderlands confirms Ramble's assessment that an allegiance to local identity is primary – as opposed to an articulated sense of *ethnicity*. Yet, while it is true, as Gellner notes, that "no one in Nepal is only a Nepali," people whose history and cultural practices emerge from Tibet and Buddhism are particularly marked, not only since Nepal has been designated as a Hindu state (Gellner *et al.* 1997)[6] but also because of the particular politics of Tibet vis-à-vis Nepal and China, as I discuss in more detail below. In that sense, *amchi* are historically marginalized and marked citizens. This marginalization exists at the levels of culture, language, politics, and human services. Most *amchi* and their communities exist on the literal and figurative fringes of the Nepali nation-state, from lack of government services such as biomedical health posts and schools, to the sheer distances between many *amchis'* home villages and the urban center, Kathmandu.

Here, we must consider in more general terms the ways that non-Hindus within Nepal relate to the forging of this Hindu nation-state (cf. Burghart 1984). Nepal was never colonized, but it has always struggled with what some scholars call an "internal colonization," namely, the ordering of its people along caste, ethnic, and religious lines by the high-caste Hindu ruling elite (Höfer 1979; Holmberg *et al.* 1999). During the Rana oligarchy (1846–1951) and the Panchayat political regime (1960–1990), debates over caste, religion, and ethnic identity were largely silenced. Such alterities could fragment Nepal's "imagined community" at a time when asserting the validity of Nepal's nation-state project against colonial and later republican India was critical (Anderson 1983; Gellner *et al.* 1997). And yet, hierarchies of caste, religion, and ethnicity have been confirmed and contested for centuries in Nepal, through collective and individual consciousness, social and political action (Parish 1996).

In sociological terms, ethnic classification systems – like all classification systems – are arbitrary; they are often politically expedient and yet rooted in what might be called primordial sentiment and perpetuated as conventions (Barth 1969; Weber 1978). In this sense, ethnicity exists only when people claim one source or form of identity against another, when consciousness *and* difference become a consciousness *of* difference. As such, ethnicity is a tool that can be used by people to define themselves, and implies a certain degree of empowerment and agency. But the use of the term "ethnic" and the designation "ethnic group" can mask power relations between and among people, particularly within the context of nation-state formation (cf. Kapferer 1988; Verdery 1994; Williams 1989). As much as ethnic categories might provide a way for individuals and groups to maximize their own interests, they often produce and reproduce structural inequalities. When viewed from this perspective, ethnic groups emerge in the context of nation-building projects that seek to create homogeneity out of heterogeneity (Munasinghe 2001) and to override the particulars of history through the articulation of an all-encompassing national narrative – what the historian Prasanjit Duara calls "universal history" (Duara 1996). Following this theoretical trajectory, we can observe many instances in which the creation and maintenance of ethnic boundaries in Nepal have been directly connected to improving one's political or socio-economic lot within the political system of the day (cf. Levine 1987). This is particularly apt in relation to the last seventeen years of Nepali history.

The 1990 People's Movement (Jan Andolan) was a democratic revolution that propelled Nepal to become a constitutional monarchy and the government to officially recognize the country's cultural diversity. Key to this transition was the rise of ethnic or indigenous (*janajati*) politics movements. These, along with social movements emerging against other forms of institutionalized discrimination (such as caste), were born out of the democratization process and can be considered part of a political vision that "demanded a new term for peoplehood and preservation of cultural diversity" beyond the Panchayat-era vision of "traditional communal harmony" (Tamang 2000). One of the movement's first major victories was to have

Nepal recognized as a "multicultural, multilingual, and multireligious" polity in the 1990 constitution (ibid.). Nepal's various *janajati* organizations have also engaged in the (re-)invention of tradition in order to cement their "indigenous" legitimacy in the present – a classic social and political strategy (Hobsbawm and Ranger 1983).

But where do *amchi* professionalizing efforts fit into this picture? As we have seen, neither *amchi* nor the communities from which they hail fit neatly into an *ethnic* category. As an illustration of this, one could cite the dearth of *janajati* organizations that claim to represent Tibetan-speaking populations from Nepal's high mountains. Rather, we can say that *amchi* from Nepal form an *interest* group, one whose identities are joined in certain ways and yet still distinguished by region and dialect. Yet Nepali *amchis'* strategies for social organization and social change share something with the articulation of ethnic identity, particularly in relation to how *amchi* are presenting their case for recognition and support to Nepali government institutions. In short, organizing professionally along lines of culture and tradition implicates them in contemporary discourses about national identity and ethnicity in Nepal (Gellner *et al.* 1997). The HAA frames aspects of their struggle in terms of being a collective of underserved *bhote* communities whose particular traditions and practices have been marginalized by, for lack of a better term, the high-caste Hindu hegemony. While the HAA's organizing goals certainly diverge from those of, say, the Mongol National Organization (MNO) or other powerful *janajati* lobbying groups, the points from which *amchi* begin to articulate their marginalization is similar – at least at the level of rhetoric – to those of a number of Nepal's ethnic and indigenous rights movements.

Perhaps most significantly, in framing themselves as an interest group with a case worthy of state recognition, *amchi* often begin by invoking the trope, and the reality, of their practice as "indigenous knowledge" and as *amchi* as purveyors of a tradition that is illustrative of Nepal's cultural diversity. To this end, the issue of language is central. While the *amchi* who make up the HAA do not necessarily share a common *spoken* language – they are divided by regional dialects, some mutually intelligible and others quite distinct – they are united *in their identities as amchi* by literary Tibetan language. The need to master written Tibetan as part of what it means to be an *amchi* or to transmit Sowa Rigpa knowledge to younger generations remains key to how the HAA understands its struggle to improve the quality of *amchi* education and practice in Nepal. Likewise, the historical unwillingness of the Nepali government to engage with the need and desire for literary Tibetan to be a part of government school curricula in the districts from which *amchi* hail fits neatly within one of the key lobbying points made by *janajati* organizations, namely the demand that "mother tongue" education be allowed in self-defined ethnic communities. And yet, while most *janajati* politicking around this issue of mother tongue education centers on basic literacy and spoken language, the *amchis'* articulation of the need for literary Tibetan is also a claim to a higher order of literacy and access to an "exclusive" language – a language, if you will, not of community or cultural identity but of science.

The legacy of Nepal's "universal history" and the reframing of Nepal as inherently diverse also bears on understandings of the politics of health development in Nepal, and *amchis'* places within this, particularly when one understands Nepali nation-state formation as integrally linked to international development aid. It is fair to describe this dynamic as symbiotic: a state-development apparatus that is also a regime of knowledge and power (Battachan 1994; Des Chene 1996; Ferguson 1994). The Nepali state maintains a longstanding alliance with, and dependence upon, foreign aid, including health care-related initiatives. The centralized Panchayat state introduced biomedicine to Nepal on a broad scale, with capital and expertise provided by foreign aid organizations (Justice 1986). This introduction of health-related development programs marked a watershed moment in conceptions of science and medical efficacy in both local and national Nepali discourse. The social symbolism of healing in Nepal also included the framing of local healing practices as belief rather than knowledge, as "backward" and opposed to *bikasi* or "developed" (Pigg 1996).[7] Today, despite shifts in development policy and practice toward validations and appropriations of "ethnomedicine" or "traditional healers" in some instances (Pigg 1997), and a more general and widely deployed set of terms about rights and advocacy that derive from international NGO "culture," if you will, Nepal's state-development apparatus still focuses on incorporating such healing systems as complements to biomedical health care, rather than as valid systems in their own right.

The HAA describes itself as a Nepali non-governmental organization whose mission is: to gain recognition and support for *amchi* from the government of Nepal, institutes of Tibetan medicine in India and China, and international non-governmental organizations; to conserve medicinal plants used by *amchi* and help to design and implement conservation and management initiatives for medicinal plants at local, regional, and national levels; to facilitate knowledge exchange between *amchi*; to provide sustainable, culturally appropriate, and high-quality health care in their communities; and, as such, to protect and revitalize Tibetan medical practice in highland Nepal. The HAA also aims to support Tibetan medical schools and clinics, provide additional education opportunities for novice *amchi*, conduct their own research on *amchi* history and practice as well as medicinal plant identification and status, and eventually propagate needed medicinals for commercial sale and individual use.[8] As in other parts of the world, the HAA's agenda as a body representing marginalized citizens as well as practitioners of ethnomedicine is framed as an appeal for the preservation of "indigenous knowledge" and "tradition" as a matter of national pride and world heritage. HAA's literature also acknowledges an increasing global interest in and market for "alternative" medicine in general and Tibetan medicine in particular. In these respects, the formation of the HAA can be seen as a reflection of – or reaction to – newly emerging professional interest groups, medical institutions, and international development organizations that have taken up the notion of "medical pluralism," as well as the drive to link "tradition" and "nature" with "modernity" and "science."[9] In sum, these aspects of *janajati* politics are also inverted, or complicated, by *amchis'* struggles to be recognized and supported within the national Nepali context and yet, ideally, not to be bound to it.

The HAA was registered as an NGO in 1998, but this official recognition was a long time in coming. As one board member of the HAA describes it:

> We first went to register in 1996. We had the papers. We'd even made stamps. But the Nepalis in the office, they saw us as *bhote*. "What is this *amchi*?" they said. "Is it like a *jhankri*?"[10] They did not know what "*amchi*" meant. I explained that *amchi* are not *jhankri*. We have texts, and make medicines from plants. I tried to explain our history – how Sowa Rigpa comes from the Buddha and from Tibet, but that it is also here in Nepal. The men behind the desks said that if we talked about Tibet we wouldn't get permission – Nepal is so scared of China, you know. So we made new papers that only said "*amchi* medicine" and "Himalaya" instead of "Tibet." Still, it took two more years to get permission.

This vignette provides a clear example of the ways individual *amchi* and the HAA must manage cultural identities, navigating between the strictures of the Nepali nation-state and their own senses of self and organizational purpose.

As part of their efforts to improve educational opportunities for novice *amchi* and network with other practitioners of Sowa Rigpa, the HAA forged connections with institutions of Tibetan medicine abroad, in China and India as well as in Mongolia and Bhutan. As such, members of the HAA are part of a growing network of practitioners of Tibetan medicine whose frame of reference is not only national but also linked to a concept that I might describe as "Tibetan medical cultures" or "satellite Sowa Rigpa communities." Here, I would locate practitioners of Tibetan medicine from Ladakh, Spiti, and Sikkim, in India, as well as those from Bhutan, Mongolia, and parts of the former Soviet Union, particularly Buryatia. As necessary and accurate as these labels are in one sense – it is undeniable that connections between Tibetan medical practice have experienced a renaissance of sorts throughout South and Central Asia, as well as Eastern Europe, particularly since 1989 – such categories are also awkward and unsatisfying. They reinforce a sense that these places are somehow inferior in relation to "high" Tibetan culture, either the Chinese or the diasporic varieties. They also silence the impacts of modern nation-state formation and nationalism on the diverse practices that constitute what we generically call Tibetan medicine in the contemporary context.[11]

In the Nepali milieu, Tibetan medical institutions and individual practitioners exist within an array of agendas, often at odds with each other. The politics of culture and development, as well as distinctions between science and religion at the state level, continues to frame the terms of these interactions.[12] The ways *amchi* are situated in Nepal reflect Nepal's status as a nation-state in relation to India and China. Although *amchi* is a Tibetan word (actually derived from Mongolian), it operates *against* and acts as a replacement for the signifier "Tibetan" within the context of Nepal, when used to describe these individuals' identities as medical practitioners. This is due in part to the political pressure China places on Nepal not to harbor "splittist" Tibetan nationalists.[13] To maintain good diplomatic and economic ties to China, Nepal must continue to prove that it sides with China on the "Tibet Question."[14] But the fact that Tibetan medicine as practiced in Nepal must not be named as such is also attributable to a Nepali nationalism that at once attempts to encompass and capitalize on "Tibetanness" while simultaneously marginalizing culturally Tibetan border communities as "backward" and "undeveloped" high-mountain peoples.[15] In this context, both the practitioners with whom I work and I myself understand the category "*amchi*" as both confined within the Nepali nation-state and transcendent of it. It is then worth asking how *amchi* from Nepal might cultivate a unified voice that can be heard by others – from whom they want support and recognition – and at the same time be attentive to their own cacophony of hopes and needs, histories and practices.

As an example of this interplay between individual experience and organizational ambition, I highlight the biographies of two people. Although the HAA has grown and changed since it was founded, becoming more diverse and democratic in its operations, the role of these two *amchis* – their professional contacts, personal rivalries, and activist visions – should not be underestimated. The first, Tshampa Ngawang, is an *amchi* originally from the Muktinath Valley in Mustang District. The second, Gyatso Bista, is an *amchi* from Lo Monthang, the walled city in the restricted region of Mustang that is also known as the kingdom of Lo.[16] Both Gyatso and Tshampa Ngawang are *ngags pa*, tantric householder priests, who identify strongly, though not exclusively, with the *rnying ma* or "old" school of Tibetan Buddhism. Their identities as *amchi*, indeed their efficacy as healers, are closely tied to their *rgyud*, or lineage, as well as their skill: both had fathers who were particularly renowned healers. Both can be considered members of noble families – specific examples of the more general claims to social status, respect, and authority often enjoyed by *amchi* in Tibetan society. Gyatso, like his father before him, serves as the royal physician of Lo.[17] Tshampa Ngawang claims ties to the aristocratic families of the Dzar-Dzong region of Muktinath Valley.[18]

Tshampa Ngawang was the chairman of the HAA from its founding until December 2002, when, during the HAA's Third National Conference, he was made "honorary chairman" and Gyatso Bista, the former General Secretary, was elected the new chairman. But even before the HAA was ratified as an NGO, these two worked to form and register an *amchi* association with Mustang District authorities. During this time, Tshampa Ngawang and Gyatso Bista visited other high-mountain areas of Nepal and other regions of the Himalayas (Ladakh, Dharamsala, Darjeeling, Tibet). At different times, they both served as consultants for the World Wildlife Fund Nepal Program and UNESCO People and Plants Initiative. In this capacity, these two Mustang *amchi* served as ethnobotanical experts in the creation and implementation of a WWF/UNESCO-sponsored conservation and development program for Shey Phoksundo National Park in Dolpa District, west of Mustang.[19] Through this opportunity, these two Mustang *amchi* cultivated relationships not only with international and national NGOs, but also with *amchi* from neighboring regions. Each in his own way, they also deployed a narrative that, although Dolpa was rich in medicinal plants and home to a few highly skilled *amchi*, it was a region more poor and "backward" than neighboring Mustang: people were dirtier and the quality of life was worse.[20] Along with the foreigners and other Nepalis involved in the WWF/UNESCO People and Plants Initiative, they encouraged *amchi* in Dolpa to organize, helping to create the momentum that has helped to carry the HAA through these past few years.

In this sense, a shared concern between "insiders" and "outsiders" about the future of Tibetan medicine as practiced in the Nepal Himalayas, if not a shared vision of a professionalizing strategy or ideal future, has helped to found and fund the HAA.[21] The HAA held its first conference and ran its first refresher training course for thirty novice *amchi* in 2001 – events that have continued for three consecutive years and that have made such training accessible to more than 100 novice practitioners. By the end of 2002, four district-level *amchi* associations, in Mustang, Dolpa, Mugu, and Gorkha, were registered with the Nepali government; they have begun to facilitate communication between individual *amchi* and the HAA. Despite the HAA's more than 120 members (including senior and novice *amchi* alike), its success as an organization has depended, to a great degree, on the work of a few people, such as Tshampa Ngawang and Gyatso Bista, who have chosen to pursue connections in Kathmandu and abroad, sometimes at the expense of meeting local health care needs – a key trope of medical professionalization in other cultural contexts as well (cf. Last 1996; Starr 1982). Some have also faced disapproval from community members who see their efforts on behalf of the HAA as mere exercises in social advancement.

The HAA's literature[22] articulates a particular narrative about why *amchi* medical practice has come to a crisis in Nepal. It highlights the political, economic, and social forces which are deemed largely outside of the control of individual *amchi*, as well as these practitioners' "nested identities" vis-à-vis Nepal and Tibet (cf. Duara 1996). According to this narrative, villagers used to trust *amchi* and the efficacy of their medicine implicitly. An *amchi*'s authority rested on lineage, reputation, and affiliations with centers of medical knowledge in Tibet. *Amchi* occupied elevated positions in society, alongside lamas and clan or village leaders, and were generally considered of a higher status than *lha pa* and *lha mo*, oracles. Their work as healers was also imbedded in a narrative of altruism and compassion. Although theoretical medico-religious precepts dictated that *amchi* not charge directly for services, payments were negotiated in culturally and economically appropriate terms: a sack of grain, the use of a draught animal, a few rupees. When the Nepal/Tibet border closed after 1959, trade in medicinal plants, as well as knowledge exchange between *amchi*, was disrupted.[23] Further, the introduction of state and foreign aid-sponsored biomedical clinics in rural Nepal also directly impacted *amchi* practice by, in some cases, challenging its efficacy and, at the least, offering alternate visions of what healing could mean and what health-seeking behaviors, motivations, and practices could be employed by patients. Today, negotiations between subsistence and cash-based economies have complicated the acquisition of *materia medica*, compromised the quality of medicines, and curtailed incentives for younger generations to train as *amchi*. While medicinal plants are still collected locally, bartered for, or bought, the terms of this exchange have changed. Furthermore, the creation of national parks and protected areas has meant that *amchi* have come into contact – and sometimes conflict – with conservation agendas aimed at monitoring and limiting the use of and trade in flora and fauna (Lama *et al.* 2001).

The HAA also articulates a relationship between *amchi* practice and biodiversity, as well as the political economy of health care and notions of "development." As Gyatso Bista has written:

> Within the Nepal Himalaya, the health of the majority of people has depended on *amchi*. Therefore, for the purpose of the health of all these people, Nepal Himalayan *amchi* need to see progress, advancement. But at this time, because there has been no development, *amchi* medicine is degenerating . . . Foreign medicines have become popular, but this means the wealth of [Nepal] is spent in other countries, to buy these foreign medicines. [Sowa Rigpa] is like a precious jewel that has been neglected. Yet, it is vital to local health and culture . . . If we can get herbal ingredients and. . . make good medicines, then we can foster a skilled culture . . . Compared with other people, *amchi* feel more strongly about the plants and herbs. *Amchi* can protect the herbal medicines as best as possible. But if we say 'as best as possible' and there are no medicinal plants left, from what should we make medicines? If there are no medicines, what are *amchi* to do?

> (Bista 2001[24])

This quote can be read in several ways. On the one hand, it can be seen as a product of the *amchi* elite and their interactions with foreign donors and conservation agendas (cf. Pordié 2001). On the other hand, it can be read as a more emic realization of the changes in availability of plants and the shifting socio-economic and cultural status of *amchi* and their medicine. Of course, these two readings are difficult, if not impossible, to disaggregate. They inform each other. Is there use or validity, for instance, in trying to pinpoint the moment when an *amchi*'s exposure to international conservation agendas ends and his sensibility about the collection of medicinal plants – the need to be attuned to taste, timing, and smell, the need to collect with the "right motivation," as stipulated in Tibetan medical texts – begins? Although very little research has been done to prove or disprove the "sustainability" of *amchi* harvesting practices, this trope of "indigenous knowledge" and "sustainability" is used as both an argument for the preservation of "traditional culture" and a justification to reform "backward" or non-scientific practices in regard to resource use and politics (cf. Li 2000). This tension is not lost on the HAA. Their organizational position emerges as one that systematically connects the regional and global proliferation of biomedicine with a discourse of cultural and ecological survival.[25] As stated in English in the HAA's first published pamphlet: "This traditional art is a wealth of many medical practitioners of our country and [the] Himalayan region. This art is a pillar of [the] life cycle for the Himalayan people."[26] Here, we should also understand that the notion of "tradition" as something that can be isolated – something that can exist outside of daily praxis – is a product of modernity itself.

And yet the HAA's literature tends to focus on what it identifies as external forces of change – development regimes, altered social and political economies – rather than to articulate a more nuanced dialectic between cultural change and continuity, between local and global forces as well as between generations. The degradation of Tibetan medicine in Nepal, as discussed in HAA literature, presents a teleology of decline that is perhaps too simple, in that it only vaguely addresses the choices and constraints made by *amchi* and their patients, which have also contributed to the diminishing socio-economic status of *amchi* and their medicine in Nepal. For example, HAA literature acknowledges the presence of biomedicine at village and national levels, but it does not speak to why many people in these *amchis'* communities now routinely choose biomedical treatment in addition to, or as a replacement for, seeking out an *amchi*, even if at a great personal expense. Although individual *amchi* know that both patients and healers move across the divides between biomedicine and Tibetan medicine, the HAA often has a difficult time articulating this pluralistic reality, partially because its hope for support rests on the notion – or image – of preserving a "traditional" practice (cf. Bode 2002; Ernst 2002).

With this background, one can understand "*amchi*" as a charged signifier – marginally Nepali and surreptitiously Tibetan, scientific and yet marked as a "traditional art." It can also be seen as a strategic winnowing of the complex social world in which *amchi* from Nepal live and work into a professional identity *by these individuals themselves*. The HAA has made the term "*amchi*" comprehensible to the Nepali state, thereby creating a means through which individuals might reap material and social benefits at the national level.

Yet the category "*amchi*" condenses – or in some cases silences – a great deal of cultural, medical, economic, and even linguistic difference internal to this group of people. Despite the HAA's professionalizing project, *amchi* are never just *amchi*; they are often more immediately and consistently identified as people from a particular community, affiliated with a distinct geographic location, religious tradition, and lineage, as well as socio-economic position. In addition, although most people who call themselves *amchi* have some background in the theory of Sowa Rigpa, many who have joined the HAA are specialists in one kind of medical practice – accomplished in bone-setting or moxibustion, gifted with healing *rlung* imbalances, adept in the recitation of *sman ngags* (oral instruction tantras) or the production of several specific medicines – but not necessarily well rounded or highly skilled Tibetan medical practitioners. In this sense, perhaps the HAA's work *can* be viewed as the production of "*amchi*" as both a professional and an ethnic marker – creating unity out of diversity for the sake of social change.

But how is this sense of *amchi* identity forged in practice in Nepal, and what of its ambivalent nature?

Identity cards and "special guests": delimiting official *amchi* identity

On the opening morning of the Second Annual HAA Conference in January 2002, the foyer outside the conference hall was bathed in sunlight and charged with activity. A cluster of *amchi* from upper Dolpa District stood in one corner of the hall, talking about the journey south. An old *amchi* from the Nar Valley in northern Manang District sat spinning a prayer wheel, a satchel made from the pelt of a snow leopard at his side. The bag was filled with silver spoons, gold and silver moxi-bustion needles, and bundles of herbs. Just as I noticed their presences, I felt the absence of *amchi* from the far-western districts of Mugu and Humla: dire places in those days, trapped between famine and armed violence, clashes between the Communist Party of Nepal (Maoist) and the Royal Nepal Army and armed police.[27] As absences go, I counted only two young women in the convening crowd. Both were students at a new school for Tibetan medicine in Lo Monthang, and one was the daughter of the HAA General Secretary. Men dominated the HAA roster. Many HAA members were *amchi* by patrilineage as much as they were *amchi* by choice.

A few young men stuck out amidst the sea of red cloaks and worn mountain faces. They wore jeans and baseball caps, their hair cropped short. These were the new *amchi* recruits from Rasuwa District, just north of Kathmandu, who had been invited by the HAA General Secretary after he made a field trip to the area. The young men spoke no Tibetan and they seemed bewildered. I asked them why they had come, what interest they had in *amchi* medicine.

"In our village, we don't know much about these old traditions, but we want to learn," said one of the young men.

> We are closer to Nepal than these other people, but *amchi* medicine is important. Now, we go to government health posts. But they're no good. The medicines are expired and the doctors don't come. If people are really sick in our villages, they go to Kathmandu or sometimes call a *jhankri* or die.

The other young man offered:

> My grandfather remembers *amchi* coming to our areas from Tibet. He learned something from them. When [the HAA General Secretary] came to our villages, we said we were interested in learning *amchi* medicine. He said HAA would pay for our food and lodging if we came, and that we could get some training.

When I asked the General Secretary about his motivation for choosing these two young men from Rasuwa, he replied that they seemed smart and sincerely motivated. They also knew about the trade in medicinal plants in Nepal – a major part of Rasuwa's economy.

"If we can help to train young people from these areas," the General Secretary explained, "then hopefully we will benefit the health of local people and conserve some of the medicinal plants. Right now, medicines are just going from these areas." By recruiting these young men as novice *amchi*, the HAA was not only attempting to swell its ranks, thereby further legitimating *amchi* medicine as a Nepali profession in the eyes of the state and international organizations, but also making a connection between professionalization and the economics of resource use. Taken together with the HAA's stance on medicinal plant conservation, as well as the acknow-ledged shifts in the forms and structures of *amchi* education, this strategy also points to their attempts at counteracting the increasing separation between those who collect medicinal plants, those who produce medicines, and those who treat patients – a reality that *amchi* from Nepal have witnessed, albeit from a distance, in the examples of institutes of Tibetan medicine in Dharamsala and Lhasa.[28]

Significantly, this effort at recruitment also expands on the definition of "*amchi*" as a professional marker. These young Rasuwa men did not lay claim to lineage or classical Tibetan language, yet they could potentially be transformed by Sowa Rigpa, a practice that they viewed as socially and culturally valuable, if also somewhat removed from their everyday experiences. More importantly, from the perspective of the HAA, they could be transformed from outsiders to insiders.

Over the previous year, the HAA had been compiling Amchi Profile Data sheets for each member – an attempt to record *amchi* life histories and information about their medical practice. These data sheets also included questions such as: Which diseases do you diagnose and treat most frequently? How much do you spend on buying and transporting medicinal ingredients each year? Do you ever use biomedical treatments or recommend a patient to the hospital? Although theoretically a trove of information, these questionnaires had been written up in English by one of the HAA's non-Tibetan-speaking foreign advisors and then translated into Tibetan. As a result, many of the questions did not make sense, either to the individual *amchi* who were supposed to fill them out or to the HAA staff who helped non-literate healers record their Amchi Profile Data. For instance, when asking about an *amchi*'s use of Western biomedicine, or allopathy, the word "allopathic" was simply transliterated into Tibetan script, but the important questions to which it referred were devoid of meaning. This example is both interesting and disturbing, in that English signifiers have now gone such a long way in delimiting knowledge claims across the world and framing the terms of the discussion (Pigg 2001).

The chairman of the HAA spent several hours that first morning of the conference monitoring the filling out of Amchi Profile Data sheets. He was most concerned with delimiting "real" from "fake" practitioners. "Since the WWF People and Plants project came to Dolpa, many people from there are now saying they're *amchi*, just so they can get the benefits of working on a *project*," he said.[29] "But we can't just have everyone who knows a plant or knows one place to put a moxibustion stick calling himself an *amchi*. Then, the quality of medicine will not get better. We won't have development."

Taken in conjunction with the presence of the Rasuwa recruits, this issue of determining professional authenticity seemed at once contradictory and apt. Revitalizing the practice of *amchi* medicine in Nepal would require new recruits and novice practitioners. Yet the presence of people who could "pass" as *amchi*, by virtue of their physical appearance and language, became cause for alarm. Much like a guild or a fraternity, the HAA was determined to screen its members as well as recruit young minds.

As the chairman presided over Amchi Profile Data, the treasurer of the HAA sat at another table registering new members and handing out identity cards once they paid their Rs. 500 annual membership fee. Though not an insignificant sum, this fee was minimal compared with the benefit most *amchi* saw in retaining the HAA identity card.

"I wish I'd had this when I was traveling last week, through Gorkha," said one *amchi* from Nubri. "The police stopped me and took all the plants I was going to bring here, to share with others and for teaching."

"These cards are protective amulets [*srung ba*] but against the army and police and Maoists, instead of demons!" said another *amchi*. I found this metaphor prescient. These laminated professional accouterments served as individual and collective protection. Although they might not always work, they had the potential to deflect harm and misfortune. They made *amchi* recognizable. These card-carrying *amchi* could prove their authenticity to outsiders, such as police, when asked. In this context, the efficacy of an *amchi*'s medicine seemed secondary to the process of formalizing *amchi* identity. Here, efficacy was not charted by a patient's recovery or the years an *amchi* had spent studying medical and religious texts. Rather, efficacy was social and political in nature – that which works not to heal but to render visible an *amchi*'s role as a healer.

While *amchi* were registered and interviewed, the conference's "special guests" milled about in the courtyard, passionately discussing the South Asian Association for Regional Cooperation (SAARC) convention that was occurring simultaneously.[30] None of the *amchi* seemed particularly concerned with these efforts at high-level South Asian diplomacy. As one *amchi* put it, "The Nepali government is only concerned with impressing big people."

Of much more immediate concern to many *amchi* who had gathered for the conference was the upcoming Kalachakra initiation in Bodh Gaya, India: ten days of Buddhist instruction and empowerment presided over by the fourteenth Dalai Lama.[31] After making the trek to Kathmandu, many *amchi* were seizing this opportunity to attend the Kalachakra ceremony. Their concerns highlighted the ambivalent position many of them occupy as Tibetan-speakers from the borderlands on the one hand and Nepali citizens on the other. Again, the ambivalence of what it means to be an *amchi* in Nepal was mirrored by the HAA members' motivations for coming all the way to Kathmandu. I could not help but wonder if an opportunity for pilgrimage – as opposed to crafting the future of Sowa Rigpa in Nepal – was the driving force behind these *amchis*' attendance at the conference.

Later that morning, the HAA chairman called the meeting to order. "Special guests" ascended to the stage. For the next three hours, the sixty-odd "general member" *amchi* who had traveled to Kathmandu for the conference sat in the audience as HAA board members, "special guests," and advisors, including myself, offered introductory remarks. The divide between stage and audience was stark –

as unsettling as it was predictable. Some of the *amchi* in the audience listened. Others dozed, spun prayer wheels, and leafed through the Tibetan-language publications that had been given to them by the HAA.[32] The chairman of the HAA recounted his personal lineage history and implored each *amchi* to do his part to "develop" and "care for" Sowa Rigpa in Nepal. The secretary of the All Nepal Buddhist Association spoke passionately about how the "current situation of *amchi*" was reflective of Hindu state-sponsored bias against the country's Buddhist communities. The statement spoke more directly to *janajati* politics in Nepal than to *amchi* medicine, but it was the only speech that received a spontaneous, though cautious, round of applause from the audience *amchi*. The chief guest, the member secretary of the Remote Area Development Committee, located the problems *amchi* currently face as part of the geographic and economic divides that partition Nepal. An esteemed Nepali practitioner of Ayurveda, also an advisor to the HAA, did his best to "prove" that *amchi* medicine and Ayurveda were "mostly the same." The country representative of the WWF Nepal Program and the representative of the UNESCO People and Plants Initiative both invoked *amchi* practice as indigenous knowledge and as key components of conservation. I expressed my interest in the HAA and *amchi* medicine both as a researcher focused on the history of Sowa Rigpa and the future of *amchi* practice and as a member of an international NGO that has given guidance and support to the HAA. The sum of these speeches created a web of meaning about why the HAA had come into existence and what its mandate was. Of course, the real question was, did the *amchi* in the audience feel the same?

In these opening speeches, *amchi* were revealed as both modern and traditional, at once ethnic Nepalis and harbingers of "authentic" Tibetan culture by the founders of the HAA and the motley crew of "special guests," each in his own way. They were represented as people from Nepal's most remote, undeveloped locales, as biodiversity-minded conservationists, and as practitioners of a dying art, in need of preservation themselves. Yet the *amchi* in the audience, to whom the speeches were directed, had little opportunity to actually respond to this representation.[33] Furthermore, none of the speeches articulated how individual claims to knowledge and lineage, or the character of local culture, ecology, and economics, might challenge attempts to meet the HAA's goals. Perhaps this diversity remained unvoiced in the official context because it was so readily apparent in more informal circumstances. For instance, the collective aesthetic and political statement of the HAA identity cards was matched by business cards peddled by individual *amchi* – subtly, in quiet moments – to all the "special guests," in the hopes of securing a patron or two for their personal endeavors, from local monasteries to new, private clinics.

"This is our sickness," the General Secretary said during an after-hours meeting.

> We know we have to be like one person when we talk to the government and try to get support to develop *amchi* medicine. To make schools or clinics we need to work together. But as soon as meetings end, we scatter like poplar seeds in the wind. We want the benefits that should come from the HAA, but it is our habit to look after ourselves. This is much easier than working as one.

The currency of certification: or, Who needs a piece of paper anyway?

On one afternoon of the Second Annual HAA Conference, the board members began designing a certificate that would be given by the Nepali minister of health to each *amchi* who passed the final exam for this year's refresher training course. As in the previous year, a Tibetan physician from Chagpori Medical Institute in Darjeeling, India, had come to Kathmandu to teach the course.[34] The curriculum focused on the *phyi ma rgyud*, one of the four medical treatises that form the foundation of Tibetan medical teachings (*Rgyud bzhi*). As in the previous year, the course would be taught from a condensed *phyi ma rgyud* reader that the HAA had produced.[35] Usually, the *phyi ma rgyud*, or "last tantra," and the other three texts, required a year of study and memorization each. But, all circumstances not being equal, these thirty practitioners would have a month to "refresh" themselves on this text, at the end of which they would take written and oral exams and then be offered a certificate of achievement, in accord with their rank.

Although finalizing the words contained within the certificate would prove difficult for the HAA board members, divining the aesthetics of the document was easy. All the *amchi* agreed that the certificate should be crowned with the HAA's official seal, rimmed in red ink, and signed at the bottom by both the chairman of the HAA and the Nepali minister of health. Before the start of the conference, the HAA board had asked the Chagpori Medical Institute if it would also validate this certificate with an institutional signature or seal, particularly because the instructor of the course had come from Chagpori. The Chagpori authorities had denied this request.[36]

The board members instantly agreed that the certificate should be bilingual, in English and Nepali. They unanimously chose to include no Tibetan on the document, even though the course would be conducted entirely in Tibetan and would be based on a preeminent Tibetan medical text. I asked the board members why they did not want to include any Tibetan on the document.

"You know about papers," the vice-chairman answered. "We cannot put Tibetan on here for the same reason it took HAA so long to get government approval for the HAA. They're suspicious of anything called 'Tibetan.' They're scared of China. And what can we do about that?"

"If we want to have the minister of health as our chief guest for the distribution ceremony," another board member interjected, "then we need to only have Nepali and English." The fact that the minister of health was to officiate the ceremony was a sign of HAA's success, albeit primarily symbolic: a mark of recognition, if not actual state support.

"We also need this certificate to make clear the differences between *amchi*," the chairman continued,

> because some of the *amchi* who have come for the conference are real scholars. They know Sowa Rigpa truly in their heart-minds [*sems*]. The course will be a chance for them to refresh what they already know, or to help them share their knowledge. But others are just learning. We have to separate these people,

and to mark how they passed the course. If we don't, the government will think all *amchi* are the same. We need to improve the quality of *amchi* medicine, and the certificate will help.

This conversation also signified the board members' grasp of the politics of language in Nepal and the relationship between licensing, standardization, and professional identity. Just as marked ethnic categories can be understood as a part of creating a homogenized nationalist consciousness, the forging of professional and NGO identities is implicated in and beholden to similar state-making processes. Pragmatically speaking, this discussion of certification picked up where the Amchi Profile Data sheets and HAA identity cards left off. The certificates provided one means of distinguishing practitioners of *amchi* medicine from other healers in Nepal and marking *amchi* medicine as codified and, in that sense, scientific. The certificate, if not the course itself, helped to create the image of a unified, standardized *amchi* experience in Nepal. And yet the value of certification remained ambiguous – a form of professionalization whose meaning was ambivalent and whose power remained questionable.

"There is no benefit in writing the certificate in Tibetan," another board member added, "because anybody who is truly an *amchi* knows he's an *amchi* and doesn't need a piece of paper to prove it. That rests in their lineage, in who their root teacher is, in their minds and hands." Therefore the certificate was only useful in that it legitimated the category "*amchi*" and thus provided a view towards financial support and recognition from the Nepali government. As much as collective *amchi* identity was reflected in the certificate and the circumstances under which it would be earned, an individual *amchi*'s identity and efficacy as a healer lived beyond the borders of this certificate.[37]

"This piece of paper won't mean anything outside Nepal," said the treasurer. "If we go to Lhasa or Dharamsala we will need to earn a new one."

"They probably put Tibetan on their certificates," the vice-chairman mused.

But the Men-tsee-khang in Dharamsala, or the Mentsikhang and the Tibetan Medical College in Lhasa would not care so much about this Nepali certificate, even if it did have Tibetan on it. Maybe they will say it is good, but it would not make it easier for Nepali *amchi* to be accepted into their schools. There, they care about us passing entrance exams and knowing literary Tibetan. In India they reserve some seats for *amchi* from places like we come from, but they want you to know Hindi or English. That is always a problem. Students who are good in English and proper Tibetan have grown up in boarding schools and don't want to be *amchi*. The young people who might make good *amchi* – who are from a lineage, who have a desire to learn Sowa Rigpa and have maybe already started to learn in their villages – have poor English and Nepali because the government schools are so bad.

"In Lhasa," the vice-chairman added, "it is more politically difficult. We are outsiders there. And the programs are more expensive. And you need to know some Chinese."[38]

"But in these other places the certificates are worth something more than the one we are making here, in Nepal," said the chairman.

I've been to Dharamsala, Lhasa, Darjeeling. What is Nepal to them? Small. Less developed. And because of politics we still have to choose India or China for educating younger *amchi*, since we do not have a proper school of Tibetan medicine here. We're always stuck in the middle.

"It would be best if we could make a real school for *amchi* medicine in Nepal," said the general secretary.

Then we would not have so much trouble with entrance exams. It would be less expensive. We could invite teachers from India and China if we needed to, but it would be a Nepali program. Then, the Ministry of Health and the Remote Area Development Committee would help *amchi* medicine. And maybe our certificates would be recognized by the schools in India or China.

Versions of this conversation had played out in previous HAA meetings, and exemplified the tenuous position *amchi* from Nepal occupy in relation to both the Nepali nation-state and institutions of Tibetan medicine abroad. No matter how diverse they are as a body of practitioners, *amchi* from Nepal are considered peripheral by all parties from whom they seek legitimization – except perhaps international organizations that view the *amchi*'s medical, botanical, and cultural knowledge as conservation and development resources and to whom "Tibetan medicine" and "*amchi* medicine" are synonymous. To institutions of Tibetan medicine in exile, *amchi* from Nepal remain "borderland" populations – a term that refers to the boundaries of a historic Tibetan nation that no longer exists, as such, but that is intensely conjured by Tibetan exiles. Within the Tibet Autonomous Region, China, *amchi* from Nepal can engender suspicion, in that they embody the arbitrariness of political boundaries in relation to the more diaphanous practices of language and culture. And yet, as much as being recognizable to the Nepali state is crucial for these *amchi*, it is not enough in itself. Despite *janajati* politicking, the state has yet to find an acceptable language through which to embrace Nepali cultural practices that can also be understood as Tibetan, broadly conceived. *Amchi* from Nepal stand at the interstices of these nationalist agendas, at once tied to diasporic and minority sentiment, both outside and within Nepal. And yet they are also clearly Nepali citizens, and trying to lobby for support as such – as representatives of a practice that can be conceived of as indigenous to Nepal, and at once culturally and medically valuable.

"So what should you write on the certificate?" I asked.

"Why don't you write something in English," the general secretary suggested. "Then it will sound good and we can put it into Nepali." At a certain level, this request was not surprising. I had helped to translate and edit previous HAA documents from Tibetan and Nepali to English, and I was the only native English speaker who advised the HAA. And yet, as Talal Asad reminds, "The process of 'cultural translation' is inevitably enmeshed in conditions of power" (Asad 1986).

It was easy for the *amchi* to imagine English as a starting point for this certificate: a normative yet still foreign language that could be deciphered by the Nepali government, international donors, tourists, and other potential sponsors. Nepali, as a language of officialdom and a medium of exchange, needed to be rendered in precise, politically astute terms. Tibetan remained a ghost language – living not so much between the lines of English and Nepali but beyond this exercise in certification itself.

"I can help with the English," I said. "But maybe you should write what you want to say in Nepali first." Even though Nepali was not the first language of the HAA board members, it was more familiar to them than English. They agreed.

"We need to put something about herbal medicines, and to say what *'amchi'* means. We should also include the dates of the course, how well they did on exams, and their name in both English and Nepali," the treasurer added.

"We'll say that each person has completed a training course in. . ." The general secretary paused. "What do we say the *phyi ma rgyud* course is about? 'Sowa Rigpa' doesn't make sense in Nepali, and if we just say we're teaching about *jadibuti* [medicinal plants], then how will they think we're different from Ayurveda?" This point recurred in many different contexts within the HAA's conferences and activities. Some of the Nepali botanists and doctors of Ayurveda who advised the HAA had suggested that they label their medical practice as "Ayurveda," since that term was eminently understandable to the Nepali state. Some *amchi* considered this option, not only because of its potential political expedience but also because it bore witness at another level to the historical relationship between Ayurveda and Tibetan medicine (cf. Meyer 1998). Ultimately, though, the board members decided against this, fearing that if they were subsumed by the term "Ayurveda" then they would lose opportunities for marking Sowa Rigpa as a "modern" Nepali, as well as a "traditional" Tibetan, practice – and a practice worthy in its own right of state support.

"What if we just say what is in the *phyi ma rgyud*? Making medicines from different ingredients, including herbs. Diagnosing and treating patients. Recognizing different diseases." In the end, the *amchi* settled on this option and set to the task of translating these ideas into Nepali words – most of them Sanskritic tongue-twisters that the *amchi* could hardly pronounce. I worked on the English. The *amchi* looked pleased.

Tradition, modernity, and the healing life

The tropes of "tradition" and "modernity" underlie many of the issues informing *amchi* professionalization in Nepal. Sometimes we understand tradition by thinking about what modernity lacks or has left behind. Put another way, the penchant to delimit the bounds of tradition seems like a product of living in a modern world, searching for an authentic past. When thinking about the dichotomy "tradition/modernity" in relation to *amchi* practice in Nepal, I find it most useful to examine tradition in relation to lineage – a concept that also retains cultural currency with most *amchi* themselves. Here, I delimit "tradition" not in terms of the past, but rather as a double helix of change and continuity that articulates past, present, and future. In this respect, lineage is a process by which continuity with the past is *claimed* (even if this is not historically accurate) and altered to reflect and be attendant to present circumstances. And, as we have seen, tradition can operate as a way of exerting social control and agency.

Is it possible, then, to consider "tradition" in its own right – not only as a product or reflection of modernity? Or to consider the fact that *amchi* are actively shaping their identities as "traditional" practitioners and the idea of "cultural preservation" as a way of engineering and managing social change? Perhaps this is a question not only of time but also of scale, context, and motivation. As I have stressed, the notion of tradition is often linked up with present-day presumptions about the unchanging nature of the past. I would argue, however, that this ignores the inherent dynamism in tradition and the truth that social practice is never stagnant. In relation to *amchi* professionalization, it is this dynamism that is only superficially acknowledged by the Nepali state, "special guests," and official HAA literature. Ironically, these narratives center on a radical rupture, locatable in time and space, when *amchi* entered modernity and began to suffer the consequences.

Yet the spectrum of meanings of tradition and modernity provides us with only a clue as to what is meant, in another language and another cultural context, by their equivalents. Likewise, the relationship between "traditional medical prac- titioners" and the international industry of "alternative medicine" is emblematic of this dichotomy but reducible to neither (Bode 2002; Miles 1998). Concepts such as "ethnomedicine" become key to understanding these dichotomies in action (Adams, 1999; Nichter, 1992). One of the crucial points raised by scholars like Pigg (1997), Langford (1995), Hsu (1999), Ernst (2002), and Farquhar (1994) is that medical epistemologies do not fit easily within binary oppositions: "traditional belief" and "modern scientific knowledge." Within this frame, little room remains to explore the challenges and potential of medical pluralism, to envision colla- boration between different pathways to medical knowledge, or to facilitate translation across the culturally defined boundaries of health and suffering (Ernst 2002; Good 1994). In the realm of development, locally embedded medical practices such as *amchi* medicine have often been folded into narratives of progress and the activities of health development policy. Their diversity, complexity, and even contradictions are often reduced to acronyms such as traditional medical practitioners (TMP), traditional ecological knowledge (TEK) or indigenous knowledge (IK) (Pigg 1995b). It is as if by naming these practices they will be able to stand on an equal footing with naturalized categories of biomedical knowledge and practice.

Pigg writes:

The concepts of tradition and development are key points around which reformulated views of identity are being constructed . . . Struggles over meaning emerge because development activities do more than implement a set of policies and programs, they reinforce an ideology of modernization.

(Pigg 1995a)

These insights map discursive uses of the Nepali term *bikas* onto changes in social perception and local transformation in Nepal. Pigg's argument also reaffirms for me the ways *amchi* from Nepal exist on the borders of the nation-state, as well as the ambivalent and partial nature of their professionalization. The "credible and credulous" healing systems about which Pigg (1996) writes in other Nepali contexts are at once reaffirmed by the ways *amchi* medicine is categorized by the HAA's "special guests" and legitimated by the HAA as it sets out a course for "*amchi* development." This situation is further complicated by virtue of the HAA's transnational leanings. *Amchi* from Nepal are participating in the construction of regional and global visions of biodiversity conservation, contributing to trans-national motifs of "authentic Tibetan culture" and at the same time beholden to the scrutiny of the Nepali Ministry of Health and institutes of Tibetan medicine in India and China – not to mention more local concerns: the medico-social roles *amchi* occupy within their communities.

Amchi involved in the HAA are attempting to carve out a conscious middle way, at once preserving and revitalizing their practice, protecting personal and secret knowledge, and at the same time promoting standardization (cf. Hsu 1999). Yet have they placed themselves in a double bind? On the one hand, they are recasting their practice according to the organizational models of NGOs, thereby running the risk of increasing the gaps between different classes of *amchi* and distancing themselves from their communities as a consequence of seeking legitimation in the eyes of the state and international organizations. On the other hand, they are relying on an appeal to authenticity – both as purveyors of Nepali "indigenous knowledge" and as representatives of "traditional Tibetan medicine" – to garner political and economic support for their endeavors both within Nepal and abroad.

Perhaps these *amchi* are actively shaping the organizational model of the NGO, the discourses and practices of development, the chaotic political realities of contemporary Nepal, and the cultural capital associated with Tibet, into meaningful terms and informed social action. However, the very act of creating a homogenized narrative about "*amchi* experience" is at once necessary and counterintuitive in terms of the HAA members' personal knowledge of the difference between *amchi* – distinctions charted in geographic, religious, linguistic, medical, and economic terms. Furthermore, despite their name, NGOs are still beholden to states. The HAA and the *amchi* who constitute its diverse roster resist easy classification as a product of "foreign" influences and development discourse, state-endorsed nationalism, identity politics, or diasporic yearnings. Yet neither are they recomposing their practice completely on their own terms. It is within this set of paradoxes that the social, political, and medical efficacy of *amchi* medicine is being formed, and reformed, in Nepal.

Postscript: organizational growth and change

Since 2002, the HAA has continued to organize national and international conferences, refresher training courses for novice *amchi* in the fundamentals of Sowa Rigpa, and specialized training and workshops on *amchi* medicine and public health, as well as on medicinal plant conservation and cultivation. These events have brought together more than 100 senior and novice *amchi* from Nepal, as well as Sowa Rigpa practitioners from Ladakh and Sikkim in India, the Tibetan Autonomous Region of China, Bhutan, and Mongolia. The HAA has also published four bilingual booklets based on the national and international conferences, and has overseen the creation of curricula and textbook materials for the four institutes of *amchi* education that exist in Nepal. These materials have been distributed nationally and regionally.

In 2003, the HAA opened its own clinic in Kathmandu. This clinic, staffed by member *amchi* on a rotational basis, not only provides medical care to people from remote mountain communities when they come to Kathmandu, but also provides the HAA with a source of income and a view towards organizational sustainability. It also serves as a site for clinical training and apprenticeship for novice *amchi*.

In 2004, the HAA held its first International Conference of Amchi, with delegates from Mongolia, the Tibet Autonomous Region (PRC), Bhutan, Ladakh (India), and throughout Nepal. The meeting revealed to all participants that which they held in common, as well as their differences, highlighting how the social, economic, and political circumstances of the nation-states in which they practice continue to legislate what it means to be an *amchi* and what it means to heal. Participants also discussed the historical significance of this meeting, both in the light of congresses of Sowa Rigpa practitioners such as those supposedly held in eighth-century Lhasa and in Mongolia during the height of the Mongol empire and as counterpoint to the Second International Congress of Tibetan Medicine held in November 2003 in Washington, DC. After five intense days of discussion, conference participants drafted a statement and set of resolutions, in both English and Tibetan. During the conference, Nepali and regional delegates discussed both constraints and potentials of their medical traditions and made several unanimous resolutions, in order to safeguard and develop *amchi* medical systems in the contemporary global context. They began their set of recommendations with the following:

> From 25 to 29 Jan. 2004, more than 40 Amchis (practitioners of traditional *sowa rigpa* medicine) from Mongolia, Tibet Autonomous Region (PRC), Bhutan, Ladakh (India), and throughout Nepal have gathered in Kathmandu for the First International Conference of Amchis in Nepal. Our medical practices are known as "Tibetan Medicine" in China and worldwide, "Traditional Medicine" or "Buddhist Medicine" in Bhutan, "Amchi Medicine" in Ladakh, India, "Himalayan Amchi Medicine" in Nepal, and "Traditional Mongolian Medicine" in Mongolia. In general, this medical practice is also identified by the name *sowa rigpa*, which means "science of healing" in classical Tibetan as well as in regional Himalayan and Central Asian languages and dialects. Although regional variations in medical history and practices exist, our medical traditions share a common set of theories and practices, as well as common medical texts the foremost among these being the *rgyud bzhi*, or the Four Medical Tantras, based on the work of Astangahrigaya Samhita, as well as the *bum bzhi*, and other fundamental textbooks.

Our mission as medical practitioners is to serve people altruistically and help promote health through the balance of humanity and nature, as well as mind, body, and spirit.

The *amchis* from each country then agreed to establish a coalition in order to address the five main areas listed below:

1   Governmental Recognition and Support for *Amchi* and their Practices
2   Development of *Amchi* Medical Educational Systems
3   Health Care Delivery and Quality *Amchi* Medicines in Local Communities
4   Conservation, Cultivation, and Sustainable Utilization of Medicinal Plants
5   Research and Documentation of *Amchi* Histories, Practices, and Texts

As foregrounded by these remarks, international connections made during this historic event have continued to inform HAA activities.

In 2006, after more than two years of collaboration with the Council of Technical Education and Vocational Training (CTEVT) as well as partners at the Ministry of Health – Ayurveda Council, the Ministry of Education, and offices of the Remote Area Development Committee, and nearly a decade of continued lobbying efforts, the HAA was granted initial recognition and support, through a grant from the Ministry of Education. Although this specific grant was to be used for the continued development of government-approved curricula for *amchi* education programs, this support marked a specific governmental commitment to, and prioritization of, *amchi* medicine. The corresponding degrees of *durrapa* (*Sdus ra wa*) and *kangjenpa* (*Rkang hzin pa*)[39] have been equated with the categories of "certificate in *amchi* science" and "community *amchi* assistant" respectively. These follow roughly parallel designations of community medical technician (CMT) and community medical assistant (CMA) within the Nepali government health care system. Within the HAA, there remains ambivalence about this track of standardization, but most member *amchi* believe this step toward state recognition has been, and will continue to be, beneficial to future generations of *amchi* – in great part because of their hopes that state-approved curricula and certified practitioners will also segue into financial support for *amchi* clinics in high-mountain communities, and wage-earning jobs for a new generation of *amchi*.

Today, the HAA is engaged in a number of ongoing initiatives surrounding the issue of medicinal plant conservation and cultivation. Working with supportive groups within the Nepali government and with international NGOs, the HAA is trying to promote an integrated approach to biodiversity conservation, health care, and income-generation activities based on the use of medicinal plants, in line with *amchi* knowledge and practices, local communities' needs and priorities, and, as possible, the innovative use of technology and other forms of scientific expertise. These developments raise further interesting questions about how *amchi* are being recognized, and for what. In great part, their recognition as healers and contributors to the health care of Nepal's population is being facilitated through their identification by Western and Nepali scientists and other "experts" as purveyors of environmental knowledge, not the reverse.

Acknowledgements

The research that forms the basis for this chapter has been supported by grants from the National Science Foundation, the Social Science Research Council, the Wenner-Gren Foundation for Anthropological Research, the Cornell Participatory Action Network, and the Department of Anthropology, Cornell University. I would like to thank Laurent Pordié, Davydd Greenwood, David Holmberg, Yeshi Choedron Lama, Yoji Kamata, Yildiz Thomas, and the board members of the Himalayan Amchi Association, who have all been instrumental in shaping this work. This paper is dedicated to Amchi Soma Namgyal (1927?–2002), Amchi Tashi Chösang (1927–1996), and Yeshi Choedron Lama (1970–2006).

Notes

1 Cf. Chapter 1, note 4.
2 *Tsampa*, roasted barley flour, is, along with butter, tea and meat, the ubiquitous food of the Tibetan cultural world.
3 This designation of Nepal as a Hindu polity changed with the political events of late 2006, when the decade-long civil war between Maoist insurgents and the Nepali state was resolved politically. Part of this still ongoing process of redefining the Nepali nation-state included rewriting the constitution, designating Nepal as a secular state, and dismantling many of the historical connections between the Shah monarchy (a Hindu institution) and the government. That said, the government remains dominated by high-caste Hindu Nepalis.
4 Hsu's (1999) work on the transmission of Chinese medicine – especially her discussion of secret, personal, and standardized transmission of knowledge – has been useful in conceptualizing the fragmented and yet undeniable changes that are occurring as a part of professionalizing processes among *amchi* in Nepal.
5 For more information on mountain deities and sacred geography in the Tibetan context, see also Blondeau (1996, 1998), Huber (1999), McDonald (1997), McKay (1998), and Ramble (1995).
6 See note 3.
7 Does the Nepali *bikas* signify the same set of expectations and dynamics as does the Tibetan *yar rgyas* – development, progress, improvement? From anecdotal encounters with *amchi* who speak Nepali, they seem to use these words to suit distinct purposes. Perhaps not surprisingly, the Nepali *bikas* tends to suggest governmental and non-governmental support, while the Tibetan *yar rgyas* is used to emphasize the moral and religious imperative of supporting *amchi* and their medicine.
8 HAA board members have participated in study tours where they have both seen the possibilities for medicinal herb cultivation and witnessed many of the challenges to this practice.
9 For a clear exposition of the construction of scientific knowledge and its imagined counterpart "indigenous medicine," see Ernst (2002).
10 *Jhankri* is a "faith healer," akin to, though distinct from, a shaman.
11 For instance, that which I refer to in this context as "Tibetan medicine" is called "Mongolian medicine" in Mongolia and "Buddhist medicine" in Bhutan, and, in the Nepali and Ladakhi context, known as "*amchi* medicine" – for reasons of both identity politics and nationalism.
12 See Adams (2001) and Janes (2001) for examples of this dynamic in Tibet.
13 This position can be understood as a contemporary ramification of the fact that Nepal, Mustang, to be precise, was the base of operations for the Tibetan resistance from 1960 to 1974 and that Nepal is home to many Tibetan refugees.

14 In recent years, this has included high-level diplomatic missions from Kathmandu to Beijing, and crackdowns on newly arrived Tibetan refugees in Nepal.

15 In relation to the marketability and capitalization of "Tibetanness" within the Nepali context see Adams (1996), Bauer (2004), and Craig (2001). For a discussion of the cultural capital and attendant social costs associated with Tibet in the global context, see Lopez (1998).

16 Jigme Palbar Bista is the twenty-fifth king of Lo in a lineage dating to the early fifteenth century. He is also known as the Raja of Mustang, and his territory encompasses much of what the Nepali government classifies as "upper" Mustang, a region to which foreigners have had access, on a restricted basis, only since 1992.

17 For practical purposes, Gyatso shares this position with his brother, Tenzin Sangbo, a monk.

18 It is worth noting that social status can be bestowed, or fabricated, as much as it can be inherited. Gyatso Bista's forefathers were not part of the Lo nobility by birth, but were given noble title as a result of their skill as Tibetan medical practitioners. Tshampa Ngawang claims to be the eighth in a lineage of *amchi* of noble birth; his relatives and contemporaries in Mustang often argue differently.

19 For more on this program, particularly the integration of ethnobotanical *amchi* knowledge with health care delivery and conservation training and management, see Aumeeruddy-Thomas (2001).

20 This trope of "backwardness" can be read as an internalization of development discourse by Nepalis (cf. Pigg 1996). It can also be read as a more emic assertion of difference, directly connected to the natural environment and local Tibetan vernacular. Both Gyatso and Tshampa Ngawang, upon their returns from Dolpa District, made comments to me such as: "In Dolpo, they eat the bitter buckwheat that we would only feed to our animals" or "The lands are filled with precious plants, like jewels, but few *amchi* know how to use them properly because many can't understand the medical texts."

21 The HAA founders were influenced and supported early on by the Japanese Institute for Himalayan Conservation (IHC). They have since received funding from the Japan Foundation Asia Center (JFAC), DROKPA, the WWF Nepal Program, the UNESCO People and Plants Initiative, JAITI Nepal, and other supporters.

22 This literature includes grant applications, brochures, and conference proceedings booklets, written in Tibetan, Nepali, and English.

23 I should stress that this narrative might not be historically accurate; very little research has been done on the trade in medicinal plants between northern Nepal and Tibet. Rather, there is a perceived significant decline in this medicinal herb trade tied directly to the closing of the Nepal/Tibet border after 1959.

24 Author's translation from the Tibetan.

25 See Gerke and Jacobson (1996) for a discussion of the encounter between Asian medical systems and biomedical research in India and the West.

26 From *hi ma' la ya'I em rje tshogs pa 'don spel thengs dang po*, published in 1998, with support from the Institute for Himalayan Conservation, Kathmandu, Nepal.

27 Since 1996, more than 14,000 Nepalis have died in a struggle between the central government and Communist Party of Nepal (Maoist) insurgents, who define this armed conflict as a "People's War." This conflict reached the beginnings of a political solution in late 2006, but ramifications of this conflict will continue to define many aspects of the future. At the time of the Second National Conference of Amchi, Nepal was deeply imbedded in a "State of Emergency."

28 The original Mentsikhang, or "House of Medicine and Astrology," was established under the direction of Khenrab Norbu and at the behest of the thirteenth Dalai Lama, in 1911. Today, it is the foremost state-supported Tibetan medical institution in China. However, the clinical practice of Tibetan medicine has been separated from the act of medical production, which is now the domain of the Mentsikhang Factory, a for-profit enterprise. The Men-tsee-khang, as this re-formed institute-in-exile is known, was established in

1961. It includes a teaching institution, a clinical hospital, and a factory of Tibetan medicine. Although the Mentsikhang and Men-tsee-khang function under different state and political pressure, both are increasingly concerned with the profitable marketing of Tibetan medicines, patents, standardization, and intellectual property rights. For more information on the Mentsikhang, see Adams and Li in Chapter 5. For more information on the Men-tsee-khang, see www.mentseekhang.org.

29 Here, "project" was spoken in English. Code switching between English, Nepali, and Tibetan provides another fruitful avenue for analysis of *amchi* professionalization in Nepal, and is part of my ongoing research interests. In this instance, the use of English terms speaks to what Pigg (2001) describes as one of the effects of development discourse and practice in the Nepali context.

30 The SAARC annual meeting in Kathmandu was historic, not only because of the troubled, politically charged atmosphere in South Asian politics, post-September 11, but also because of brewing tensions between India and Pakistan over Kashmir.

31 The Kalachakra initiation scheduled to begin on January 21, 2002, was rescheduled for January 2003 owing to the Dalai Lama's ill health.

32 These publications included *gangs jongs gso rig sgron me*, published in Ladakh, India, and supported by Nomad RSI, and Lama *et al.* (2001).

33 This was mitigated the following day, when most "special guests" had vanished, and the general member *amchi*, HAA board members, and a few advisors broke into small groups for discussion and knowledge-sharing exercises.

34 The original Chagpori Medical Institute was founded at the behest of the fifth Dalai Lama, and was situated on top of a hill of the same name in Lhasa. As mentioned at the beginning of this chapter, the original Chagpori was destroyed in 1959. It was reformed in exile in the early 1990s, with the guidance and patronage of Trogawa Rimpoche. Although Tibetan medical students at Chagpori must pass final exams dictated by the Dharamsala-based Men-tsee-khang, Chagpori functions as an independent institute in other respects (personal communication, B. Gerke, March 5, 2003).

35 During the third refresher training course, held in January 2003, this exclusive emphasis on the *phyi ma rgyud* was reconceptualized, and students were given select teaching from all four tantras, as well as other medical texts.

36 The Chagpori representatives said they could not authorize any such certificate because it was being given in Nepal, not India, and because they were still beholden, at the level of certification, to the Dharamsala Men-tsee-khang. However, HAA members thought the reason for Chagpori's refusal was more a product of Tibetan religious politics. Indifferent to, if not ignorant of, Tibetan religious politics, the HAA had rented office space from a supporter of the Sikkim-based Karmapa, while Chagpori, and the Tibetan government-in-exile, supported the recognition of the Karmapa from Tsurphu Monastery in Tibet, who fled to India in 2000.

37 Jean Langford's (1999) work with practitioners of Ayurveda in India provides a useful comparison in this instance, in that she takes up the issue of certification in relation to professional identity and medical efficacy.

38 Since 2001, the HAA has been exploring this option of sending good novice *amchi* from Nepal to institutes of Tibetan medicine in India or Tibet (China), and examining their curriculums as new educational models.

39 The *durrapa* and *kangjenpa* categories emerge from the history of Tibetan medicine, specifically the ranking of different Sowa Rigpa practitioners based on years of study, examination results, and the recommendations of senior teachers. In the context of the HAA's work with CTEVT, the *kangjenpa* category is a two-year three-month program that includes both didactic and clinical training, and that requires a Nepali Class 8 school certificate for entrance. The *durrapa* category corresponds to a three-year program of study, for which entrants mush have *either* a *kangjenpa* degree *or* a school-leaving certificate (SLC) and proven proficiency in the literary Tibetan and Nepali languages.

References

Adams, V. (1996). *Tigers in the Snow and Other Virtual Sherpas*, Princeton, NJ: Princeton University Press.

Adams, V. (1999). *Equity of the Ineffable: Cultural and Political Constraints on Ethnomedicine as a Health Problem in Contemporary Tibet*, Boston, MA: Foundations of Health and Equity, Harvard Center for Population and Development Studies.

Adams, V. (2001). The Sacred in the Scientific: Ambiguous Practices of Science in Tibetan Medicine, *Cultural Anthropology* 16(4): 542–575.

Anderson, B. (1983). *Imagined Communities: Reflections on the Origin and Spread of Nationalism*, London: Verso.

Asad, T. (1986). The Concept of Cultural Translation in British Social Anthropology. In G. Marcus (ed.), *Writing Culture: The Poetics and Politics of Ethnography*, Berkeley: University of California Press.

Aumeeruddy-Thomas, Y. (2001). Working with Tibetan Doctors (Amchi) for the Conservation of Medicinal Plants and Health Care Development at Shey Phoksundo National Park, Dolpa, Nepal, *Medicinal Plant Conservation* 7, New York: IUCN Species Survival Commission.

Barth, F. (1969). *Ethnic Groups and Boundaries: The Social Organization of Cultural Difference*, Boston, MA: Little, Brown.

Battachan, K. (1994). Ethnopolitics and Ethnodevelopment: An Emerging Paradigm in Nepal, *State, Leadership and Politics in Nepal*, Kathmandu: Tribhuvan University.

Bauer, K. (2004) *High Frontiers: Dolpo and the Changing World of Himalayan Pastoralists*, New York: Columbia University Press.

Bista, G. (2001). *Hi ma' la' ri rgyud du gso ba rig pa bbyung rtshul dang em rje' lo rgyus*, *Himalayan Amchi Association Nepal Newsletter*, Kathmandu: HAA with support from Japan Foundation Asia Center.

Blondeau, A.-M. (1996). *Reflections of the Mountain: Essays on the History and Social Meaning of the Mountain Cult in Tibet and the Himalaya*, Vienna: Verlag der Österreichischen Akademie der Wissenschaften.

Blondeau, A.-M. (1998). *Tibetan Mountain Deities: Their Cults and Representations*, Vienna: Verlag der Österreichischen Akademie der Wissenschaften.

Bode, M. (2002). Indian Indigenous Pharmaceuticals: Tradition, Modernity, and Nature. In W. Ernst (ed.), *Plural Medicine, Tradition, and Modernity, 1800–2000*, London: Routledge.

Burghart, R. (1984). The Formation of the Concept of Nation-State in Nepal, *Journal of Asian Studies* 44(1): 101–125.

Craig, S. (2001). A Tale of Two Temples: Culture, Capital, and Community in Mustang, Nepal, Paper presented at the New York Conference on Asian Studies, Ithaca, NY.

Des Chene, M. (1996). In the Name of Bikas, *Studies in Nepalese History and Society* 1(2): 259–270.

Duara, P. (1996). *Rescuing History from the Nation*, Chicago, IL: University of Chicago Press.

Ernst, W. (2002). Plural Medicine, Tradition, and Modernity: Historical and Contemporary Perspectives: Views from Below and Above. In W. Ernst (ed.), *Plural Medicine, Tradition, and Modernity, 1800–2000*, London: Routledge.

Farquhar, J. (1994). *Knowing Practice: The Clinical Encounter of Chinese Medicine*, Boulder, CO: Westview Press.

Ferguson, J. (1994). *The Anti-Politics Machine, "Development," Depoliticization, and Bureaucratic Power in Lesotho*, Cambridge: Cambridge University Press.

Gellner, D., Whelpton, J. and Pfaff-Czarnecka, J. (eds.) (1997). *Nationalism and Ethnicity in a Hindu Kingdom: The Politics of Culture in Contemporary Nepal*, Amsterdam: Overseas Publishers Association, Harwood Academic Publishers.

Gerke, B. and Jacobson, E. (1996). Traditional Asian Medical Cultures Encounter Biomedical Research, *Ayur Vijnana*, Vol. 1, Kalimpong: International Trust for Traditional Medicine.

Good, B. J. (1994). *Medicine, Rationality, and Experience*, Cambridge: Cambridge University Press.

Hobsbawm, E. and Ranger, T. (eds.) (1983). *The Invention of Tradition*, Cambridge: Cambridge University Press.

Höfer, A. (1979). *The Caste Hierarchy and the State in Nepal: A Study of the Muluki Ain of 1854*, Khumbu Himal, Innsbruck: Universitätsverlag Wagner, pp. 31–238.

Holmberg, D., March, K. and Tamang, S. (1999). Local Production/Local Knowledge: Forced Labour from Below, *Studies in Nepali History and Society* 4(1): 5–64.

Hsu, E. (1999). *The Transmission of Chinese Medicine*, Cambridge: Cambridge University Press.

Huber, T. (1999). *Cult of the Pure Crystal Mountain*, Oxford and New York: Oxford University Press.

Jackson, D. P. (1984). *The Mollas of Mustang*, New Delhi: Library of Tibetan Works and Archives.

Janes, C. (2001). Tibetan Medicine at the Crossroads: Radical Modernity and the Social Organization of Traditional Medicine in the Tibet Autonomous Region, China. In L. Connor and G. Samuel (eds.), *Healing Powers and Modernity: Traditional Medicine, Shamanism, and Science in Asian Societies*, Westport, CT: Bergin & Harvey.

Justice, J. (1986). *Policies, Plans, and People: Foreign Aid and Health Development*, Berkeley: University of California Press.

Kapferer, B. (1988). *Legends of People, Myths of State: Violence, Intolerance, and Political Culture in Sri Lanka and Australia*, Washington, DC: Smithsonian Institution Press.

Lama, Y. C., Ghimire, S. K. and Aumeeruddy-Thomas, Y. (2001). *Medicinal Plants of Dolpo: Amchis' Knowledge and Conservation*, Kathmandu: World Wildlife Fund Nepal Program Publication Series.

Langford, J. (1995). Ayurvedic Interiors: Person, Space and Episteme in Three Medical Practices, *Cultural Anthropology* 10(3): 330–366.

Langford, J. (1999). Medical Mimesis: Healing Signs of a Cosmopolitan "Quack," *American Ethnologist* 26(1): 24–46.

Last, M. (1996). The Professionalization of Indigenous Healers. In T. M. Johnson and C. F. Sargent (eds.), *Medical Anthropology: Contemporary Theory and Methods*, New York: Praeger.

Levine, N. (1987). Caste, State, and Ethnic Boundaries in Nepal, *Journal of Asian Studies* 46(1): 71–88.

Li, T. M. (2000). Articulating Indigenous Identity in Indonesia: Resource Politics and the Tribal Slot, *Comparative Studies in Society and History* 42(1): 149–179.

Lopez, D. (1998). *Prisoners of Shangri La: Tibetan Buddhism and the West*, Chicago, IL: University of Chicago Press.

McDonald, A. W. (ed.) (1997). *Mandala and Landscape*, New Delhi: D. K. Printworld.

McKay, A. (1998). *Pilgrimage in Tibet*, London: Curzon Press.

Meyer, F. (1998). The History and Foundations of Tibetan Medicine. In J. F. Avedon (ed.). *The Buddha's Art of Healing: Tibetan Paintings Rediscovered*, New York: Rizzoli.

Miles, A. (1998). Science, Nature, and Tradition: The Mass-Marketing of Natural Medicine in Urban Ecuador, *Medical Anthropology Quarterly* 12(2): 206–225.

Munasinghe, V. (2001). *Callaloo or Tossed Salad? East Indians and the Cultural Politics of Identity in Trinidad*, Ithaca, NY: Cornell University Press.

Nichter, M. (ed.) (1992). *Anthropological Approaches to the Study of Ethnomedicine*, Tucson, AZ: Gordon and Breach Science Publishers.

Parish, S. (1996). *Hierarchy and its Discontents: Culture and the Politics of Consciousness in Caste Society*, Philadelphia: University of Pennsylvania Press.

Pigg, S. L. (1995a). The Social Symbolism of Healing in Nepal, *Ethnology* 34(1): 17–36.

Pigg, S. L. (1995b). Acronyms and Effacement: Traditional Medical Practitioners (TMP) in International Health Development, *Social Science and Medicine* 41(1): 47–68.

Pigg, S. L. (1996). The Credible and the Credulous: The Question of "Villagers' Beliefs" in Nepal, *Cultural Anthropology* 11(2): 160–201.

Pigg, S. L. (1997). "Found in Most Traditional Societies": Traditional Medical Practitioners between Culture and Development. In F. Cooper and R. Packard (eds.), *International Development and the Social Sciences: Essays on the History and Politics of Knowledge*, Berkeley: University of California Press.

Pigg, S. L. (2001). Language of Sex and AIDS in Nepal: Notes on the Social Production of Commensurability, *Cultural Anthropology* 16(4): 481–541.

Pordié, L. (2001). Research and International Aid: A Possible Meeting. The Case of Nomad RSI in Ladakh, *Ladakh Studies* 15: 33–42.

Ramble, C. (1993). Wither, indeed, the Tsampa Eaters, *Himal* 6: 21–25.

Ramble, C. (1995). Gaining Ground: Representations of Territory on Bon and Tibetan Popular Tradition, *Tibet Journal* 10(1).

Ramble, C. (1997). Tibetan Pride of Place: Or, Why Nepal's Bhotiyas Are Not an Ethnic Group. In D. Gellner, J. Whelpton and J. Pfaff-Czarnecka (eds.), *Nationalism and Ethnicity in a Hindu Kingdom: The Politics of Culture in Contemporary Nepal*, Amsterdam: Overseas Publishers Association, Harwood Academic Publishers.

Snellgrove, D. (1961). *Himalayan Pilgrimage*, Oxford: Bruno Cassirer.

Starr, P. (1982). *The Social Transformation of American Medicine*, New York: Basic Books.

Tamang, M. (2000). Democracy and Cultural Diversity in Nepal, Paper presented at the 29th Annual Conference on South Asia, University of Wisconsin-Madison, University of Wisconsin.

Verdery, K. (1994). Ethnicity, Nationalism, and the State: Ethnic Groups and Boundaries Past and Present, *The Anthropology of Ethnicity*, Amsterdam: Het Spinhuis.

Weber, M. (1978). Economy and Society. In G. Roth and C. Wittich (eds.), *An Outline of Interpretive Sociology*, Berkeley: University of California Press.

Williams, B. (1989). A Class Act: Anthropology and the Race to Nation across Ethnic Terrain, *Annual Review of Anthropology* 18: 401–441.

4 The diffusion of Tibetan medicine in China

A descriptive panorama

Chen Hua

Tibetan medicine was formed and developed by Tibetan doctors over a long historical period, through the refinement of the folk therapies of the Tibetan plateau and the amalgamation of the medical cultures of China, India and Tazi (ancient Iran), combined with the influence of Buddhism. Tibet is therefore the original centre of Tibetan medicine, but this medical system did not remain confined to Tibet itself. As shown in this book, it has spread to the neighbouring areas of Tibetan cultural influence and beyond. However, little information is available to date on the diffusion of Tibetan medicine within the political boundaries of today's China.

The spread of Tibetan medicine in this context may be divided into two stages. The first stage was from the eighth century to the eighteenth century, with Tibetan Buddhism as the central medium of transmission. During this period Tibetan medicine spread to the Tibetan inhabited areas, such as Qinghai, Sichuan, Gansu and Yunnan Provinces, and to the Mongolian areas, as well as Fuxin of Liaoning Province and Chengde of Hebei Province, forming several secondary developmental centres. The second stage appeared over recent decades following the uneasy political transition of Tibet. In this stage, Tibetan medicine spread across rural and urban China, especially through the expanding trade in Tibetan medicines, increased intercultural contact and the influence of the media. The diffusion of Tibetan medicine has therefore been shaped over many centuries by the multiple and interlocking factors of politics, religion, economics and culture.

In this chapter, I will provide factual data on the structural and institutional development of Tibetan medicine in these regions, an enquiry which I hope will be useful for future investigations on the social nature of this development. I will mainly focus on aspects pertaining to education, medicines preparation and mass production, and clinical practice. To this end, I will first explore the past and present situations of Tibetan medicine in the Tibet Autonomous Region. I will then turn to the Tibetan inhabited areas of China, and finally examine the fate of Tibetan medicine in Mainland China.

The Tibet Autonomous Region

The Tibet Autonomous Region (TAR) as it is known today is the centre where Tibetan medicine originally emerged and developed over many centuries. While

Tibetan medicine is based on textual foundations, the knowledge was mainly trans-mitted orally, as is the case for many of the areas in the rural Himalayas. This was done through 'transmission from master to apprentice' and from 'father to son', as well as learning in medical colleges (*sman pa grva tshang*[1]) located in monasteries (Li Dinglan 1989). Before 1959, there were however two major institutions of Tibetan medicine in Tibet: Iron Hill Medical College (*Lcags po ri*) and the School of Medicine and Astro-computation (*Sman rtsis khang*), respectively established in the late seventeenth century (1696) and early twentieth century (1910).

From 1951 onwards, this medical system entered a period of dramatic change, embedded in the tumults of dramatic political transition. For over fifty years, Tibetan medicine has been greatly transformed and standardized in terms of its educational modalities, clinical practice and research (Cai 1995; Qiangba 1996). This process of transformation dates back to the beginning of the 1960s,[2] an important step of which was the founding of a technical secondary school of Tibetan medicine in Lhasa.[3] This school is sometimes considered to be the first to have provided modern medical education. Some well-known doctors of Tibetan medicine taught in this school, which trained fifteen doctors with the idea of seconding them to the Iron Hill Medical College and the School of Medicine and Astro-computation (*Sman rtsis khang*). However, these students graduated in 1962 following the merger of these two institutions – Chagpori having been destroyed – to form the Hospital of Tibetan Medicine of Lhasa City (Cp. *Lasashi Zangyiyuan*) in 1959, a period known for its political complexity. This hospital in Lhasa set up a training class of Tibetan medicine in 1963 and recruited forty-five students, most of whom went on to become well-respected doctors of Tibetan medicine.

Tibetan medicine was later drastically undermined during the Great Cultural Revolution (1966–1976). It came close to an impasse because of its relation with religion, which at the time did not match the national political agenda. Some form of controlled support did however exist and tended to rationalize Tibetan medicine, by associating it with the rudiments of Chinese biomedicine at the levels of education and practice. In 1972, a course in Tibetan medicine was introduced at the Medical School of Lhasa City (Cp. *Lasashi Weisheng Xuexiao*), with 181 students. After graduation, these students were assigned to work in different areas of the TAR in order to provide easily accessible health care in Tibet.

In 1974, the Chinese government revised its strategy towards this medical system, particularly because some aspects of it were consonant with materialism, socialism and the politics of health care in China, and began to correct what are now perceived to be past faults. In Lhasa, a research group on Tibetan medicine including mainly older practitioners was formed. These persons were in charge of collecting and systematizing the classics of Tibetan medicine, which were lost or damaged during the Cultural Revolution. They also began to summarize clinical experiences in Tibetan medicine. During this period, Tibetan medicine progressively and partially recovered and developed.

Following the 'reform and opening' in 1978, the Chinese government supported the development of Tibetan medicine by adapting policies, providing funds and encouraging the privatization of the practice. This led Tibetan medicine to move forward to a new flourishing period. Since the end of the 1990s a network of Tibetan medicine has been formed, centred on Lhasa, its service covering the majority of the Tibet region. Hospitals of Tibetan medicine have been founded in each of the six prefectures of Tibet and in seven of the seventy-five counties that constitute these prefectures. Each of the remaining counties have departments of Tibetan medicine in their county hospitals.

From 1981 to 1986, one-year training classes for advanced study in Tibetan medicine were held every year at the Hospital of Tibetan Medicine of the Tibet Autonomous Region (formerly the Hospital of Tibetan Medicine of Lhasa City),[4] with students coming from Tibet, Qinghai, Gansu, Sichuan, Yunnan and Xinjiang. The nature of the course curriculum and of the training offered marked out these courses as different from any that had previously been available. The students went back to their places of origin to work as doctors of Tibetan medicine, forming the backbone of the Tibetan medical system in China.

In 1984, following a lengthy period of consideration, the concerned government departments decided to set up an institution of higher education for Tibetan medicine in the Tibet region. This led in 1985 to the setting up of the Department of Tibetan Medicine at Tibet University (Cp. *Xizang Daxue Zangyixi*), Lhasa. Twenty-seven students, all graduates from senior middle schools, were recruited to this department. The graduates later became part of the Tibetan medical elite. In September 1989, a separate College of Tibetan Medicine of Tibet (Cp. *Xizang Zangyi Xueyuan*) was opened, as a result of the development and the autonomy of the above-mentioned department of Tibet University. This offered both secondary and higher levels of study. By 1991, there were more than 340 students in this college, which had expanded to include a substantial library, a department for foreign students, and the Research Institute of Tibetan Medicine and Astro-computation. This college provides five-year undergraduate training to students. Besides common and introductory courses, the curriculum is divided into special-ized courses in Tibetan medicine such as diagnosis (Moon King's medical diag-nosis), history of Tibetan medicine, ethics in Tibetan medicine, detoxification, details of the three basic humours (*nyes pa*), elective courses in biomedicine such as internal medicine, surgery, gynaecology and paediatrics, and elective courses in astrology.

The central Hospital of Tibetan Medicine of the Tibet Autonomous Region at Lhasa includes a large clinic, an inpatient department with 250 beds, and three subsidiary organizations, that is, a pharmaceutical factory, the Research Institute of Tibetan Medicine and the Research Institute of Astro-computation. Some services at this hospital are provided free of charge to the Tibetan people and some have to be paid for. Each year there are approximately 230,000 individual visits made to the clinic. A total of over twenty specialized departments have been established at the hospital, based in both Tibetan medicine and biomedicine. Specialized Tibetan medicine departments include: internal medicine; stomatology; ophthalmology; surgery; gynaecology and obstetrics; 'tumours'; intestinal and stomach diseases; paediatrics; and preventive health care. In addition to these are departments specializing in biomedical techniques, such as radiotherapy, laboratory testing, ultrasound, electrocardiography and gastroscopy. Doctors treat the diseases they encounter either solely through traditional Tibetan medical techniques or through a combination of Tibetan and biomedical methods. The claimed aim of this is to enrich and develop the technologies and theories of diagnosis and treatment in Tibetan medicine, although this attempt at integration faces serious technical, epistemological and social challenges.

Traditionally, all Tibetan medicines were handmade from their various components of herbal, mineral and animal origin. After the medicines were finished, monks in the monastery sometimes performed specific rituals and read Buddhist sutras aloud for seven days to bless the medicines and to 'potentialize their efficacy'[5] (Li Dinglan 1989). Today, this ritual is still performed in some places, including pharmaceutical companies, but the preparation techniques have been industrialized. There are twenty-two pharmaceutical factories of various sizes manufacturing Tibetan medicine in the TAR. An increasing number of these factories make Tibetan medications using modern pharmaceutical technologies. The medicines made in these factories are sold in the markets in new forms and varieties. The first-established modern pharmaceutical factory of Tibetan medicine in the TAR is the Pharmaceutical Factory of Tibetan Medicine of the Tibet Autonomous Region (Cp. *Xizang Zizhiqu Zangyaochang*). This factory was set up in 1964; its original name was the Pharmaceutical Factory in the Hospital of Tibetan Medicine of the Tibet Autonomous Region. By the end of the 1990s, this factory was producing more than 300 different varieties of Tibetan medicines. In September 2001, its name was changed again to the Tibetan Pharmacy Joint Stock Co. Ltd (Cp. *Xizang Zangyao Gufen Youxian Gongsi*). At present, the surface area of workshops in this company is 13,800 square metres, and the workshops are installed with automatic product lines manufacturing different forms of drugs such as pills, powders, syrups and instant mixtures.

Since the first standard of the Ministry of Public Health for Tibetan drugs was issued in 1995, Tibetan pharmaceutical production has moved towards higher levels of standardization. This standard ensures the regulation of the quality, safety and technological process of medicines manufacturing. To date, several new kinds of Tibetan compounds have been developed. Among them, forty-one types of Tibetan *materia medica* and ninety-seven types of Tibetan patent medicines come up to the national standard. Twelve kinds of Tibetan patent medicines have been classified as varieties of Chinese medicines and are therefore protected by the government (that is, the prescriptions and technological processes of these medicines), and twenty-five types of drugs recognized by national medical insurance are listed in the catalogue. At present, Tibetan medications to treat stomach diseases, rheumatoid arthritis and heart disease sell particularly well all over China. The best-selling Tibetan medications contain the medicinal plants *Cordyceps* sp., *Saussurea* sp., *Crocus sativus*, *Rhodiola sacrae*, *Swertia mussotii*, *S. franchetiana* and other *Swertia* species.

Tibetan patent medicines are made from many kinds of *materia medica* and take the form of powders, pills, creams, oils and capsules. The majority of these contain over twenty-five different medical materials, while some exceed 100. Most of the names of the patent compounds derive from the name of the principal drug followed by the total number of ingredients. Of the 300 types of commonly used compound medicines there are approximately ten that are the most frequently taken. These include: medicines for treating diseases of the digestive system, such as Twenty-five Ingredients Turquoise Pill (*g.yu rnying* 25), Seven Ingredients Saffron Medicine (*gur gum chogbdun* 7), Fifteen Ingredients Black Pill (*dagman* 15), Pomegranate Stomach Medicine (*Sabru Dansgnas*), Grub Thob White Pill (*sgrub thob ril dkar*) and *rin chen grang sbyor*; medicines for treating diseases of the brain, heart and blood vessels, such as Seventy Ingredients Pearl Pill (*mu tig* 70), Twenty-five Ingredients Coral Pill (*rin chen byu dmar* 25, or *rengqing chumar* 25), Twenty-five Ingredients Pearl Pill (*mu tig* 25, or *Mutik* 25); and tonics, such as the trademarked 'Tibet Tonic' (Cp. *Xizang Buwang*).

Tibetan inhabited regions of China

The Tibetan people in China are predominantly distributed across the vast Qinghai-Tibet Plateau. In addition to those residing inside the TAR, there are concentrations of Tibetan people in the ten Tibet autonomous prefectures and the two Tibet autonomous counties in Qinghai, Sichuan, Gansu and Yunnan Provinces. Tibetan people residing in these areas also use Tibetan medicine to prevent and treat diseases, but Tibetan medicine developed in these areas under different conditions and in different ways from those inside the TAR.

Qinghai Province

Qinghai Province has the highest concentration of Tibetan people outside the TAR. The *Sku 'bum* (*Ta 'er*) Monastery, located in *Ru gsar* (Huangzhong) County, is a famous Tibetan Buddhist Monastery with a celebrated medical college (*sman pa grva tshang*). The monastery was first built in 1560 and it was one of the key developmental centres of medical knowledge for Tibetan medicine. The medical college of *Sku 'bum* Monastery has long played an important role in the training of Tibetan doctors and in providing medical treatment. It also collected, preserved and arranged classical medical literature and published medical books.

In the past, the training of doctors of Tibetan medicine was largely carried out in the medical colleges. Besides *Sku 'bum* Monastery, medical colleges were attached to *Guanghui* (Cp.) Monastery (Serkhog Gonpa [Tsenpo Gon Ganden Damcholing]?), *Xiaqiong* (Cp.) Monastery (Jakhyung Shedrubling in Hualong Hui Autonomous County), *Lajia* (Cp.) Monastery (Rabgya Gonpa [Tashi Kundeling] in Maqen County) and others.

The number of doctors trained by these monastery medical colleges was small, but they were seen to have a higher medical level than those taught by other methods, and some of them went on to become famous and well renowned doctors of Tibetan medicine.

After 1949, the development of Tibetan medicine in Qinghai began to move away from the basis of the *Sku 'bum* medical college towards new forms of institutions. At first, a few scattered clinics of Tibetan medicine appeared. By 1978, departments and clinics of Tibetan medicine had been set up in a number of the larger hospitals. In 1979, a hospital dedicated to Mongolian-Tibetan medicine was founded in Haixi Mongolian-Tibetan Nationalities Autonomous Prefecture. Following on from this, hospitals of Tibetan medicine began to be founded in different parts of Qinghai.

A course in Tibetan medicine was offered at the Medical School of Huangnan Tibetan Nationality Autonomous Prefecture (Cp. *Huangnan Zangzu Zizhizhou Weisheng Xuexiao*). Between 1981 and 1990, 313 doctors of Tibetan medicine were trained on this course. From 1988 to 1991, the Society of Tibetan Medicine of Qinghai Province held six training classes for doctors of Tibetan medicine, attended by over 600 people.[6] Qinghai College of Tibetan Medicine was set up in 1987 in Xining, and by 1992 it was recruiting students from all over China. In the college, 60 per cent of the courses are based on traditional medicine and 40 per cent on biomedicine, with optional courses in English and computing also available. The college requires its students to study Tibetan medicine, Han medicine and bio-medicine to a high level, on the basis that incorporating the strong points of different schools of medicine furthers the overall development of the Tibetan medical system.[7]

By 1990, twenty-three hospitals of Tibetan medicine had been founded at the Qinghai province and prefecture levels, and a large number of smaller clinics had been established in the villages. The hospitals of Tibetan medicine have an organized system that provides detailed medical records of all aspects of the diagnosis and treatment of patients.

Sichuan Province

The main centres of Tibetan medicine in Sichuan Province are in *Dkar mdzes* (Ganze) Tibetan Nationality Autonomous Prefecture and *Rnga ba* (Aba) Tibetan and Qiang Nationalities Autonomous Prefecture. The influence of Han medicine on the development of Tibetan medicine in these areas of Sichuan was very strong, owing to the significant contributions to medical knowledge that came from *Sde dge* (Dege) and *Ser shul* (Shiqu) counties. In the middle of the eighteenth century, during the time of the eighth Dalai Lama, the classical works of Tibetan medicine became widespread in the Tibetan inhabited areas of Sichuan. During the same period Dilmar geshe (*dil dmar dge bshes bstan 'dzin phun tshogs*), a doctor of Tibetan medicine from *Sde dge* (Dege) County, completed the classic Tibetan pharmacopoeia *Crystal Pearl* (*Shel gong*, Cp. *jingzhubencao*), written on the basis of his systematic research into the *materia medica* of Sichuan and other areas. Shortly thereafter, the Tibetan doctor Sedu Qujiu (*Si tu chos (kyi) 'byung (gnas)*) incorporated into Tibetan medicine four methods of diagnosis and various elements of treatment said to originate from Han medicine. He wrote the medical books *Enweng, Hard Understanding of the Rgyud-bzhi, Qimailuocheng* (Cp. phonetically transcribed from Tibetan) and *An Explanation of the Crystal Pearl of Materia Medica*. Doctor Seduo Qingxianliangle (Cp. phonetically transcribed from Tibetan) corrected mistakes and updated a number of books on Tibetan medicine, in addition to writing his own medical books *Daduo* [Tiger Bag] and *Renduo* [Leopard Bag].

In the eighteenth century, a xylographic printing house was set up in *Sde dge* (Dege) County and went on to become an important academic centre of Tibetan medicine in Sichuan. It produced a large number of medical books in the Tibetan language, some of which are still in use today.[8] *'Ju mi pham rgya mtsho* (Ji Mipangjiacuo in Chinese literature), a nineteenth-century scholar from the Shiqu area, wrote five medical volumes, including seventy pieces of writing, and taught twenty-one disciples. He became known as the modern founder of Tibetan medicine in Garze Prefecture.

Tibetan medicine in Sichuan belongs to the Southern school. It is characterized by a special proficiency in treating diseases of the spleen and stomach, warm-natured and hot-natured diseases, oedema and 'high blood pressure'. It also has special therapies for rheumatic diseases caused by high altitude. Other distinguishing features of this school are the presence of large quantities of medicinal herbs in one prescription and the frequent use of bloodletting to cure diseases. After 1950, the national medical organizations employed some practitioners of Tibetan medicine from the Tibetan inhabited counties of Sichuan Province as formal medical personnel. The government encouraged doctors of Tibetan medicine to teach disciples – in a rather materialist approach – and to set up collective clinics within the government planning socialist frame. At the same time, a department of Tibetan medicine was established in the People's Hospital of Ruoergai County and a hospital of Tibetan medicine was prepared for construction in *Sde dge* (Dege) County. Several training classes for students of Tibetan medicine were held in *Sde dge* and other counties, providing a trained group of primary personnel. After 1969, more than 100 medical stations offering Tibetan medicine were set up, and nearly 200 Tibetan 'barefoot doctors' were trained to work in them.

In the late 1970s, four-year courses in Tibetan medicine were established at the medical schools of *Rnga ba* (Aba) and *Dkar mdzes* (Ganze). By 1984, 173 doctors of Tibetan medicine had graduated from these schools. The local government of *Dkar mdzes* (Ganze) prefecture cooperated with Akong Tulku Rinpoche (Rokpa International) to open a school of Tibetan medicine in *Sde dge* (Dege). This school began recruiting students in 1991, offering a nine-year course that taught students to a very advanced level. By the end of 1992, there were 219 high- and middle-level doctors of Tibetan medicine in the province. By this time, the Hospital of Tibetan Medicine of Ruoergai and the Hospital of Tibetan Medicine of *Dkar mdzes* (Ganze) prefecture had been established, and departments of Tibetan medicine and of Han-Tibetan medicine were in operation in twenty-three county-level hospitals. Hospitals of Tibetan medicine were also planned for construction in *Rnga ba* (Aba) Prefecture and in other counties.

Gansu Province

Tibetan medicine in Gansu Province is mainly concentrated in the *Gan lho* (Gannan) region, where there are many Tibetan Buddhist monasteries. Medical establishments in the monasteries of *Gan lho* (Gannan) include the medical college of Gongba Monastery at Benba Gully in *Co ne* (Zhuoni) County, the Buddhist Palace of the Medical Master in Langmu Monastery in *Klu chu* (Luqu) County, and others.[9] The most famous, however, is *Bla brang* Monastery located in *Bsang chu* (Xiahe) County. Constructed in 1784, this monastery has a well-known medical college which played the roles of both a centre of learning and a clinic of Tibetan medicine. A lot of medical xylographs were also stored in this monastery.

Historically, the *Gan lho* (Gannan) region has produced large numbers of famous doctors and scholars of Tibetan medicine. For example, the thirteenth-century doctor Jige (Cp. phonetically transcribed from Tibetan) from the Jicang of *Klu chu* (Luqu) is known to have discussed, while in the Amdo region of Tibet, the religious doctrines of Buddhism and the wisdom of medicine with *'Phags pa*. The latter went on to become the Yuan Dynasty emperor's adviser. When the famous doctor Nianchang Kalongmanjia[10] (Cp. phonetically transcribed from Tibetan), an assistant to the fifth Dalai Lama Ngawang Lobsang Gyamtso (*Ngag dbang blo bzang rgya mtsho*), had an audience with Emperor Shunzhi, he cured the emperor's disease using Tibetan medicine and was rewarded generously.

In *Gan lho* (Gannan), as in other regions, the second half of the twentieth century saw education in Tibetan medicine go through the methods of Chinese modernity. In 1979, a medical school was set up in *Gan lho* (Gannan) region offering a one-year course in Tibetan medicine to a class of ten students. The school continued to recruit students in ever-increasing numbers each year and by the end of 1990 had trained over 150 students. In 1989, a Department of Tibetan Medicine was established at the College of Traditional Chinese Medicine of Gansu Province (Cp. *Gansu Sheng Zhongyi Xueyuan*) in the *Gan lho* (Gannan) region. Prior to this, Gansu Province had trained its doctors of Tibetan medicine by selecting students and sending them for training in Tibet and Qinghai. With the development of local infrastructures, formal training became possible without the need to send students elsewhere, and modern hospitals of Tibetan medicine began to be set up. In 1970, the Hospital of Tibetan Medicine of *Bsang chu* (Xiahe) County was opened. Following this, hospitals of Tibetan medicine were gradually opened in other counties, including: the Clinic of Tibetan Medicine in Langmu Monastery in *Klu chu* (Luqu) County; the Hospital of Tibetan Medicine in *Klu chu* (Luqu) County; the Hospital of Tibetan Medicine in *Rma chu* (Maqu) County; Malu Hospital of Tibetan Medicine in *Co ni* (Zhuoni) County; and the Hospital of Tibetan Medicine and Traditional Chinese Medicine in *Co ni* (Zhuoni) County.[11]

Yunnan Province

Tibetan medicine is also practised in the Tibetan areas of the Yunnan Province. The above-mentioned great pharmacopoeia *Crystal Pearl* (*Shel gong*) has also recorded many varieties of Tibetan medicinal plants found in this province. In 1957, after the founding of the *Bde chen* (Diqing) Tibetan Nationality Autonomous Prefecture, several famous doctors of Tibetan medicine from this area became members of the national medical organization. A number of research books, such as *Tibetan Herbs in Diqing* (Cp. *Diqing Zangyao*) by Yang Jingsheng and Chuchen Gjiangcuo (1987), *The Essence of the Clinic in Tibetan Medicine* (Cp. *Zangyi Linchuang Jingyao*) and others, were published in Yunnan. It is notable also that bloodletting and moxibustion are both very popular in the Tibetan inhabited areas of Yunnan.

Mainland China

In the thirteenth century, the political and military control over Tibet by the Yuan Dynasty favoured the merging of Tibet with the territory of China in 1270. The influence of the Tibetan religious masters on the Yuan royal court enabled some cultural and religious aspects of the Tibetan tradition to spread throughout China. Tibetan Buddhism, supported by the royal courts, developed rapidly during the Yuan, Ming and Qing Dynasties (Tao 2000; Xian 1999). This laid the foundations for the diffusion of Tibetan medicine to other areas of China, outside what is today the TAR.

Later, in the sixteenth century, the classic works of Tibetan medicine were translated into Mongolian. Alongside Tibetan Buddhism, Tibetan medicine became established in these Mongolian regions, which later became part of the Chinese Empire during the Qing dynasty. The diffusion of Tibetan medicine into these areas played an important role in the subsequent development of Mongolian medicine. By the seventeenth century, the institution of monastic medical colleges was being used to teach medicine in Mongolian areas. Famous medical colleges include those of Aerbasi Mountain in Etuoke Banner; Ruiying Monastery in the present Fuxin County of Liaoning Province; Budala of Rehe (Chengde of Hebei Province); and Kulun Monastery in what is today Mongolia.

In recent years, great efforts have been made to develop Tibetan medicine and to extend its influence both in China and abroad. To achieve these ends, the Research Centre of Tibetology of China (Cp. *Zhongguo Zangxue Yanjiu Zhongxin*) cooperated with the *Lho kha* (Shannan) Hospital of Tibetan Medicine in Tibet to establish the Beijing Hospital of Tibetan Medicine (Cp. *Beijing Zangyiyuan*) in Beijing in 1992. This hospital uses complementary methods, offering Tibetan medicine as the primary method of treatment and backing it up with tests and examinations based in biomedicine. Specialist departments at this hospital include a department of blood vessels of the heart and brain, a department of atrophic gastritis, and a department of diseases of the liver and gall bladder. There is also a treatment centre of Tibetan hydrotherapy. By 1999, this hospital had diagnosed and treated over 300,000 patients from China and abroad, and seems, according to an earlier work of Li Jixiang (1994), to have obtained good social relevance. The founding of this hospital is the result of cultural interaction, although at times uneasy, between people of Tibetan and Han ethnic origins, and these interactions have played an important role in the diffusion of Tibetan medicine in China.

With the successful marketing of Tibetan medicines in many areas of China, knowledge of Tibetan medicine and pharmacology has spread across the whole country. In 2000, the Guangdong Office of the Foundation for the Development of Tibet (Cp. *Yuanzhu Xizang Fazhan Jijinhui Guangdong Banshichu*) set up a Store of Tibetan Drugs from the Snow-Covered Area (Cp. *Guangzhou Xueyu Zangyao Zhuanmaidian*). To date, three branches of the store have been established. The stores sell several hundred varieties of Tibetan medicines in a range of different forms (pills, powders) originating from five of the main Tibetan inhabited areas, namely the TAR, and Sichuan, Qinghai, Yunnan and Gansu Provinces. The store regularly invites famous doctors of Tibetan medicine from the Tibetan areas to work in their head office and their branches. The doctors diagnose diseases and treat their patients using medicines, moxibustion and other techniques free of charge. Not only do the patients consult the doctors of Tibetan medicine in the store, but some doctors of traditional Han medicine and biomedicine also consult them for their knowledge on Tibetan medicine. Over a period of one year, these stores have served approximately 100,000 customers, from both China and overseas.

Accompanying a period of 'reform and opening' and the efforts being made to hasten the economic development of the west of China, the production of Tibetan drugs has rapidly become a mainstay of industrial progress in the Tibetan region. A significant proportion of the Tibetan patent medicines manufactured in the twenty-two pharmaceutical factories in the TAR are sold at outlets scattered across thirty provinces, municipalities and autonomous regions of China. In addition to this, travellers from different parts of China often purchase precious pills (*rin chen ril bu*) or patent medicines from the scenic spots and tourist sites in the Tibetan inhabited areas. A fair number of Tibetan patent drugs may also be found in the catalogues of commonly used medicines in over 600 hospitals across Mainland China.

Finally, publications, academic interest, education and the media play important roles in the diffusion of knowledge concerning Tibetan medicine. Two recent books, *Chinese Tibetan Medicine* (Cai 1995) and *Tibetan Medicine in China* (Qiangba 1996) examine the basic theories and the historical development of Tibetan medicine. Periodicals such as the *Chinese Journal of Ethnomedicine and Ethnopharmacy*, the *Journal of Medicine and Pharmacy of Chinese Minorities* and others often publish papers on Tibetan medicine. In courses on the history of traditional Chinese medicine taught in the colleges of traditional Chinese medicine and those on medical anthropology taught in the departments of anthropology, teachers will offer at least an introductory knowledge of Tibetan medicine in the classes, while some offer more in-depth study (Yu 1983; Chen 1998). Newspapers and the internet also frequently publish information on Tibetan medicine, available to an enormous readership.

Conclusion

The development of Tibetan medicine in China involves an increasing amount of biomedical research. This is primarily concerned with basic research on Tibetan medicine,[12] the clinical observation of a variety of treatments and research on the histology, chemical components, pharmacology and toxicology of medicinal plants. More recently, the research industry has explored newly patented Tibetan medicines and health nutritional supplements. The existing Chinese literature on the subject, most often written in non-Western languages, shows the enormous interest in biomedical research that has been inspired by Tibetan medicine in China. This contemporary trend of research actually echoes the diffusion and increasing popularity of Tibetan medicine throughout the country and represents another medium, albeit highly specialized, through which the development and promotion of this medical system is taking place. Chinese economic development and the increasing exploration of the western regions of China have also contributed to the spread of Tibetan medicine throughout the country.

However, the further development of Tibetan medicine faces a number of difficulties. First, Tibetan medicine has its own theoretical medical background, which makes contemporary research a major epistemological challenge. Moreover, scientific research on Tibetan medicine suggests the need for improvements, both technical and in terms of orientation, in particular regarding the effectiveness and safety of certain procedures. For instance, the method of making *btso-thal* (*zuotai* in Chinese literature) by washing and smelting mercury (*dngul chu*) is a traditional Tibetan technology of pharmacy. In this method, *btso-thal* is supposed to be extracted from mercury and then used as a 'guide' for various precious Tibetan compounds. Some doctors and patients worry about the consequences of the accumulation of heavy metals such as mercury and lead in the body from the use of such medicines. Some research appears to have proved that taking these drugs will not cause an accumulation of heavy metals in the body, but the reliability and validity of such studies need to be rigorously questioned.

Second, Tibetan medical knowledge is predominantly recorded in the Tibetan language, the translation of which poses challenges (physiology, diseases and so on). This appears to be a limiting factor in the diffusion of Tibetan medicine to the Han inhabited areas.

Finally, the increasing popularity of Tibetan medicine and the subsequent overexploitation of raw materials, particularly medicinal plants, is putting increasing pressure on the environment. The Qinghai-Tibet Plateau is the highest plateau in the world, with a very fragile and delicate ecosystem. Unsustainable harvesting has led to a situation in which certain species of medicinal plant are today endangered. As a result of the resource deficiencies facing Tibetan *materia medica*, some Tibetan pharmaceutical products do not contain the required quantity of medical components. The quality of some drugs is therefore said to be decreasing, and certain new types of Tibetan medicines can no longer be produced. A comprehensive range of measures must therefore be taken at the national, regional and local levels to address these problems, which have directly resulted from the development of Tibetan medicine in China and abroad.

Notes

1 Otherwise mentioned as Chinese pinyin (Cp.), the transcriptions are taken from Tibetan.
2 Yet it was greatly heterogeneous in terms of both teachings (quality and methods) and level of practice.

3 This school might have been set up around 1959 but the available literature in Chinese makes no mention of either its date of creation or its name in Tibetan.
4 The Hospital of Tibetan Medicine of Lhasa City was renamed the Hospital of Tibetan Medicine of the Tibet Autonomous Region in 1980.
5 While this ritual existed at the Iron Hill Medical College (*Lcags po ri*) and the School of Medicine and Astro-computation (*Sman rtsis khang*), it was most probably not common among individual practitioners.
6 The exact place where these training sessions occurred is not known.
7 There are debates surrounding such combinations of medical teaching, but they are beyond the scope of this descriptive chapter.
8 More than sixty volumes of medical books including 1,200 pieces of writing printed by this publishing house remain in existence.
9 The Tibetan names for Gongba, Benba Gully, the Buddhist Palace of the Medical Master and Langmu were not available for this research.
10 No record has been found of where this doctor is from.
11 *Co ni* (Zhuoni) County has therefore two distinct hospitals. The former offers the practice of Tibetan medicine and biomedicine, whereas the latter offers both Tibetan medicine and Han medicine together with biomedicine.
12 These research activities actually focus on the arrangement of the basic theories, the methods of diagnosis and treatment, and the preparation of medicines. The research also includes research on a comparative level regarding the basic theories of Tibetan medicine to contrast with or to complement those of traditional Han medicine and biomedicine.

References

Cai, Jingfeng (1995). *Zhongguo Zangyixue* [Chinese Tibetan Medicine], Beijing: Kexue Chubanshe [Science Press].

Chen, Hua (1998). *Yixue Renleixue Daolun* [An Introduction to Medical Anthropology], Guangzhou: Zhongshan Daxue Chubanshe [Publishing House of Sun Yat-sen (Zhongshan) University].

Li, Dinglan (1989). Xizang Jindai Yixue Jiaoyu Chuyi [My Humble Opinions on Education of Medicine in Modern Times in Tibet], *Xizang Yanjiu* [Research on Tibet] 2: 104.

Li, Jixiang (1994). Beijing de Hui, Meng, Zang Zu Yiliao Jigou [The Medical Institutes of Hui, Mongol, Tibetan Nationalities in Beijing], *Zhongguo Keji Shiliao* [China Historical Materials of Science and Technology of Chinese Medicine, Science and Technology] 15(1): 66–70.

Qiangba, Chilie (1996). *Zhongguo de Zangyi* [Tibetan Medicine in China], Beijing: Zhongguo Zangxue Chubanshe [Chinese Tibetology Publishing Company].

Tao, Ke (2000). Lun Zang Chuan Fojiao Dui Hanzu de Yingxinag [On the Influence of Tibetan Buddhism on the Han Nationality], *Gansu Shehui Kexue* [Social Science of Gansu] 2: 83–86.

Xian, Ba (1999). Yuan, Ming, Qing Shiqi Zang Chuan Fojiao Zai Qing Gan Ning Diqu de Xingshuai [The Rise and Decline of Tibetan Buddhism in the Areas of Qinghai, Gansu and Ningxia during the Period of the Yuan, Ming and Qing Dynasties], *Qinghai Minzu Xueyuan Xuebao (Shehui Kexue Ban)* [Journal of the National College of Qinghai (Social Science Edition)] 3: 36–41.

Yang, Jingsheng and Chuchen, Gjiangcuo (1987 [1989]). *Diqing Zangyao* [Tibetan Herbs in Diqing], Kunming: Yunnan Minzu Chubanshe [Yunnan Nationality Publishing House].

Yu, Shenchu (1983). *Zhongguo Yixue Jianshi* [Brief History of Chinese Medicine], Shanghai: Fujian Kexue Jishu Chubanshe [Science and Technology Publishing House of Fujian].

Part II
The politics of knowledge

5 Integration or erasure?

Modernizing medicine at Lhasa's Mentsikhang

Vincanne Adams and Fei-Fei Li*

As most readers of this volume will already know, Tibetan medicine has been integrative, from the outset. Tibetan medicine, or what is sometimes called *Rgyud bzhi* medicine, emerged out of a multi-century effort to integrate elements of Indian, Persian, Chinese, and indigenous shamanic with Buddhist scriptural insights on the relationship between health and the body (Meyer 1981, 1992; Dummer 1988). Moreover, since at least the seventeenth century, Tibetan medicine was based, at a minimum, on the textual forms of the Four Tantras (*Rgyud bzhi*) but also the important commentaries written by skilled medical practitioners in the centuries before and after (Zhurkar, Lodri Gyalbo, Desi Sangye Gyatso, and the like) which surely modified these texts (intentionally or not) in the process of selective elaboration, exclusion, and clarification in relation to folk and village-level beliefs and religious practices. Even with textual resources, the transmission of medical teachings varied from region to region, monastery to monastery, one family of practitioners to another. In some instances, family-based lineages of practitioners derived much of their knowledge of pharmacopoeia and medical practice from oral instruction and visual observation alone, a tradition that debatably contributed to more integrative outcomes in relation to varied folk practices when it came to medicine.[1] In this essay, we do not attend to the history of integration within Tibetan medicine, but focus instead on that which has resulted from Tibetan medicine's exposure to what is called Western scientific medicine or "biomedicine."[2]

A few orienting points are offered at the outset. First, an account of the history of encounters between biomedicine and Tibetan medicine begins long before the period of time of the greatest impact of this encounter. During the era of British colonialism in India, Tibetan doctors were known to travel to northern India and throughout the Himalayan region in search of potent medicinal ingredients. In India, Nepal, Bhutan, and Sikkim, Tibetan doctors were exposed to British and American physicians and surgeons, and some amount of cross-cultural exchange of medical knowledge occurred (Adams and Dovchin 2000; McKay 1997).[3] During the reign of the thirteenth Dalai Lama, members of noble families were sent to study science and technology, including medical sciences, in Britain. They brought back knowledge and techniques of medicine practice that formed a foundation for integration of Tibetan and Western medical ideas. The first efforts at modernization of the formal state-run system of training of Tibetan doctors was initiated by the government of Tibet in 1916 with the building of Mentsikhang, an alternative to the monastic medical institution called *Lcags po ri*, built in the seventeenth century (Rechung 1973). Our focus is on the current moment of engagement that began in the 1960s and has intensified in the years since then.

Second, although we focus in this essay on the interface between Tibetan and biomedical practices, giving the impression that the two "systems" of medicine are discrete, there is a long history of mutual implication in each other's traditions that precedes their current moment of engagement and continues to influence the ways "integrated" medicine is carried out today. Tibetan doctors have borrowed from and incorporated elements of other medical systems from the outset, including biomedical traditions, just as Western medicine has absorbed elements of non-Western medical thought and practice throughout the period of colonialism and after (Marglin and Appfel 1990; Harding 1998). However, practitioners who have been trained primarily in one or the other medical tradition today tend to act, in practice, as if their traditions were and are discrete, and often incommensurable, despite their ability to integrate them in the care of patients. We focus on the moments of "integration" in which it is clear that either distinguishing between the traditions becomes a priority or incommensurability becomes an obstacle to effective medical care.

We also note, at the outset, that Tibetan doctors tend to refer to the practices of biomedicine as "outside" (*phyilu'i*) or "Chinese" (*gyami'i*) medicine or as "Western medicine" (in English). In this essay we use the more analytic term "biomedicine" for the collection of practices referred to by these labels. These practices should not be taken as forming a coherent and essential whole that is uniformly practiced in ways that are universally standardized. Just as biomedicine within the United States and European nations is normatively diverse in its execution, even with procedures putatively labeled the same way (Berg and Mol 1998), biomedical practices throughout the TAR, and in China more generally, often bear little resemblance to the biomedicine practiced in its countries of origin.

Finally, the data for this essay are derived from research collected at Lhasa's traditional Tibetan medical hospital, the Mentsikhang (Medical and Astrology Institute), and, to a lesser extent, from faculty and students at its new TAR Tibetan Medical College. These are the TAR's premier medical institutions for study and practice of Tibetan medicine. Our information from the Medical College comes from interviews with professors who currently teach at the college and current students or recent graduates of the college. Within Mentsikhang, our observations are drawn from interviews, observations, and publications in relation to three divisions: the women's division, the liver division, and the digestive division. Integration took different forms in each department. In the women's division, doctors trained in either biomedicine or Tibetan medicine worked side by side. In the digestive and liver divisions, integration was not introduced by way of practitioners of biomedicine who were assigned to these wards but rather by way of requirements on the part of the hospital that the division follow certain biomedical diagnostic and treatment protocols that were presumed to be effective. Encounters between biomedical doctors and Tibetan medicine doctors were observed in all divisions over the course of research. Tibetan doctors in all three divisions were all formally trained in Tibetan medicine, and to varying degrees within each ward all of the doctors had been taught some biomedicine in the course of their medical training.

Integration occurring by way of the training of physicians was limited. In general, Tibetan medical physicians received different amounts of exposure to and training in biomedicine. A much older generation of physicians had very little training in biomedical concepts or practices and came to know them solely through their participation in socialist reform programs (some were trained in the methods of barefoot doctors and sent to the countryside, for example) and through their work in the ever-changing Tibetan medical hospital and college. As elaborated below, those trained during the Cultural Revolution had much more exposure to biomedical ideas in at least a rudimentary primary health care orientation, including basic biomedical disease lists, primary biomedical treatment regimens, and basic theories of biomedical etiology and pathology (Janes 1995). These doctors also received the least formal training in traditional theories of Tibetan medicine. Doctors trained from the late 1970s onward have been offered coursework in anatomy, physiology, and the basic pharmacology of biomedicine.

Historical contexts for integration

Although Tibet appears as a special case within China because of its history, the phenomenon of integration saw its birth in China and its Asian neighbors in the early nineteenth century. After the series of military defeats with Western powers starting then, China and its neighboring societies underwent a "reformation" that prioritized an embrace of Western sciences while consciously or subconsciously rejecting their own Eastern scholarly fields of knowledge. Even decades before the communist government, the Kuomintang government encouraged the study and practice of Western medicine. Many early twentieth-century Chinese intellectuals who were among the elite group given opportunities to go overseas majored in the study of Western medicine. Chinese medicine came to be seen as marginal and backward in a rather voluntary way by cultural and political Chinese elites long before the time of the communist revolution. In Tibet, exposure to Western medical sciences appeared to have brought fascination but no rejection of traditional medicine in the manner seen in China.

By the time of the revolution that brought communist forces into Tibet, the rejection of traditional indigenous culture and knowledge in favor of that from Europe (especially in the sciences) was already articulated as a prime target of Chinese revolutionary politics. At first, the communist government favored the development of biomedicine, but then led a campaign against the high-technology, high-specialization forms of biomedicine that had been steadily growing in mainland China. During the Cultural Revolution, the communist government recognized the practical utility and efficacy of Western medicine (Li 1994), articulating an ambiguous position that rejected what it saw as imperialistic medicine while simultaneously laying the foundation for a new "communist" model for public health that relied on many biomedical concepts, eventually inspiring the global primary health care movement inaugurated at Alma Ata in 1978. Making good on the promise of building a Chinese nation on Chinese foundations and following the gradual path in socialist reformation, they established the "barefoot doctor" program emphasizing an integration of traditional medical practices (those officially recognized as medical traditions of the minority populations, *minzu*) with basic training in rudimentary biomedicine.

From the perspective of Chinese and Tibetan histories of the contemporary era, Tibetan medicine's exposure to and integration with biomedicine is recent, from the period of time just prior to the onset of Maoist socialism and the arrival of the People's Liberation Army to the Tibetan Plateau in the early 1950s.[4] The most profound effects of exposure to biomedicine came with socialist reform policies and the eventual construction of biomedical hospitals in Tibet's major cities (in part to service military personnel). The first large-scale effort to integrate Tibetan and biomedical resources occurred during this period, in the 1960s, when Tibetan medicine was given official status as a traditional medical system (like that of what is now called Zhongyi or Traditional Chinese Medicine) and made to serve the anticolonial impulse of the revolution. Tibetan medical doctors were trained in the methods of "barefoot doctors" (Janes 1995; Adams 2002) and variously sent down to the countryside for rural service using whatever resources they could to sustain a healthy population and proselytize the benefits of socialist reforms.

The barefoot doctor campaign laid a foundation for support of existing indigenous medical traditions in part because these medical practices were politically useful and because they were recognized by the state as empirically effective. However, under these reform programs, efforts were also made to eliminate the religious and superstitious elements of indigenous medical practices, including (if not particularly) those found within the religious components of Tibetan medicine. These elements were thought to be residual features of a feudalistic social order and not an essential part of medical efficacy. Such policies resulted in efforts to simplify Tibetan medicine into simple disease and treatment lists, and either to ignore theory altogether or to strip it of any of its "superstitious" features, including reference to karma, spirits, tantric physiological principles, and the like (Janes 1995). Theoretical disjunctures between Tibetan and biomedical perspectives that emerged from this effort to combine basic forms of both systems were largely swept under the rug, as fears of recrimination for advocating more traditional theoretical approaches paralyzed many of Tibet's most knowledgeable medical scholars. This trend has persisted, post-Cultural Revolution, for different reasons today (described below), but with slightly less severe outcomes (Adams 2001). In China's minority region of Tibet (Xizang), this history of "integrated medicine" nevertheless laid a foundation for a thriving set of practices that do "integrate" the two traditions in Tibet today, though not entirely smoothly or unambiguously.

In the post-Mao eras of liberalization throughout China, greater emphasis has been placed on revitalizing some aspects of traditional Tibetan medicine, witnessed in part by the construction of a new inpatient hospital and a new college for Tibetan medicine. However, these innovations have also been based partly on a desire to remake these medical traditions into a form that resembles biomedicine, in clinical and practical aspects. Official policies toward the revitalization of Tibetan medicine have also failed to overcome political suspicions of "religious" elements in Tibetan medicine, resulting in efforts to transform medical theory into something that is more compatible with biomedical models. In the decades since liberalization, there has been a steady push for a more "integrated" medicine, as seen in the requirement that Tibetan medical students take courses in biomedical theory and that hospitals make use of specific biomedical diagnostic, treatment, and record-keeping techniques, as if there were an automatic or simple way to translate between the two systems, linguistically and practically.

The underlying pretext for policies of integration is that Tibetan medicine must emphasize its "scientific" foundations over its "religious" foundations in order to compete with other medical modalities in the modern world – an assumption that both requires Tibetan doctors to adopt Western scientific techniques and epistemological practices and also fits conveniently with official government policies regarding religion among Tibetans. A younger generation of doctors at Mentsikhang has been taught in basic biomedical theory, and they are familiar with basic germ theories, use of antibiotics, and anatomical and physiological models of biomedicine. However, many of these scholar physicians have sought to enrich their knowledge and understanding of Tibetan medical theory from the most senior generation of physicians through private tutorials and apprenticeship. They do so on the grounds that Tibetan theoretical foundations form the "scientific" roots of Tibetan medicine. As the older generation of scholarly physicians passes, younger scholars find themselves somewhat worried about their ability to maintain and pass down the full knowledge of Tibetan medical theory and practice from an older generation that still fears open disclosure of knowledge that the government deems "religious" and therefore superfluous to effective medicine.

In addition to official policies toward integration, there are other social pressures that indirectly contribute to integration of biomedicine and Tibetan medicine in the urban context. The government does not subsidize Tibetan medicine as much as it subsidizes its government biomedical facilities, making it more possible for the Tibetan hospital to add staff trained in biomedicine than in Tibetan medicine when the government will pay salaries for these positions. At the same time, because Tibetan medicines and treatments are less expensive than those offered at biomedical facilities, this means that poor Tibetan clients are often more likely to seek Tibetan medical treatments than biomedical ones, even if they would prefer to seek biomedical care (Janes 1999). But this also means that the majority of Mentsikhang's clientele are the least likely to be covered by government insurance programs and the least likely to be able to afford the services they get (meaning they ask for reduced-rate or subsidized care from the hospitals).

In tension with this trend is the problem of inequity in policy regarding medicines. Biomedicines are much more profitable than Tibetan medicines in Tibet and so, for hospitals that are more and more pressured to survive on reduced government subsidies as reformation of the health system deepens across China, more pressure is put on traditional medical hospitals to offer biomedicines to make a profit. Under the current Chinese health care system each medicine or treatment procedure, whether Western or Tibetan or Chinese, is assigned a specific price range by the government. In these lists, both Chinese and Tibetan medicines are much cheaper than biomedicines. Thus, for any given illness, even if there are highly effective Tibetan medicines, "the hospital is pressured to prescribe biomedicine because it has to feed this many doctors and staff," says a senior officer at the Mentsikhang. Thus, Mentsikhang administrators recognize that, when they can charge patients who can pay for services, they receive more for biomedicines and use of biomedical technologies than Tibetan. In the end, these trends mean that Tibetans who wish to use Tibetan medicines because they are less expensive find it harder and harder to obtain Tibetan medicines even when they are preferred. This is particularly true in rural areas (Janes 2002). Nevertheless, the bulk of Tibet's poorest citizens can only afford to seek Tibetan medicine.

Financial pressures from having a client population that is least able to pay for services results in greater financial strain on the hospital. This, in turn, results in greater efforts on the part of Tibetan medical staff to commercialize in ways that will mass-market their treatments for the local, national, and international medical markets. This generally means making their medical services and pharmaceutical products look more like those of biomedicine, even while appealing to a consumer interest in "traditional" medical alternatives to biomedicine. Preparation and packaging of medicines now most frequently occurs in a manner that is standardized according to Western biomedical measures, as understood by the Chinese state, to make them more commercially attractive and to accommodate demands for greater standardization of ingredients and mode of delivery in the international market.

Economic, social, and political pressures also compel Tibetan medical scholars to undertake research programs that aim to establish the validity and efficacy of Tibetan medicine by way of biomedical research techniques and standards. The desire to participate in discussions about the efficacy of Tibetan medicine (at conferences, in scholarly publications, and in research projects) often results in efforts to "integrate" medical practices and theories, which almost always means forcing Tibetan medicine to conform to biomedical standards rather than the reverse, even while publicly advocating and advertising the "alternative" qualities of Tibetan medicine.

Another reason there is pressure on Tibetan medical doctors to standardize both preparation and packaging of their medicines is the particular way that issues of intellectual property have been played out in China. Before aggressive commercialization and marketing practices entered Tibet, the idea of medical intellectual property was virtually non-existent. Prescriptions were widespread and often transparent from doctor to doctor, clinic to clinic, and hospital to hospital. Remedies were not uniformly standardized, although compounding ingredient lists were often shared, and were taught as curricular subjects at the medical hospitals. But as China, along with the rest of Asia, opened its market to the world and increasingly participated in globalized medical exchange, intellectual property became a more and more pressing issue. Tibetan doctors and hospitals soon found their own medicine prescriptions scooped by visionary businessmen (often Chinese) and that the commercialization of their products profited these entrepreneurs more than the Tibetan hospitals or doctors. In order to catch this wave of profit making, Tibetan medicine hospitals and pharmaceutical factories (traditionally affiliated with the hospitals) have now joined in the process of patenting their own prescriptions. Again, however, this process is overseen by government agencies that require standardized methods of preparation and packaging that are almost exclusively developed according to biomedical protocols.

These internationalization and commercialization trends are consistent with government policies that advocate greater integration in the delivery of hospital services. Pressure from within the medical infrastructure, both from the Health Bureau and from the Communist Party representatives (in the Health Bureau and assigned to the Tibetan medical infrastructure), is toward making greater use of biomedical resources to expand and improve services offered by the hospital. Such pressure is also placed on doctor-scholars who have attempted to undertake research and publication about their areas of specialty (Trinlay 1998).

Integration efforts have resulted in a variety of practices that are worth describing for what can be learned about the conflicts, resolutions, successes, and failures of integrated medicine. In this locale, integrative medicine is carried out by practitioners who have learned to incorporate bits and pieces of one another's traditions, but we note again that doctors tend to position themselves vis-à-vis "foreign" practices as practitioners of one or the other tradition, rather than as "integrated" practitioners. It is, of course, at these moments of both conjuncture and differentiation that incompatibilities become more obvious and therefore, perhaps, more provocative of discussion about what integrated medicine really means in this locale. In what follows, then, we will illustrate "integrated medicine" as it appears in and through its achievements and ongoing tensions in three areas: diagnosis, treatment, and outcomes. Our title, "Integration or erasure?," refers to the ways we might read these encounters as tensions over these two possibilities. Integration in its best possible sense results in the sharing and exchange of knowledge and practices, as opposed to its opposite: the substitution and erasure of one for the sake of incorporating the other.

Integration in diagnosis

In many wards of Lhasa's Mentsikhang, it has become customary to examine patients not only by way of pulse, urine, tongue analysis, questioning, and physical palpation but also by way of the use of thermometers, blood pressure cuffs, ultrasound machines, and laboratory assays. A wide variety of data gets produced through these techniques of diagnosis, and doctors with varying types of training are expected to make use of them to come up with effective treatment plans for their patients. Few Tibetan doctors are able to make full use of the kinds of information that all of the biomedical resources provide, in the same way that few biomedical doctors practicing within Mentsikhang pay much attention to the descriptions of the pulse, urine, or tongue that Tibetan doctors use to ascertain disorders. For a number of Tibetan doctors in the women's division, for example, the presence of biomedical lab results, ultrasound reports, temperature readings, and blood information often served as little more than "filler" information for diagnostic charts that the hospital required. They were of little use to the Tibetan doctors in their determination of actual treatment programs. In contrast, this information was crucial to the biomedical physician working in the ward. Young Tibetan-trained physicians working with biomedical doctors in the ward increasingly made use of this information as well. In the digestive department, we saw a different trend: endoscopic measurements are often of tremendous importance to Tibetan doctors for at least certain groups of patients. That information helped them determine Tibetan-named diagnoses. In the liver department, we also observed that use of the hepatitis blood test was considered mandatory even among Tibetan-trained doctors.

As would be expected, younger Tibetan doctors who had received more training in biomedical methods used biomedical data more substantively. Often, they would attribute this to the relative ease of using biomedical techniques over Tibetan. It takes many years to learn how to use pulse diagnosis effectively or how to read urine, they would say, but one could learn in a very short time that the presence of white blood cells in a lab report indicated infection or that an ultrasound reading that showed a growth in the ovary of 3.1 centimeters indicated it was filled with fluid – something that only the best Tibetan doctors could "see" using pulse, urine, and palpation methods. Tibetan doctors maintained that this was one reason Western-trained doctors were largely incapable of incorporating Tibetan methods into their own diagnostic repertoire. One Tibetan doctor put it this way: "As for Western medicine, it is very easy to just follow the manual, but for Tibetan medicine it is very hard to start from scratch and learn anything within a short time."

The more compelling question than what diagnostic instruments were used in diagnosis was how doctors, in some cases working side by side with the same patients, gave names to the disorders they saw. Given that in each medical tradition different names are given to various medical disorders or clusters of symptoms, and given that these correspond to different ways of not only naming disease but also viewing the body and the causes of disease, how did doctors in this integrated medical environment decide how to name diseases?

In the best circumstances that we viewed in Lhasa's Mentsikhang, doctors were able to come up with diseases lists that mapped exact correspondences between biomedicine and Tibetan medicine. This did not necessarily mean that practitioners had a shared conception of single diseases, but that a simple linguistic translation could be deployed as a placeholder for assumptions about a shared perception of symptoms. Correspondences emerged from deciphering a "match" of the most obvious forms of symptoms related to differently named diseases described by a patient. Eradication of symptoms using either Tibetan medicine or biomedicine confirmed this shared assumption about disease label translatability.

In the digestive unit, doctors generally used only Tibetan diagnostic categories and names. But when a research project was initiated by a Western researcher whose methods were primarily informed by biomedical referents for symptoms believed to be associated with infection from *Helicobacter pylori* (HP) found in common biomedical literature, the doctors had to begin the lengthy process of mapping correspondences for a set of similar disorders that were named in both systems. Thus, they learned that *powa lengta* could be translated as acute gastritis on the basis of symptoms of acute abdominal pain, distension, diarrhea and vomiting; *mashuo ningba* was chronic superficial gastritis on the basis of shared perceived symptoms of distension, stomach pain, decreased appetite, and eructation; *bu ru* was chronic atrophic gastritis; *Pomu tomey* was erosive gastritis; and *badken mobu* was peptic ulcer, and so on.

In the women's division, a biomedically trained physician worked alongside Tibetan doctors. Among these doctors we observed an easy mapping of one set of names for disorders onto others. For example, of the nine types of growths in women's reproductive tract, there were seven that corresponded to known biomedical conditions: cervical cancer, fibroids, ovarian cyst, endometriosis, polyps, ectopic pregnancy, and molar pregnancy. But two named types of growths in the Tibetan system had no biomedical equivalents, although one biomedical doctor proposed that one of them could be "retained products of conception" as it was known in biomedicine, even if the Tibetan doctors dissented from this view. In this case "matches" were found on the basis of symptom description in Tibetan medical textbooks as compared with photographs of the appearances of the growths found in biomedical textbooks. The non-matched diseases were considered so rare that they were largely ignored. The effort to match diseases was, in this division, prompted by our research inquiry, in which a biomedical physician showed photos of disorders from a Chinese medical textbook to Tibetan doctors in order to elicit the Tibetan terminology that was used to describe these cases. In most of these cases, Tibetan medicine doctors noted that these names were taken from, and symptoms describing these diseases were found in, the *Rgyud bzhi*.

The process of co-naming was not something that doctors in any of the wards endeavored on a daily basis, in part because patients were "assigned" to one or another doctor on initial admission. In the women's division, the biomedical physician would offer disease names for her patients, and Tibetan doctors offered Tibetan labels for their patients. When conferring about co-treatment of patients, however, both doctors assumed the interchangeability of disease labels. Biomedical names offered by the biomedical physicians were generally in Chinese, but we found that in a number of cases the biomedical doctor would use the Tibetan name interchangeably because for certain diseases it was presumed that there was an exact correspondence between disease labels. On most hospital records, Tibetan disease names were used, including those that were "known" in Tibetan medicine and seen as having equivalents in biomedicine, and those that were "new" to Tibetan medicine – disorders that were identified by biomedicine and given a Tibetan translation. When a biomedical label was given, usually in Mandarin, that label was kept on the record for the course of treatment. Hospital administrators did not seem to mind having two different naming systems at work in their records.

In cases where practitioners saw an easy translation between disease labels for the same biological conditions, practitioners said they benefited from a feeling of "confirmation" from the other tradition. This effect was heightened when the diagnostic technologies from one tradition were used to confirm the diagnosis in the other tradition. For example, Tibetan medicine uses pulse, urine, and interrogation to determine the presence of an ulcerated bleeding stomach. When endoscopy was used to make visible the bleeding stomach, confirming a "peptic ulcer," it had the effect of legitimizing Tibetan medical diagnostic techniques. When the Tibetan condition *badken mobu* was given the disease name "peptic ulcer" in biomedicine, it gave the Tibetan doctors a sense that their methods of diagnosis were effective in a universal, scientific sense. Similarly, when a Tibetan diagnosis of *sha skran pembo* (flesh growth in the ovary) was made using pulse, urine, and interrogation methods and then when ultrasound examination produced an image of fibroids in the ovaries, Tibetan doctors said that the ultrasound confirmed the accuracy of their own methods. In cases like these, the names were assumed to be interchangeable: the condition described by the term *sha skran pembo* was taken as the same as that described by the term "fibroids"; *badken mobu* was "peptic ulcer," and so on.

One of the side effects of this dual diagnostic process in which "matching" occurred was the increased borrowing of ideas about pathology and etiology, wherein whole categories of phenomena from one system were seen as interchangeable with the other. Thus, Tibetan medicine uses the idea of "*bu*," or bugs, worm, small creature, as a source of symptoms for various disorders. When biomedical doctors explained that the cause of various gastric diseases was bacteria or a virus they would colloquially refer to this as "a bug," but not in the sense of it being borrowed from the Tibetan concept. Nevertheless, the ability to switch between the Tibetan term "*bu*" and the Western terms "bacteria" and "virus" (and even "bug") was made easy by this linguistic slippage. Conceptually, it meant the same thing to Tibetan doctors whether one referred to a pathogen as a bug or bacteria, or a virus, since all were categorically similar in that they were external living pathogenic agents. The fact that Tibetan understandings of these "*bu*" upon closer inspection did not always map neatly onto the category of either "bacteria" or "virus," let alone that the linguistic move also merged "bacteria" with "virus," thereby erasing the distinction of great importance in biomedicine, was seldom addressed. Only among a younger generation of Tibetan doctors, who had more training in biomedicine, did the distinction between "bacteria" and "virus" become important. This subtle difference suggests that, in the process of piloting integrative medicine, the more familiarity doctors had to both systems, the less obvious it was to them how to integrate, since they understood on a more theoretical and practical level how difficult it is to map some concepts to each other in a straightforward manner across the two traditions.

Along the same lines, another outcome of the validating and matching process is that doctors often transferred knowledge about etiology and treatment from one system to the other once it was assumed that the disease was, for all intents and purposes for them, the same "biological" thing in each tradition. For example, biomedical knowledge surrounding etiology, pathology, and prognosis for "peptic ulcer" was seen as expanding upon Tibetan knowledge about "*badken mobu*." Tibetan doctors adopted the idea that peptic ulcers can be caused by external pathogens (bacteria = *bu*), expanding their recognition of the role of poor diet in causing this condition. In addition to food and behavioral causes of *badken mobu*, Tibetan doctors also now understood that *Helicobacter pylori* could play a role in causing peptic ulcers/*badken mobu*. But integrating knowledge between the systems in this way also posed challenges. In both Tibetan medicine and biomedicine, poor diet is considered one cause, among others, of peptic ulcer/*badken mobu*. However, the types of foods that are considered "causative" of disease in each system are not always the same. Similarly, Tibetan conceptualization of the proximate cause (internal humoral imbalance) leading to *badkan mobu* did not map easily onto biomedical conceptualizations of anatomical and physiological disruptions of digestive biochemistry that lead to peptic ulcers. As we will see later, the question of whether doctors chose to identify *badken mobu* or "peptic ulcer" made a difference in conceptualizing not just the condition of the disease but also the best treatment approach to it.

In the women's division, similar patterns emerged. Biomedical conceptions of the bacterial and viral bases of sexually transmitted vaginal and reproductive diseases are now being adopted by Tibetan doctors who would not have historically considered sexual relations to be involved in some diseases. That Tibetan doctors now recognize that the spread of papilloma virus is a cause of cervical cancer in some women is an example of this. The development of cancers in the cervix, uterus, and/or ovaries was generally understood in the context of various long-term humoral imbalances, in turn related to reproductive history, diet, and climate. At the same time, that these Tibetan medicine doctors identified the locations of these growths in discrete reproductive organs, such as the ovaries, already reflected a borrowing from biomedical anatomical maps. Growths in the reproductive tract (of which the Tibetan condition translated as "cervical cancer" was one) were often attributed to stagnated menstrual blood, weakened downward expelling winds (*thursel rlung*), and prolonged exposure to cold (environmental, dietary, internal). Reproductive history played a role in the development of growths/*skran* also, since traumatic birth experiences, miscarriages, or abortions contributed to problems that could result in stagnation of blood leading to development of growths in the reproductive tract. But, historically, sexual history was not generally considered a cause of growths.[5] When the biomedical terms were substituted for Tibetan terms, however, a transfer of knowledge was assumed to be possible. When the term "fibroids" was substituted for *sha skran pembo*, or *skran 'dre* was called "cancer," it was assumed that biomedical knowledge was able to "expand" the horizon of knowledge for Tibetan medicine, bringing it new understandings of etiology and pathogenesis that could be deployed in preventive efforts as well as in research on the development of medicines.[6]

Among Tibetan doctors it was sometimes assumed that biomedical knowledge is more complete in its physiological detail than Tibetan medical knowledge. Therefore, the direction of transfer was almost always toward the use of biomedical knowledge to expand Tibetan understandings. Seldom was there a reverse move to assume that Tibetan concepts ought to expand biomedical knowledge. This expansion was always presumed to be improving Tibetan medicine, rather than erasing it, although some Tibetan doctors who steadfastly resisted incorporating biomedicine suggested that the latter was in fact occurring.

A rare exception to this directionality of knowledge transfer was in the way that the biomedical doctor in the women's division made use of information about hot/cold relations in regard to diet and medicines. We found that women with high blood pressure during pregnancy were advised to avoid certain heating foods that would augment the potency of their *mkhris-pa* (bile) and worsen their high blood pressure. Similarly, in the women's ward, the biomedical doctor made use of Tibetan treatment priorities. Women suffering from uterine infections and weak digestion would, when treated by Tibetan medicine doctors, often be prescribed medicines for their digestion before taking medicines for their infection. So, when doctors knew that a disorder could be eliminated by use of antibiotics, but that the patient with weak digestion would not be able to properly absorb antibiotics (because Western medicines are stronger than Tibetan), they would first be treated with medicines to improve their digestive function and then eventually given medications for their uterine infection. The biomedical doctor working in the women's division had incorporated the idea of the validity of this approach into her daily practices with patients, and on a rare occasion actually made this sort of determination independent of Tibetan medicine physicians. The openness of this doctor could perhaps be attributed to the fact that this biomedical doctor was reared by two Tibetan medicine doctors and was, we were told, more sympathetic to Tibetan medical approaches than other biomedical doctors in the hospital. In general, biomedical doctors working in the Mentsikhang (as either visitors or permanent staff) did not make great efforts to use Tibetan medical strategies in the absence of Tibetan doctors. The direction of knowledge transfer was usually to substitute new and "better" biomedical knowledge for what was perceived as "incomplete" or rudimentary Tibetan knowledge – a trend, again, opposed by more senior Tibetan physicians who had great expertise and great understanding of medical theory.

Complications in integrated diagnoses

One of the most difficult practices of integrated diagnosis was establishing correspondences between diseases when matching symptoms was not straight-forward or was downright impossible. For example, in the liver division doctors could find no single equivalent for hepatocirrhosis, a set of symptoms that corresponded to three different Tibetan disorders: 1) *cinca mobu gye-ba*; 2) *cinya truton*; and 3) *cinnya ton tabu*. Similarly, in the women's division, we found that "bile-related womb disorder" (*mngal nad mkhris gyur*) was one of the most common disorders among female Tibetan patients. When we asked the resident "biomedical" doctor for the name of this disease, we were told it was "PID, pelvic inflammatory disease." However, when a second foreign biomedical physician was asked to diagnose patients with *mngal nad mkhris gyur*, she found that it corresponded to not just pelvic inflammatory disease (some with cervical or tubal inflammation/infection and some with both), but also various vaginal inflammations/infections (related to yeast infection and early-stage STDs) and also to menstrual irregularities and pain (with no other biomedical disease) and to ovarian cysts – a much larger category of disorders than would have fallen under the rubric "PID" in her Western hospital. Finally, there were some disorders named in biomedicine that had no Tibetan equivalent (for example, some of the sexually transmitted diseases).

The problem arising from not having exact correspondence of diseases was that it made visible both how closely linked disease names were to ideas about etiology and treatment and how different these ideas were across medical systems. In research efforts, for example, this problem presented enormous difficulties in determining which diseases would be evaluated for outcome efficacy – the Tibetan diseases or the biomedical – as well as in determining what treatment models would be pursued for evidence of successful or failed clinical outcomes.

In clinical practice, the problem of not having exact correspondence of diseases produced ambiguity that sometimes resulted in confusion over treatments. For example, patients with the disease of "diabetes" occasionally came to the Tibetan medical hospital with that disease label, having undergone treatments at a biomedical clinic that were intended to increase the insulin capability of the body, or to reduce sugar consumption. But for a Tibetan doctor, whose diagnosis placed the patient into one of several different disease categories (all of which correspond to biomedicine's diabetes), the effort to increase insulin or reduce sugar intake would not necessarily be seen as appropriate in all cases. In some cases, it would be seen as counterproductive to take this course of action. In this case, lack of one-to-one correspondence between named disorders led to some confusion over whose disease labels were the appropriate ones for pursuit of therapy.

The process of "naming" a disease thus can result in extraordinary confidence-building on the part of practitioners in each tradition but it can also result in confusion over whose diagnostic categories should be treated as valid at a given point in time with a given disorder. "Naming" was not just about different names for the same biological conditions; it was a process of determining different approaches to bodies, disorders, etiology, and treatments. And the decision about how to "name" a patient's condition was deeply intertwined with the kinds of diagnostic tools that doctors relied on to come up with a named condition. The existence of biomedical techniques created an environment wherein they occasionally became seen as shortcut routes to diagnosis. In the sense that there were differently skilled practitioners, biomedical techniques of diagnosis sometimes became a crutch that was overused. From the perspective of skilled Tibetan doctors, a diagnosis made using only biomedical technologies was insufficient; letting biomedical technology be the ultimate source of diagnostic information was a sign of insufficient skill in using Tibetan techniques of diagnosis to their full potential. Experienced Tibetan doctors suggested that relying on biomedical tests alone would lead to incomplete diagnostic information and therefore insufficient knowledge of how to determine the best treatment.

This too was disputed. From the perspective of those doctors who relied more heavily on biomedical instrumentation for diagnosis, use of biotechnological instruments was important because it was, for them, the best way to affirm objective empirical information. The instruments simply made it possible to see and confirm the presence of diseases that were much more elusive to the touch of pulse, or the alterations in urine or mucous. For more traditional Tibetan doctors, however, this logic was flawed. Biomedical tests, for example, missed key distinctions between patients. These doctors stressed that different diseases or disorders might give rise to equal or very similar "numbers" using the biomedical instruments or assay tests, but Tibetan diagnoses would clearly identify them as different diseases that manifest in different ways that were "visible" in different pulsations, urine consistencies, tongue patterns, and subjective reporting of symptoms. Thus, while biomedical diagnostic techniques were frequently used in Mentsikhang, and some are mandatory, we also found some distrust of the results that were produced by these tests. In practice, most doctors went through the motions of collecting both types of diagnostic information, but in the end relied mostly on one type of information over the other (Tibetan over biomedicine or vice versa) in "naming" the disease.

As more pressure was put on Tibetan doctors to use biomedical instruments and medicine, we found that it was more often the Tibetan diagnostic approaches that were left behind in favor of use of biomedical instruments for making diagnoses. Sometimes, Tibetan diagnostic information was either not collected or not used because it was too difficult to conceptually translate the type of information from one system into that of the other. For example, Tibetan medicine places great emphasis on disorders involving the wind system *rlung*. *Rlung* is seen as responsible for all movement in the body: from breathing to corporal movement, to the flow of fluids such as blood and lymph into, out of and throughout the body. As well, *rlung* function is closely associated with emotional and perceptual phenomena such that changes in perception are believed to produce subtle changes in such things as the flow of blood, the beating of the heart, and the distribution of fluids. Eventually, alterations in a person's *rlung* can produce changes in the digestion of foods, the ability of the body to absorb and use the nutrients in foods, and the functioning of the organs. In diagnosis, Tibetan doctors are able to grasp that a wide variety of behavioral, social, and even religious circumstances may play a role in perceptual experiences of the patient, and in this way have a physiological effect on the body. Although we realize that Tibetan medicine treats the subject of open discussions of emotional disruption with patients with a great deal of caution (for fear of upsetting patients), we suspect that efforts to make sense of the complex layering of relationships between emotions and physiology was increasingly being left behind in doctors' efforts to maximize their patient load in a day, or to complete their paperwork and rounds in ways that accommodated biomedical and Tibetan framings of disease.

More problematic was the cleavage in understanding basic principles of physiology between Tibetan-trained and biomedically trained physicians. To the biomedical physicians we spoke with, the concept of *rlung*, along with many others related to the bile or phlegm systems, was considered religious or philosophical. It was a concept that did not correspond to any empirical physiological reality that they knew of or that could be measurable with biotechnologies now available. Broken into various physiological effects (blood pressure, heart rate, etc.) it could be translated. But as a coherent physiological system, it did not make scientific sense. This lack of correspondence of basic ideas about physiology and anatomy between the systems created potential for disagreements between physicians attempting an "integrated" method of diagnosis. To avoid these disagreements, in an environment in which Mentsikhang required use of these biotechnologies, Tibetan physicians often resorted to a shedding of information about Tibetan diagnosis. We found a willingness to minimize and eliminate those aspects of Tibetan medicine that seem to be outside the purview of biomedicine and to foreground and legitimize only those aspects of Tibetan medicine that could be shown to have biomedical equivalents in "visible" physical terms.

Mixed use of diagnostic techniques resulted from this underlying potential for contestation over whose diagnostic criteria were prioritized in determining treatment regimens. Resistive Tibetan doctors or those who were less well trained in biomedicine were sometimes tempted to disregard many of the tests used and required by the government administration for record keeping (e.g. white blood cell counts, hourly or daily blood pressure measure, liver function tests, etc.), presuming they were irrelevant to diagnosis even if the test information was produced. But different assumptions about the relevance or priority of different diagnostic tests occasionally resulted in perceptions of inadequate diagnostic information to make a correct diagnosis. For example, when a biomedical doctor was not involved in the initial diagnosis of a patient, she would sometimes find after the fact that information from ultrasound or blood tests was incomplete because the "relevance" of that sort of information was not apparent to the Tibetan doctor performing the initial diagnosis. There was no way to "backtrack" and obtain initial diagnostic measures once treatment regimens were started, once they had begun to have an effect.

The presence of two contrastive systems diagnosis thus created the potential for struggle alongside opportunities for growth in each system. The prevailing trend, however, even when the opportunities for "growth" were realized, was for Tibetan medicine to be viewed as if it were "behind" biomedicine and that it could "catch up" by making use of diagnostic tools and disease labels even when they did not integrate in any straightforward way with Tibetan conceptualizations of disease or approaches to diagnosis. In summary, the prevailing tendency was to adopt the biomedical label and tests even when they were not well understood or appropriately used by Tibetan doctors, such as when test information was not completely recorded, or when information relevant to a biomedical diagnosis was left out. Along with this, there was sometimes a tendency among younger doctors to shed Tibetan medical information because it did not fit well with biomedical conceptualizations, despite a certain resistance to this tendency among older physicians. This was more often the case when the mid-level and younger generation of Tibetan doctors did not themselves feel skilled enough in pulse, urine, and tongue analysis to make accurate Tibetan diagnoses, and when they could use biomedical instruments whose reliability tended to remain largely uncontested in the broader urban environment of patients and medical administrators. Coupled with an increase in public faith in biomedicines (from intravenous injections to diagnostic technologies), and a willingness to try to please patients that is built into Tibetan approaches to healing, the trend toward greater reliance on biomedicine was increasing. We found this to be the case even when Tibetan patients came to the Tibetan hospital specifically after being disappointed with their care in biomedical facilities.

Integration in treatment and the problems it presented

With the number of areas of contestation that were visible in attempts to integrate Tibetan and biomedical approaches in diagnosing patients, it is surprising that there were not more conflicts over decisions about appropriate treatment regimes. As with practices of biomedicine, Tibetan doctors often began a course of therapy on the basis of preliminary symptoms, bypassing the need to actually debate disease labels in any formal sense. In most departments, the range of disorders was minimal, with most patients presenting with the same disorders. With more complicated and unusual cases, closing in on a specific disease name often only occurred after a course of successful treatment.

However, in some wards, whether or not there was direct correspondence between Tibetan and Western diseases, it was common for practitioners to assign both biomedical and Tibetan treatments in the assumption that each treatment would target the specific kinds of symptoms perceived by each system's diagnostic repertoire. Thus, in the women's division patients who arrived with any accompanying symptoms of fever were almost always given intravenous antibiotic treatments (gentamycin, penicillin, and metronidazole were the most common) along with a full course of Tibetan medicines. This was also true for patients who came with some infection or inflammation in the digestive and liver divisions. An archival study in the liver division indicated that, for most hepatitis patients, their initial phase (three to seven days) of hospitalization nearly always consisted of intravenous use of penicillin.[7] When asked, all the doctors explained that they believed biomedical treatments were most effective at treating acute-stage emergency medical situations. Standard practice was thus to use IV antibiotics along with Tibetan medicines for the first stage of hospitalization to suppress the acute symptoms and then afterward to use Tibetan medicines to eradicate the "root" cause of disorders.[8] By "root cause" they generally meant the imbalanced state of the body – the fertile field – that enabled disorders to develop in the first place.

In keeping with this assumption, Tibetan physicians also described biomedical treatments as having a much more rapid effect – eradicating initial symptoms much faster – than Tibetan treatments. However, they also maintained that, with biomedical treatments alone, a patient's symptoms were likely to return equally rapidly because the root cause that enabled the disease to form in the first place had not been altered or improved by biomedicine alone. Thus, to many Tibetan doctors, biomedical treatments were only able to treat superficial symptoms, not underlying disease foundations. Evidence that this was the case was found, they maintained, in the fact that many of their patients came to the Tibetan medical hospital only after taking an unsuccessful course of biomedical therapies at one of the many biomedical facilities in Lhasa. In almost all of these cases, the patients claimed that they felt better initially after biomedical treatments, but as soon as they came home their symptoms returned. They came to the Tibetan hospital because they had been told by friends or relatives that Tibetan medicine would be able to eradicate their disease for good.

We also collected stories from doctors that patients explained that their symptoms were too elusive or "atypical" to enable doctors to provide them with a disease label in biomedicine. Prior to coming to the Mentsikhang, some of these patients received minimal treatment or very partial treatment because there was hardly any protocol to follow for such cases in biomedicine. One doctor from the digestive division commented that the reason biomedicine could not treat these patients was because it could not "go down to the root" of the problem, and surface symptoms were just too elusive for them to draw any conclusions that would guide them toward a specific course of therapy. Tibetan medicine had the ability to diagnose more subtly, therefore to "see" disorders that evaded the biomedical gaze. This was not true for all Tibetan physicians, some of whom were more eager to point out that, in most cases, failure to cure in biomedical facilities had as much to do with poor quality of medicines and poor biomedical skill as it did with a failure of biomedicine per se.

To biomedical doctors working within Mentsikhang, there was also a dissenting view: one biomedical doctor stated that Tibetan medicines were relatively weak in contrast to biomedicines, if not ineffective in many instances, even if the brand of biomedicines available in Tibet might be less potent than those available elsewhere, like Beijing, Hong Kong, or the United States. Thus, patient improvement in most cases could be attributed primarily to effective use of biomedicines. Recurrence of diseases, when this occurred, was attributed to the problem of patients being non-compliant (and failing to complete full courses of treatment) or to the fact that patients often re-infected themselves with or re-exposed themselves to pathogenic agents before completing their therapy. In the case we explore in more detail below, over interpretation of the success, or lack thereof, of Tibetan treatments for *Helicobacter pylori*, this was exactly what happened. It was argued that Tibetan medicines failed to eradicate the root cause of this disease in a way that only use of antibiotics could.

For biomedical doctors working within Mentsikhang, Tibetan medicine can look unsystematic and idiosyncratic. Some Tibetan diagnoses indicate need for different treatments in two different people who, in Western medicine, are seen as having the same disease. Moreover, it is common for Tibetan medicines to be altered as they go through various stages of recovery. From the Tibetan perspective, the biomedical approach of giving the same treatment to all patients with the same disorder was only justified when the patients all had exactly the same diagnosis, cause, and constitutions. Tibetan doctors maintained that, in most cases, patients with one similar disease had accompanying diseases or causes that made one patient's case very different from the other. For example, all "bile-related womb disorder" (*mngal nad mkhris gyur*) patients would get intravenous metronidazole and combinations of different Tibetan medicines because the biomedical doctor maintained that the infection would be best treated with this strong antibiotic. However, some Tibetan doctors in the ward maintained that, while it probably would not hurt these patients to have antibiotics, it did not necessarily help all of them. Some of these patients had the disease by way of overactive bile, while others became sick with this disease because of weakened wind, and so on. Even if the antibiotic helped to reduce the patients' fevers, it would do little to improve the long-term strength of the wind or decrease the bile. For these patients, a variety of different Tibetan medicines was needed depending on the other specific symptoms of the patients.

In some cases, the presence of different views of treatment approaches posed potential conflicts over treatment. As with the case of weak digestive function described above, when biomedical treatment of infection in the uterus called for antibiotics, Tibetan doctors would occasionally see this as counterproductive in a patient whose digestive function was weak from the body being "too cold." In these cases, the doctor's perception that the bile needed "heating" in order to properly digest medicines would lead to prescription of "heating" medicines, not medicines that would reduce the function of the bile. The increase of "bile" can in turn generate fever. In one system, the approach is to reduce fever but in the other it is to increase heat. In order to avoid open conflict about this, and in the absence of explicit efforts to coordinate such theoretical discussions into their practices, doctors in most departments simply offered both treatments simultaneously. But this effort required that the doctors did not try to communicate about potential counter-indications or try to reach consensus about the physiological processes and therapeutic needs in any detailed manner.

In fact, from the appearance of actual treatment practices, one would get the impression of a seamless integrated whole, a unified field of empirically valid engagements between patients and doctors of both traditions in the Mentsikhang. From a distance, Tibetan and biomedical practices appear to be deployed in great complementarity and with relatively high rates of effectiveness. In fact, Tibetan and biomedical doctors seldom openly disagreed about the utility of using both biomedical and Tibetan treatments together, and it is this sort of engagement that most represents, for many of them, the practice of "integrated medicine." However, the smooth appearance of a complementary set of practices began to break down the moment questions were asked about the attribution of effectiveness and the attribution of failure. Even though practitioners of each tradition attributed effectiveness to their own medicines, there was little open discussion of this sort in the wards of the Mentsikhang beyond those about the use of antibiotics for infections as a primary course of treatment before Tibetan medicines. In fact, most doctors, when asked, said that it is the "dual" action of the medicines that had the most potent effect, in the sense that they believed there was a "division of labor" of the medicines, again with biomedicine being useful for acute symptoms and Tibetan treating chronic imbalances. But, if patients themselves arrived with stories of the failure of biomedicine, or Tibetan medicine, then doctors were quick to substantiate these critiques that mirrored the stories of their patients, affirming their view that the two treatments together were better than single approaches alone.

Despite this view, we also found that the lack of confrontation over attribution of effectiveness led to a sense among some Tibetan doctors that medicines could be substituted for one another without causing damage to either tradition. We found a willingness on the part of Mentsikhang doctors, for example, to try new biomedical treatments for conditions that already have Tibetan remedies. In other words, Tibetan doctors did not use biomedical medicines only for those aspects of disorders for which they felt Tibetan medicine was ineffective or too slow to produce effects. They increasingly used biomedicines instead of Tibetan treatments even when they had Tibetan medicines that they previously relied upon solely for treating diseases. This was in part a response to the epistemological stance many of them had adopted – in which they recognized the equal utility of either medical treatment. It also stemmed from their perception of patient desires and a tendency within Tibetan medicine to prioritize patient desires over their own. Patients often requested biomedical intravenous drips for their disorders in the belief that these drips would serve as "magic bullets" with fast remedies for any ailment they might have. Doctors often offered these drips, whether or not they felt these patients' diseases required such treatments, because they felt that giving patients what they wanted would produce ameliorative effects even if it wasn't precisely what their disease warranted. This was also true when patients were not paying out of pocket for their treatments but were being remunerated by their work unit or other insurance programs.

The trend toward using more biomedicines was also in response to some Tibetan doctors' perception that many Tibetan medicines have lost their potency over the years, owing to a variety of factors (from environmental degradation to lack of proper tantric empowerments by skilled lama-physicians), and that some biomedical treatments were now generally more potent than Tibetan. In addition, the increasing financial strain that we mentioned before also prompted increasing use of bio-medicine, because they noted that patients cannot stay in the hospital as long as they used to (since privatization schemes have required them to engage in more cost recovery of their own). With patients spending less time in the hospital, doctors perceived that they must get them better more quickly than was historically possible with use of Tibetan treatments alone. Tibetan medicines simply take much longer to show an effect than biomedicines.

In the end, the easy deployment of both biomedical and Tibetan treatments for most patients has led to a gradual slippage in doctors' confidence in Tibetan medi-cines and increasingly greater use of biomedicine. Few patients receive only Tibetan medicine at Mentsikhang today. However, in the absence of sustained discussions about the evidentiary bases for making treatment decisions which are shared across medical traditions, the potential for overusing and misusing biomedicines was large, as was true for much of rural China, where doctors regularly over-prescribed antibiotics, and patients often failed to continue with a full course of treatments, following the standards more rigorously enforced in other countries like the United States. Biomedicines in general were not regulated within China, and patients were able to receive intravenous injections of many drugs from street vendors with little or no training in any medical tradition. Mentsikhang doctors also offered IV antibiotic treatments for short-term (outpatient) visits for even the most minor symptoms. The possibility of medicines producing counter-effects that were dangerous for patients was seldom broached in the wards of Mentsikhang, as little to no research on the active ingredients and physiological effects of these medicines was carried out and a great many Tibetan doctors had not received full training in appropriate use of antibiotics. This danger was posed not only by the way that biomedicines were used but also by the way that biomedicines were used in conjunction with Tibetan medicines with little or no research on possible counter-indications.

Finally, doctors involved in attempts to conduct research on clinical efficacy found that, without collaborative efforts to establish mutually agreed upon protocols for evaluating benefit or lack thereof (or counter-indications) of integrated treatments, there was little consensus about making the case for sustaining sole use of one type of treatment over another. Physicians followed idiosyncratic treatment protocols, based on simple observation of patient outcomes and treatment patterns learned by apprenticeship with more senior doctors. Although also true for biomedicine, it was not recognized as a strength of biomedical practice. Randomness and idiosyncrasy of practitioners were part of the reason American physicians were now calling for "evidence-based" medical training and practice. The tendency toward a "lineage-based" model of medical practice was more pronounced among Tibetan doctors than biomedical doctors.[9] For Tibetan doctors, the fact that each doctor treated a disease in a unique way – or, as one physician explained, "each doctor treats that disease in his or her own way" – was taken as a strength of Tibetan medicine, providing a level of specificity for patient and of practitioner that maximized the skill of practitioners and prioritized the needs of the individual patient. For biomedical doctors, however, this idiosyncratic pattern was taken as a weakness – a sign that Tibetan medicine was not scientific. When discussions about suitable research methods for evaluating the benefits of one treatment over another were broached, the models for research were being largely imported from biomedical models that discredited the idea and the practice of "lineage"-based idiosyncratic patterns of treatment.

In summary, Tibetan medicines were being used, often because physicians and patients had more confidence in Tibetan than biomedical treatments, but increasingly Mentsikhang patients were provided biomedicines in addition to, and even sometimes without, Tibetan medicines. The tendency to supply biomedicines to raise money for the hospital was cross-cut by the tendency to offer Tibetan medicines to less wealthy patients because they could not afford biomedicines. Coordinated efforts at integration of treatments were primarily focused on assumptions about the speed with which biomedicines worked, coupled with perceptions that Tibetan medicines would take longer but get to the "root" of the problem. While the emphasis among many Tibetan doctors was to establish a basis for legitimizing Tibetan medicines, the epistemological ground for legitimizing their sustained and continued sole use of Tibetan medicines within the hospital was being rapidly eroded. Few Tibetan doctors questioned whether or not the addition of biomedicine to treatment protocols for so many patients, and the commensurate decline in use of Tibetan medicines solely for treatment, would have a negative impact on Tibetan medicine. But, as Janes (1995) pointed out, we suspect that this pattern was gradually eroding Tibetan doctors' confidence in the potency of Tibetan medicines as "stand-alone" resources for producing effective cures.

Integration of outcomes

How are outcomes negotiated within Mentsikhang's integrated medical environment? Although there was little contestation over attributions of efficacy since such attributions were usually made on the basis of existing practices of integrated medicine, with credit applied to both medicines as opposed to controlled trials that would isolate the benefits of each treatment, when such discussions were opened the question of how to interpret outcomes posed serious difficulties. Despite the fact that patients were regularly discharged on the basis of consensual agreement about amelioration of symptoms, if not eradication of disease, the question of what evidence existed as affirmation of effective treatment was in a number of cases the subject of some debate. A few case examples illustrate this pattern.

In the study of Hp carried out within the digestive division, researchers found that outcomes were debated in terms of the relative weight doctors chose to place on each tradition and, again, on the "naming" of the symptoms as an identified disease. In this study, Hp-positive patients were identified by biomedical measures, C13 UBT test before and after treatment, and traditional Tibetan diagnostic methods, including pulse reading, tongue reading, urinalysis, and questioning.[10] Eight significant clinical Hp symptoms were chosen for evaluation: abdominal pain, abdominal distension, borborygmus, diarrhea, acid regurgitation, vomit, dyspepsia, and constipation. Hp-positive patients with significant symptoms were treated with traditional Tibetan medicines. Two separate areas in Lhasa prefecture were involved in this study, one before another in time. Treatment lengths in various medication groups did not exceed eight weeks in total. A five-month follow-up survey was also performed for twenty-one of the patients in the groups that received earlier treatment. The research found that, of the Tibetan medicines used, none was able to eradicate Hp bacteria infection. However, significant improvement of most debilitating symptoms was shown. Reported improvement for the eight categories of symptoms ranged from 83.3 percent to 100 percent in the first population and from 76.3 percent to 94.1 percent in the second population. Furthermore, eradication rates within the improvement category ranged from 50 percent to 100 percent for all symptoms except one in the second population. In the five-month follow-up group, there was no statistically significant Hp symptom recurrence. Other research suggests no spontaneous symptom relief for symptomatic patients with Hp infection. Moreover, patients reported uninterrupted and moderate to severe symptoms in these populations for a period of from five to twenty years prior to the study. A year later, preliminary re-study data collected in the study communities revealed similarly high rates of continuous symptom relief since the Tibetan treatments. However, the findings from this study also showed that Tibetan medicines were incapable of bacteria eradication in any of the study groups. The symptoms were eliminated, but the Hp was not.

Doctors involved in this study could have used this evidence to raise questions about *whose* outcomes were supposed to count, a question that ultimately leads, once again, back to problems of "naming" the disease being studied. Were the collections of symptoms named as the set of some six disorders in Tibetan medicine the "disease" being studied? If so, then Tibetan medicine cured them. Or was infection with Hp the disease, therefore ongoing infection evidence that Tibetan medicine ultimately did not work to cure these patients? This study raised a considerable amount of confusion within the research group, forcing the Western researchers to reconsider what constituted a "cure" in this instance. Tibetan doctors along with patients clearly saw the positive effect of symptom control using Tibetan medicines. But the Hp C13 UBT test continued to show, at least on the surface, that there was no improvement whatsoever in terms of the disease that biomedicine calls "Hp infection." So on the one hand "*powa ching cha mu bu*," along with several other "Tibetan diseases," was cured, but, when the disorder was called Hp, in the terms of biomedicine Tibetan medicines proved to be ineffective. Tibetan doctors could have asked questions about how we evaluate effective outcomes in terms that were mutually consistent within each tradition. But they didn't. Instead, they adopted a position of defeat in the research. The director of the digestive division stated that the research was a failure for Tibetan medicine because it showed that Tibetan medicine did not work.

Similarly, but with a different outcome, we found that doctors in the women's division sometimes contested evidence of outcomes for Tibetan treatments of growths in the reproductive tract. Biomedical doctors used evidence from ultrasound reports to note that, in one case, Tibetan medicine had failed to reduce the size of ovarian growths in a patient. For these doctors, the ultrasound image was sufficient evidence that Tibetan medicine had not worked. But Tibetan doctors told us that ultrasound evidence was not sufficient to determine whether or not the treatment was successful since, by Tibetan diagnostic procedures and patient reporting, the "disease" causing the growths had been cured. For the Tibetan doctors, the disorder had been cured at its humoral "root" and therefore the cause of the growths was removed. Pulse, tongue, urine, and patient reporting of a subsiding of all symptoms were the evidence of this. The residual evidence of growths in the ultrasound could be read as something akin to "scar tissue" that would eventually either go away or remain in that stabilized state and therefore not an indication of active disease. This is not to say that Tibetan doctors did not also use evidence of growth reduction made visible in ultrasound reports to show that Tibetan medicine did work. But, they insisted, lack of evidence of such reduction in ultrasound reports was not sufficient to state that it did not work. Just as in the case of "naming" the disease, the same empirical evidence can be read and interpreted in different ways in biomedical and Tibetan traditions. In this case, Tibetan doctors did not legitimate biomedical views, but rather maintained that there were other ways to read the evidence generated by biomedical technologies.

Thus, beyond the surface appearance of a seamless complementarity of integrated Tibetan and biomedical medical practices in Mentsikhang there was a sustained potential for small rifts in epistemology and empiricism. In order to function as an integrative team of doctors with different approaches to the meaning of empirical evidence, doctors had to avoid discussions that would lead to outright disagreement, especially in front of patients. However, the fact that there was potential for what appeared to be a "misreading" of the evidence in the eyes of each other's traditions, and the fact that this was not often openly discussed, was sometimes a basis for negative outcomes for patients. In some cases, patients who were being given one set of medicines based on the biomedical model were being given Tibetan medicines whose effectiveness Tibetan doctors believed was blocked by the powerful effect that the biomedicines produced. The overuse of biomedicines, or malprescription of them in the absence of qualified biomedical doctors in every ward where they were being used, was also a trend that led in some instances to negative outcomes for patients. Finally, the compromise of Tibetan medicine because certain information had to be excluded in the therapy management because of the overwhelming presence of biomedical evidence produced in things like ultrasound, X-rays or lab tests meant that Tibetan medicine was even mis-practiced by its own practitioners.

Even with these potential drawbacks, the prevailing perception was that more was to be gained from integrated medicine than lost. Cases, such as one we witnessed, helped affirm this perspective. In 1998, Tibetan doctors in the women's division diagnosed a patient with bile-related womb disorder on the basis of her symptoms of high fever and severe abdominal pain as well as pulse and urine analysis. The Tibetan doctors were later criticized by biomedical doctors brought in from another ward at Mentsikhang for having failed to identify that this patient was suffering from severe end-stage tuberculosis, but more importantly for not recognizing that they should have called the biomedical doctors to the case sooner.[11] Although the Tibetan doctors were treating the patient with medicines that had some effect on bringing down fevers, by the time they were confronted with the alternate biomedical diagnosis – late-stage tuberculosis – the patient was failing rapidly. She was quickly moved to Lhasa's main tuberculosis hospital, but died a few days later. Herein, the possibility of reading symptoms differently in each tradition was, ultimately, not a source of contestation, since the Tibetan doctors in this case quickly acknowledged that the biomedical diagnosis was more correct than theirs and that, in any case, Tibetan medicines were less useful for this disease than biomedicines. Discussions about appropriate integration here were not pre-existing; they emerged out of a crisis scenario. In part to avoid future crises like these, especially in labor and delivery services, the women's division hired a full-time biomedical physician. As a result, the women's division considers itself fully integrated today.

Conclusion

The director of the Mentsikhang in Lhasa knows very well that the future and survival of traditional Tibetan medicine in Tibet depends on his ability to advocate the benefits of Tibetan medicine while also incorporating, quickly and somewhat unsystematically, biomedical techniques, technologies, and knowledge. He recognizes that the legitimacy and integrity of Tibetan medicine depend in large part on being able to distinguish the unique contributions of Tibetan medicine prior to and in the absence of biomedical knowledge and practices. But, in reality, this delicate dance of integration requires efforts that first define differences but then erase them for the sake of practical medical clinical encounters and decision-making in the face of sometimes tremendous physical suffering.

In practice, the effort to integrate in Lhasa's Mentsikhang most often means adopting biomedical standards and authority and eliminating perceptions that Tibetan medicine is capable of advancing on its own, by its own rules or standards. This occurs when the hospital requires new kinds of record keeping that map physical bodies and pathological states using biomedical diagnostic tests, and ways of tracking patient outcomes that are standardized for biomedical hospitals. It also occurs when areas of contestation over knowledge and technique are ignored or effaced by an underlying awareness that things could be debated, but they are not, for the sake of maintaining an appearance of complementary integration. Finally, it occurs when Tibetan doctors who otherwise have great faith in Tibetan medicine are compelled to abandon their methods under the weight of evidence that suggests biomedicines work better, faster, or more cost-effectively than Tibetan medicines. Using the Tibetan medicines alone becomes, in this environment, a second-best option – effective but limited, inexpensive but time-consuming.

Sometimes, integration mutually enhances each tradition, as when efforts are made to define ways that biomedical knowledge can further Tibetan understandings of disease, or when Tibetan conceptualizations of disease classification and approaches to treatment are incorporated into biomedical treatment programs. However, the overall trend that we witnessed in Lhasa's Mentsikhang was more toward substitution of Tibetan with biomedical options in a process of *bio-medicalization*.[12]

Tibetans in the TAR in general are riding a new wave of modernization in which Westernized culture emerges by way of Beijing and Hong Kong as attractions of modernity. These attractions are not just for new knowledge and technologies but for new ways of organizing and transferring knowledge, of thinking about bodies, and pathogenesis, and about how to be modern in medicine. As in other parts of the developing world, this process often breeds an inner sense of inferiority about indigenous forms of knowledge, and this is certainly true within Tibetan medicine despite government efforts to also advertise and support this indigenous medical system. The government's idea is to put medicine on the "right track" and this symbolically gets deployed through demands that require standardization of all medical institutions in China, the majority of which are biomedical institutions. These are both bureaucratic and cultural demands in the sense that they create the possibility for official tracking and scientific research, but also in their ability to map the future in ways that are already defined by the cultural systems that come with these biomedical institutions. When the head of the women's ward was asked why so few of her patients received only Tibetan medicine during their stay in the women's division, she told me "This is integrated medicine" but then added in the same breath: "We must run to catch up with Western medicine." When I offered the suggestion that sometimes it seems as though Tibetan doctors should just run in the opposite direction, she told me: "That is impossible, because Western medicine is now everywhere in the whole world." Ironically, efforts on the part of the government, the Health Bureau, and the administration in Mentsikhang to "globalize" Tibetan medicine also force Tibetan medicine into packages (both epistemological and practical) that are already designed by biomedicine.

Integration in the United States is considered a relatively new phenomenon. Popular use of alternative therapies is enormous, but actual integration within established biomedical institutions is still fairly rare and, therein, use of non-Western medical alternatives is even more uncommon (with the exception of acupuncture). Where it is found, the pattern of integration is generally that bits and pieces of the alternative modalities are broken off from the "mother ship" and incorporated into a biomedical therapeutic regime. It is virtually impossible to find "integrated" medicine that enables an even exchange of two medical knowledge systems and approaches, something that might be labeled a "balanced integrated medicine." The biomedical viewpoint has the uncanny ability to absorb and transform non-Western medical ideas in ways that often undermine the integrity of the non-Western system.

In the Tibetan Autonomous Region, the potential for the opposite is made possible. Within Tibetan medical institutions such as Mentsikhang, it is bits and pieces of biomedicine that are added onto Tibetan medical practice. But even here it is not clear that such integration results consistently in a kind of absorption in which Tibetan medicine transforms and incorporates biomedical practices and "makes them into their own." In fact, the opposite often occurs. Sometimes, Tibetan medical practices become displaced by biomedical resources and, even with bits and pieces of biomedicine being brought into Mentsikhang, they have a gradual effect that is slowly transforming Tibetan medicine in ways that, we fear, may undermine the theoretical basis for its approach to health, the body, and healing. We would call this a precariously balanced integration, at best. The more training in biomedicine the younger generations of Tibetan doctors get, the greater tendency they have to rely on biomedical routes to diagnosis and treatment and evaluation of patients' outcomes and the less they rely on strategies to perfect their skill with traditional Tibetan medicine. The best practitioners of Tibetan medicine within Mentsikhang know that Tibetan medicine has a great deal to offer patients, on its own or integrated with biomedicine, but the ability for these doctors to take leadership roles in the processes of modernizing Tibetan medicine by way of integration is limited. Hopefully, this trend will be reversed as a younger generation of committed Tibetan medical scholars comes of age in the Tibetan Autonomous Region.

Notes

* The authors would like to acknowledge the support of Princeton University, the National Science Foundation, and the Lhasa Mentsikhang for partial support and research collaboration that enabled the collection of data upon which this paper is based.

1   Debatable, because in many cultures (including Tibetan) it is believed that oral instruction provides a more reliable means of transmitting knowledge incorruptibly than written forms.

2   Use of the phrases "Western medicine" and "biomedicine" is problematic in two ways. First, although both refer to the medical system that dominates in Western industrialized countries, there are other forms of medicine (alternative medicines) that play an increasingly important role in these locations. Second, the phrases are problematic because the forms that "Western medicine" or "biomedicine" takes in China in general, but particularly in remote regions like Tibet, frequently make it unrecognizable as Western or biomedicine in contrast with its practices in Western countries.

3   For example, in one account a famous female Tibetan doctor skilled in techniques of eye surgery learned about biomedical surgical techniques in India but was advised not to attempt such surgeries in Tibet because of the risks posed by septic conditions.

4   For a more complete history of the institutional development, support, and suppression of Lhasa's Mentsikhang, see Janes (1995), and for complementary ethnographic descriptions of the processes of integration with biomedicine, see Janes (1999, 2001, 2002).

5   Although there was one sort of growth, unidentified in the biomedical system, caused by the problem of women having sex at too young an age and too frequently, before they were mature.

6   Another example is the use of the biomedical phrase "sexually transmitted disease" as a label for disorders that are thought to neatly map *Trichomonas* onto the Tibetan name *marutse* and candida onto the Tibetan name *asolika* (two disorders found in the *Rgyud bzhi*). These disorders were considered to be caused by external bugs, *srin-bu*, but associated with hygiene and water contamination, not necessarily sexual relations.

7   Survey conducted by Fei-Fei Li in 2000.

8   An exception to this was when women's division patients were put on medicines to improve digestion before taking strong antibiotic treatments.

9   Farquhar (1994) describes the epistemological foundations for this sort of pedagogically based medicine for Zhongyi.

10 This study gathered data on the curative benefits of traditional Tibetan medicines for treatment of symptomatic patients with Hp-positive infection. Our research questions were two-fold: 1) Can Tibetan medicine eradicate Hp infection; and 2) What is its effectiveness in relieving symptoms putatively related to Hp infection? The research was conducted on two populations (n = 86) in rural Lhasa prefecture, Tibetan Autonomous Region, P.R. China. The two study populations showed infection rates of 82 percent and 93 percent respectively among those reporting known gastric symptoms prior to medication.

11 At that time, there were no biomedical physicians assigned directly to the women's division.

12 Janes (1995) provides more detail on this from an institutional historical perspective, noting that one Tibetan doctor feared that Tibetan medicine would become "a shallow form of herbalism" (like traditional Chinese medicine), also following Margaret Lock's analysis for East Asian medicine in Japan (1990).

References

Adams, V. (2001). The Sacred in the Scientific: Ambiguous Practices of Science in Tibetan Medicine, *Cultural Anthropology* 16(4): 542–575.

Adams, V. (2002). Establishing Proof: Translating "Science" and the State in Tibetan Medicine. In Mark Nichter and Margaret Lock (eds.), *New Horizons in Medical Anthropology*, New York: Routledge, pp. 200–220.

Adams, V. and Dovchin, D. (2000). Women's Health in Tibetan Medicine and Tibet's "First" Female Doctor. In Ellison Banks Findly, *Women's Buddhism/Buddhism's Women*, Cambridge, MA: Wisdom Publications.

Berg, M. and Mol, A. (eds.) (1998). *Differences in Medicine: Unraveling Practices, Techniques and Bodies*, Durham, NC: Duke University Press.

Dummer, T. (1988 [1994]). *Tibetan Medicine and Other Holistic Health-Care Systems*, New Brunswick, NJ: Routledge (New Delhi: Paljor Publications).

Farquhar, J. (1994). *Knowing Practice*, Durham, NC: Duke University Press.

Harding, S. (1998). *Is Science Multicultural? Postcolonialisms, Feminisms, and Epistemologies*, Bloomington: Indiana University Press.

Janes, C. (1995). The Transformations of Tibetan Medicine, *Medical Anthropology Quarterly* 9(1): 6–39.

Janes, C. (1999). The Health Transition and the Crisis of Traditional Medicine: The Case of Tibet, *Social Science and Medicine* 48: 1803–1820.

Janes, C. (2001). Tibetan Medicine at the Crossroads: Radical Modernity and the Social Organization of Traditional Medicine in Tibet Autonomous Region, China. In Linda H. Connor and Geoffrey Samuel (eds.), *Healing Powers and Modernity: Traditional Medicines, Shamanism, and Science in Asian Societies*, Westport, CT: Bergin & Garvey.

Janes, C. (2002). Buddhism, Science, and Market: The Globalisation of Tibetan Medicine, *Anthropology and Medicine* 9(3): 267–289.

Li, Z. (1994). *The Private Life of Chairman Mao*, New York: Random House.

Lock, M. (1990). Rationalization of Japanese Herbal Medication: The Hegemony of Orchestrated Pluralism, *Human Organization* 49: 41–47.

McKay, A. (1997). *Tibet and the British Raj: The Frontier Cadre 1902–1947*, London: Curzon Press/London Studies on South Asia (SOAS).

Marglin, S. and Appfel, F. (1990). Smallpox in Two Systems of Knowledge. In Frederique Appfel and Stephen Marglin (eds.), *Dominating Knowledge: Development Culture and Resistance*, Oxford: Oxford University Press.

Meyer, F. (1981 [1988, 2002]). *Gso-Ba Rig-Pa, Le Système Médical Tibétain*, Paris: Editions du CNRS.

Meyer, F. (1992). Introduction. In Y. Parfionovitch, G. Dorje, and F. Meyer (eds.), *Tibetan Medical Paintings: Illustrations to the Blue Beryl Treatise of Sangye Gyamtso (1653–1705)*, London: Serindia (reprinted by Harry N. Abrams, New York, 1992).

Rechung, R. (1973). *Tibetan Medicine*, Berkeley: University of California Press.

Trinlay, P. (1998). *Bod Lugs Gso Rig Gyi Rgyun Mthong Mo Nad 'Gog Bchos Bya Thabs* [Health Measures for Commonly Seen Sicknesses of Women], Lhasa: People's Publishing House.

6 Hijacking intellectual property rights

Identities and social power in the
Indian Himalayas

Laurent Pordié

The exploitation conducted by Western pharmaceutical groups of certain
indigenous medicinal plants sparked off a strong reaction in India regarding
intellectual property rights and biological heritage. The affair of the neem tree,
Azadarichta indica, was one of the main factors in this reaction and became the
subject of serious controversy (Kocken and van Roozendaal 1997). This pesticidal
tree, from which an American pharmaceutical company, W. R. Grace, patented
the extraction process of an active substance in 1992, has changed the relation India
has to its biological resources, or at least the means established to promote their
protection. The neem tree is today a symbol of the fight against 'bio-pirates'. These
are persons sponsored by foreign industrial groups who study (one speaks of bio-
prospecting), patent and illegally exploit, or hijack, natural substances of particular
interest for the activities of the industry concerned (mainly medicine, cosmetology
and agro-industry). India responds to the issues underlying the industrial
exploitation of biological resources by positioning itself in the economic, political
and legislative arenas of the international scene. To this end, India frames its policy
and attempts to implement international laws and agreements bearing on the use,
protection and preservation of phytogenetic resources and the related knowledge
(Challa and Kalla 1995; Dutfield 1999; Subramanian 1999). Indigenous assets
and knowledge, according to Amita Baviskar, are 'a common courtesy in conservation policy in India today' (2000: 101). The establishment of environmental
and legal policies generates conflicts of interest between politicians and communities, and is highly questioned by specialists (Busch 1995; Dhar and Chaturvedi
1998; Kothari 1999).

This national movement has repercussions throughout the land, including the
regions where the so-called scheduled tribes[1] are found. This is the case in Ladakh,
a semi-autonomous district in the State of Jammu and Kashmir. However, although
the local protagonists agree to follow this national policy, they also redefine its
meaning and purposes. This chapter analyses the local reinterpretations and the
social uses of intellectual property by the Ladakhi *amchi* elite.[2] This research departs
thereby from the classic framework of studies on intellectual property, which
constitute an abundant literature but which are usually concerned with the juridical
and legal dimensions, ethical and economic issues, globalization and development,
with inequality between countries or between cultures and with the formidable

aporias which autochthonous populations come up against in their defence of traditional knowledge (see Aubert 2002; Brush 1999; Coombe 1998; Dutfield 2000; Juma 1999; Lanjouw 1997; Swanson 1995).

The ethnography of diverse structures of *amchi* medicine makes it possible to understand according to which modalities and which issues the simple idea of a possible pharmaceutical investigation crystallizes the discourse on intellectual property and the potential loss of a biological heritage. Intellectual property rights (IPRs) bear strong symbolism, which is used by the practitioners to strengthen or affirm their social status, both within and outside their community. In the particular ethnic and political context of this region, IPRs also appear as a theme of major importance in the assertion of ethnic and medical identities. These social phenomena are to be understood in a climate in which biomedicine largely dominates the therapeutic field (Kuhn 1994) and in which, along with wider socio-economic changes, it has greatly affected the social and medical conditions of the *amchi* (Pordié 2002).

This situation is certainly complementary to the concern which the *amchi* express towards the ecological challenges pertaining to IPRs, and their social repercussions should not always be presented as completely intentional. Nevertheless, the *amchi* make use of a variety of strategies, which refer to subjects (including institutional subjects) who claim a place of their own, a base from which relations with an exterior target or threat can be managed (de Certeau 1980). These strategies are at the same time echoing the ecological scenario of IPRs and a conscious local social practice. This chapter therefore examines and unravels the logics at play in the social expression of intellectual property rights. Although the IPRs' context is dictated by international agendas and is embedded in the national policies and politics of the Indian state, viewing IPRs from the local perspective entails a shift of the analytic lens from these macro-concerns to the immediate relations of the *amchi* elite, located primarily in the medical world. This chapter does not disregard the broader context, but circumscribes its expression to the fundamental elements perceived and experienced daily by the *amchi*: the issues occurring within their own community, the challenges to their medical system in the national society and their collective social relations with other institutions and medical practitioners, especially the exiled Tibetans. In short, the study of the social use of IPRs makes it possible to respond to two fundamental questions: How does the medicine of the *amchi* locally appropriate new issues? How does it integrate external rhetoric so as to generate its own social dynamics?

This research was mainly conducted between 1998 and 2002, although more recent data are also included. It focused primarily on the core group of the urban *amchi* elite from Leh, the regional capital, in particular the leading individuals of two influential institutions. These are a minority who hold some form of power or influence, expressed or symbolized within the *amchi* community and beyond. They are today the driving forces who elaborate the institutional narratives of Tibetan medicine in Ladakh and who represent the Ladakhi *amchi* in the regional political scene and at the national level. Despite the relative heterogeneity of this group and a certain lack of coordinating efforts, they are the main agents in the social redefinition of urban Tibetan medicine, mainly through decision-making, exemplarity and the diffusion of representations and ideologies. The ethnography conducted in such a locale is indicative of the contemporary trend of the medical system in institutional settings, notwithstanding the existence of micro-resistance and the fact that it is today limited to a specific group.

The course of intellectual property rights in Ladakh

The official demand for the protection of intellectual property rights pertaining to traditional medical knowledge and resources dates back to 10 September 1994. Sh. P. Namgyal, former Union Minister of State, and Dr S. T. Phuntsog, Project Officer at the Amchi Medicine Research Unit (Government of India),[3] Leh, wrote and issued a petition then addressing the matter. The signatories were two persons having notable influence in Ladakh and who continue today to occupy roles in the political scene and beyond, i.e. an active role in the Ladakhi demand for Union Territory status, for the former, and functions at the highest level of institutional biomedicine, for the latter. S. T. Phuntsog is said to be the first trained Ladakhi biomedical doctor. He is also partly educated as an *amchi* and belongs to an *amchi* family lineage (*brgyud-pa, syn. rgyud-pa*). Although he does not practise as an *amchi*, he is very much involved in this medical system and is well integrated into the corresponding community. He is both an eminent representative of the biomedical profession[4] and a leading figure of the *amchi* community. The *amchi* elite regularly seek his advice and tend to follow it. This petition therefore received an overwhelming welcome and was further encouraged. It officially expressed the *amchi*'s situation in a new framework and contextualized their knowledge and practice within society as a whole. This medical system was said to need protection and support for both public health matters and cultural survival, while it was presented as threatened by biomedicine and Western society. The petition has been the main element in shaping contemporary discourse on IPRs and related issues, as shown in the following quote:

> The indigenous Amchi system of medicine needs to be promoted and protected in the interest of both the health needs of the population and in retaining a vital part of Ladakhi cultural tradition . . . The sources, the products, the processes and the skills of the Amchi community in preparing the various formulations. . . are a separate and distinct body of knowledge inherited from their ancestors and modified and refined over the centuries to form an effective medical system . . . While there is no secret in the practice of Amchi medicine, there is certainly a group of collective ownership of the entire indigenous system of medicine. . . which, in modern terminology, can be termed as 'intellectual property'. In the international scenario of public health and the treatment of disease, the allopathic system of medicine[5] with its scientific and technological base, has captured the world market . . . These multi-national [pharmaceutical] companies conduct or sponsor commerce-oriented scientific

research . . . Their attention is increasingly turning to various indigenous systems of medicine all over the world.

(Namgyal and Phuntsog 1994)

The petition was addressed to several central Indian authorities[6] on behalf of the Ladakh Amchi Sabha (LAS). This is the oldest, most influential association of Ladakhi *amchi* and was (self-)designated as the community's representative body for IPRs. The petition states that 'the intellectual property of the indigenous Amchi system belongs collectively to the Amchi Sabha and may be termed as a "Collective Intellectual Property" over which the Amchi Sabha possesses the complete, total and absolute rights' (ibid.). Since that time, the LAS has been responsible for securing 'Collective Intellectual Property', but not much has happened to date.

Earlier, in the first week of September 1994, some *amchi* and prominent Ladakhi citizens met at the office of the Ladakh Ecological and Development Group (LEDeG) to discuss IPRs issues. The HIMEX ECO-ENV team, sanctioned as such by the Indian Ministry of Defence, facilitated the meeting. The HIMEX project comprised 'eco-environmental' studies on the *amchi* system of medicine, which included IPRs. According to a participant, Tashi Norbu,[7] the meeting aimed to 'persuade the *amchi* to refrain from playing into the hands of interested commercial organizations which might approach them under the garb of research and development'. On 9 September 1994, the day before the petition was issued, the matter of IPRs was broadcast on All-India Radio, Leh, in the form of a discussion between the two authors of the petition. Another official meeting took place in late 1994 at the head office of the Ladakh Amchi Sabha, and 'propounded and strengthened the same views' (Tashi Norbu). Later on, in 1995, Major-General S. G. Vombatkere, from the Directorate of Discipline and Vigilance, Army Head-quarters, also team leader of the HIMEX project, released his final report, which showed that British nationals were collecting plants and herbs in Ladakh under the directive of a consortium of organizations. This was the first time the *amchi*'s medical heritage was officially proven to be threatened, and clear details were given about the foreign bio-prospectors.[8] It was then strongly recommended that the local representatives take action. This initiative was followed by a great deal of informal and official internal correspondence,[9] eventually leading to the expulsion of a number of foreigners involved in plant collection, but it did not lead to any process of policy-making (Pordié 2005). In the spring of the same year, the matter was made public through an article published by the co-authors of the petition in the local journal *Ladags Melong* (cf. Namgyal and Phuntsog 1995). In the summer of 1995, Dr P. K. Hajra, Director of the Botanical Survey of India, informed the *amchi* that they should avoid giving information or specimens of plants to foreigners. At that time, the television company Doordarshan prepared a documentary on the *amchi* which was supposed to cover collective intellectual property rights. The *amchi* had hoped that this would further the case of IPRs in Ladakh and increase awareness among the population. However, the documentary only contained very basic information on the *amchi*'s practice and, according to an *amchi* interviewed by the Doordarshan crew, 'it did not touch on the issues of IPRs'.

Following this period of intense activity, the practical concern fell from favour and IPRs remained for several years no more than a regular topic in the local discourse about pharmacopoeia and medicine, and occasionally appeared in the minutes of meetings, mentioning the need for their protection but not specifying any progress (see for example 'News Bulletin', 22 September 1998). Nearly four years passed and there were no further activities until, in 1999, the France-based organization Nomad RSI (Recherche et Solidarité Internationale) launched an IPRs project which was included in a broader research and development programme on *amchi* medicine. Its intention was to help in setting up some pre-legal activities on the subject, but the results have been very limited. The organization appointed an international lawyer from Mexico[10] who, depending on local goodwill and authorization, could not interact with his Ladakhi colleagues. This drastically limited his work to the reactivation of the previous contacts established by the *amchi* representatives in 1995. His main *amchi* counterpart alleged repeatedly for three months that the local law enforcement officials were on holiday. This had to be construed as an effort to prevent him from meeting the people concerned. The reasons invoked were then legitimated by the *amchi* and understood by the lawyer, owing to the great sensitivity of the issue of IPRs, thus concealing their social aspect. In 2001, a young French political scientist helped the local Nomad RSI team to design an information campaign on IPRs. This work resulted in the publication of a special issue of the journal *Gangs Jongs Sorig Dron Mai* (*gangs jongs gso rig sgron me*)[11] in January 2002, in close collaboration with several *amchi* representatives, who received informal training on IPRs, and media broadcasting of the subject. One of the focal points of Nomad RSI was to strengthen the organization of the representative body for IPRs at the Ladakh Amchi Sabha, but internecine conflicts among leading *amchi*, IPRs legal limitations and the social challenges they represent undermined the initiative (cf. Pordié 2005).

Yet IPRs are still at the centre of the discourse pertaining to *amchi*'s pharmacopoeia. What use, then, is made of IPRs in Ladakh if their practical implementation remains scanty? In other words, what are the challenges and motives that give IPRs a social existence?

IPRs as a platform for social power

Bio-prospecting and IPRs telescope individual and collective fields. Concerned with juridical matters, rooted in modern natural sciences and biomedicines, and largely based on the international capitalist economy, they shed light on social transformation and, in particular, on social power at the micro-level. In spite of the relevance of many of the contemporary works on IPRs, most of them present more or less explicitly the indigenous community, or a concerned minority thereof, as a homogeneous body facing external interests (e.g. Timmermans 2003). They thus overlook intra-community variations, their heterogeneity and the multiple possible uses of IPRs. Yet the social uses and modulations of IPRs in the two ethnographical cases I will present as examples show a fundamental bipartition opposing the community to the individual within the group. This opposition further questions individual social legitimacy, and highlights assumptions about bio-prospecting and the West, as if today the pirates were roaming the high mountains. Intellectual property rights are retranscribed as a reason for power; their plasticity permits the assertion of power for the benefit or the disadvantage of a single person, while systematically encapsulating the presumed community interests.

Individual negotiations for individual power

Intellectual property rights appertain to three main registers of power. These are social powers, moral influences and political authorities (Léonard 1981). IPRs involve a number of protagonists, including an *amchi*, N.T., who occupies a governmental position that gives him a certain degree of responsibility within Ladakh. This *amchi* is today perceived by his counterparts as the most virulent defender of intellectual property rights. This virulence surpasses the mere level of discourse and is expressed at various times in his radical decision-making. On two occasions, he was involved in the departure of foreigners from Ladakh. The two British bio-prospectors mentioned earlier left the region in this way in 1995. However, they had worked in collaboration with N.T. before the latter, newly appointed to his post, decided to forgo their services. He was simply respecting the policies of his patron institution, which is under the jurisdiction of the central government. The *amchi* was thus exhorted to scrupulously adhere to national, or indeed nationalist, protective policies. He therefore avoided collaboration with foreigners. He did, however, comment benevolently on this subject:

> They stopped the project because they could not convince the *amchi*. It was also a social project so they did not want to continue it without the *amchi* approval. To be frank, I feel sorry for them; there was lots of politics around.

In 1999, a Dutch charitable organization, the Plant Foundation, devoted to the conservation of medicinal plants, underwent the same fate. This organization was directed by a retired woman who had converted to Buddhism and followed the recommendations of her Tibetan master, who advised her to take in hand the conservation of certain medicinal plants in Ladakh. Not having any practical experience in this domain, she erred only on the side of incompetence. She achieved no tangible results despite three years spent in Ladakh, notably in the Sengi-La area. N.T. nevertheless suspected her of harming the indigenous medical system by undertaking to 'steal' its resources for the profit of an imaginary pharmaceutical group. One of the *amchi* belonging to the institutional elite told me in 1998: 'If she takes notes all the time when I speak with her, it is because she knows nothing. In this case, how can she help us? She is suspect.' This *amchi* was not directly involved in her expulsion, but he does express this fearful tendency in Ladakh, at times brought into people's minds by IPRs' narratives.

These two episodes were also embedded in personal relationships and brought to light the importance of common courtesy in Ladakh. In both cases, basic social values were seen to be lacking.[12] The departure of foreigners occurred rapidly in all cases, not as a result of legal procedures, but through the mere diffusion of rumours by the security agencies. The foreigners were unable to resist the social pressure surrounding IPRs. They were harassed, either on the pretext of a refusal on the part of the *amchi* to cooperate or by verbal threats alluding to difficulties with the law. These foreigners working on tourist visas found themselves in a sufficiently worrying situation to decide to immediately take the first plane out. I myself was seriously intimidated at the start of my work in Ladakh by N.T., before he accepted me as a collaborator, but always subject to negotiation. Without going into further detail, we see that the power with which N.T. found himself vested stems from a new order: the defence of intellectual property and the preservation of flora. My interlocutor therefore understood the social issues correlated to the virulence of his discourse on intellectual property long before understanding the complexity of the legal meaning.

Furthermore, this *amchi* became a leader in this domain in Ladakh, as he is in charge not only of an institution which is supposed to be active in the defence of IPRs, but was also related to a former regional leader of the Bharatiya Janata Party (BJP).[13] He then himself joined this party. What is important here is the conjunction of factors favourable to the social positioning of N.T., combining his political orientations, the mandate of his institution, which is directly dependent on national policies, and his perspicacity in making the defence of intellectual property rights an important priority.

I have chosen to present this case to support my argument because of N.T.'s major role in the domain, but there are other individuals, notably some of those brought together in associations, who have taken up the same type of logic. Today, an *amchi*'s commitment to the new subject of intellectual property pertaining to medicinal plants ensures or confirms his status in the community of practitioners, as he finds himself vested with the influence and functions of a representative of the defence of his counterparts' rights.[14] It is also this very social power which potentially lends him the means to achieve the implementation of this defence. In short, the social uses of pharmaceutical research by certain practitioners of the *amchi* elite confer on them a power which nurtures itself as it is applied. Further, this power never rests only on constraint or habit. As Didier Fassin states, 'to be completely efficacious, it has need of a broad base of recognition on the part of those who are subject to it, and it is to this that the person or persons who exercise that power devote themselves' (1996: 171): to obtain the recognition of their power and to use this power to acquire greater recognition.

IPRs are to be considered as a platform on which power is both exhibited and gained. They help to build a social legitimacy and to consolidate it by the regular reactivation of a number of elements, which can possibly be seen as rituals (cf. Abélès 1997), such as attending and taking a firm position in official meetings, organizing IPRs-related activities, drafting letters and correspondence, and threatening foreigners. Furthermore, such individual social practices are idio-syncratic and deeply embedded in the institutional environment.[15] These two parameters denote the possibility of a stringent discourse on IPRs emerging and are indispensable for its transformation into actual social power.

Representing conflicts: IPRs as a collective motto

The discourse on intellectual property rights can be geographically represented by a circle with the capital of Ladakh at its centre.[16] The nearer one comes to the periphery, namely the villages, the more moderate the discourse becomes, to then entirely disappear in the most remote areas. This schematic description tallies with the distribution of social power in the *amchi* community which, apart from a few exceptions, is concentrated in the urban zones and is consubstantial with the institutionalization of Tibetan medicine in Ladakh. The *amchi* who hold institutional positions may stir up their ardour and improve their knowledge through regular contact with representatives from Delhi, and the local and international NGOs. The narratives on intellectual property are today a systematic warning to foreigners interested in plants in Ladakh. Those aspiring to defend IPRs see in each visitor a potential danger, and exhort their community to 'be very careful [because] sometimes [the foreigners] say they just like plants, but they can be working for multinational companies. If they could patent the plants, they would take our knowledge without even saying thanks', says one *amchi*. However, this position, generally considered as legitimate by the *amchi*, is at times directed to stigmatizing individuals in their own community, for a variety of reasons that have little to do with the preservation of biological heritage. Intellectual property rights thus serve as a motive for contouring collective issues of a social nature. They have brought a new set of problems while defining and developing old tensions.

This applies to the case of S.D., an *amchi* from the Indus valley who belongs to the Ladakhi elite. This *amchi* was very active for about a decade in the development of his medical system in Ladakh until the mid-1990s, and since then has managed his own association. S.D. also has various Ladakhi and, in particular, non-Ladakhi (international) relations that reinforce his social status. He is in open conflict, however, with many institutional *amchi* based in Leh regarding quarrels dating back several years which concern the allocation of funds by donators, *chindak* (*sbyin bdag*). His categorical refusal to be more closely integrated in the central group of *amchi*, around and within Ladakh Amchi Sabha, marginalizes him.

For the past few years he has spent the winter in Europe and, according to local rumours, runs a clinic there from which he earns a substantial amount of money for each consultation. Whether or not this is true, this *amchi* has aroused the jealousy of certain of his counterparts. He sometimes welcomes groups of foreigners to Ladakh, to whom he sells theme excursions on medicinal plants and 'Tibetan medicine'.[17] He leads his guests on medicinal plant tours in the mountains, showing them various plants and explaining the fundamental principles of his medicine. This is not an evil in itself, since he manages to put into practice what many other *amchi* would have wanted to do, and his income is said in part to benefit his programmes. His attitude nevertheless gives rise to comments and fosters tensions. On 28 July 1999, a general circular was issued by the secretary of the LAS in which this *amchi* was implicitly called to order:

> It [has come to be known] that foreigners are dealing with and collecting plants from various mountains of this region, which is strictly objectionable, as most

of the rare and important plants are already almost [extinct] and endangered
. . . Those *amchi* who are involved in such activities may please inform this
association well in advance. Otherwise the matter will be brought to the notice
of the District Magistrate and Forest Dept. All are hereby [asked] that any
foreigners. . . collecting or identifying medicinal plants may be brought to the
notice of this association [LAS] for necessary action.[18]

There are other *amchi* who occasionally agree to accompany tourists on a hike,
or even to discuss in detail with them their *materia medica*. However, the official
nature of S.D.'s excursions and his differences with some influential members of
the *amchi* elite have played a crucial role in furthering his marginality. An *amchi*
having institutional responsibilities said to me in August 1999: '[S.D.] does. . .. We
don't really know what [S.D.] is doing. He stays in his village. He is hiding himself.
We are quite suspicious.' This suspicion concerns the association of foreigners with
medicinal plants, but it is used to signify other problems.

In such cases, the central elite community mobilizes IPRs to support an accu-
sation against single individuals, based solely on assumptions, and to foster their
stigmatization. The situation is thus reversed: IPRs become an instrument to target
a fellow *amchi* and not to be directly used for individual purposes, as the previous
section has shown. Whether used individually or collectively, IPRs are always
accompanied by a *movement of power*, for better or for worse, and discursively
invoke community interests. Their social manipulations tend to provoke or
accentuate the demarcation of individuals from the group in a manner very rarely
seen otherwise. However, this type of social negotiation does not preclude the fact
that the *amchi* are worried about the possible exploitation of their plant resources
or that they see bio-prospecting as a threat to their system. They pragmatically use
IPRs in a variety of situations to mediate, conceal or delimit social issues pertaining
to both medicine and its actors.

IPRs encapsulate contemporary international challenges of traditional medicines
and issues of indigenous knowledge; to the concerned elite *amchi* they represent
a crucial and very new aspect of Tibetan medicine in Ladakh.[19] IPRs are thus
exceptional in the medical field, straddling various sectors such as biology, ecology,
medicine and politics. This characteristic overlapping of different sectors permits
a series of hijackings, such as the juxtaposition of the IPRs agenda with *amchi*
medical and ethnic identities.

Intellectual property and identities

Both IPRs and *amchi* identities oscillate between medicine and society. Their social
convergence sheds light on ethnicity, the environment and the relations between
various branches of medicine. Intellectual property and the production of *amchi*
identities are framed by *medical objects* (āyurveda and biomedicine) or *social
objects* (local politics, development of the medical system and encounters with non-
Ladakhis). Conceptually, the social dynamics of IPRs allow a decoding of various
shapes and shades that identity can take and which are revealed by the way the

amchi position themselves in relation to the Western, Indian (non-Ladakhi), Tibetan and Ladakhi spheres. This will highlight *centripetal* and *centrifugal* processes pertaining, respectively, to the dynamics orientated towards the community itself and to those directed towards elements external to the community. To elucidate this point, medical and ethnic identities will be first distinguished so as to expose clearly their multifaceted expressions and to later facilitate the understanding of their imbrications in the case of the Ladakhis' uneasy relationship with Tibetan exiles. However, before considering how IPRs are translated in identity, it would be expedient to briefly present the main contemporary elements which contribute to the emergence of 'modern' identities in Ladakh – that is, an internal political logic and the influence of, and interaction with, external actors. These elements will contribute to a better understanding of the context which fosters and nurtures itself on the social and political uses of IPRs.

The emergence of contemporary identities in Ladakh

Since 1947, when Ladakh was annexed to the State of Jammu and Kashmir in newly independent India, the Ladakhi political space has been characterized by a series of demands regarding the creation of regional autonomy.[20] These autonomist movements, however, have never been directed against the Indian Union, but against the administration of Ladakh by Muslim Kashmir (Bray 1991; van Beek 1998). The local representatives' disapproval of the political and administrative management of Ladakh has led to various Buddhist agitations, among which was a particular and very violent conflict between the Buddhist communities and the police forces in 1989. These agitations were orchestrated by the Ladakh Buddhist Association (LBA), a sectarian group very involved in Ladakhi social and political life (cf. Aggarwal 2004; Mills 1999; van Beek and Bertelsen 1997). Their religious nature, which is presented as communal,[21] disseminated a set of representations regarding the relations between the different religious groups in Ladakh and, to a certain extent, exacerbated those relations. A series of negotiations with the central government followed and allowed a partial autonomy for Ladakh, ruling out, however, the coveted Union Territory status. This autonomy assumed its present form on 3 September 1995, at the time of the first elections to the Ladakh Autonomous Hill Development Council, Leh (LAHDC).[22] However, the constitution of the LAHDC did not improve the social climate, since the populations are fragmented (e.g. religious minorities, isolated populations) and new tensions have arisen (van Beek 2001). These events have been retranscribed in the field of identity. On the one hand, they socially (or, better, politically) produced a homogeneous 'virtual' Ladakhi identity situated in political and ideological discourse.[23] This identity embodies what Georges Balandier has described elsewhere as 'the staging of power' (1980). On the other hand, they concealed religious particularisms (nearly 50 per cent of the population is Muslim) and heterogeneity of identities.[24] In the contemporary political context, this manoeuvre is inclined to project the image of a unified Ladakh to the outside world. As Marc Abélès recalls:

the protagonists in the political game present themselves as having received a mandate from the entire society. The legitimacy, whether based on immanence or on transcendence, is a quality assumed by power. The task of this power is to reflect the image of coherence and cohesion of the collectivity which it embodies.

(Abélès 1997: 247)

And it is indeed to this effacement of differences which current political leaders still relate. On 25 August 2002, in an unprecedented event in Ladakh, most regional and national political parties were suspended in order to create the Ladakh Union Territory Front (LUTF), a single non-sectarian regional party which advocates the objective of liberating Ladakh from Kashmir.

One must also consider the tourism industry, to a great extent centred on 'ethnic' or 'cultural' tourism, which serves to promote and sell ethnicity and (Buddhist) culture to both national and international tourists. Certain features of Ladakhi 'culture' are brought to the fore (e.g. folklore, monastic environment) and others are systematically glossed over. This marketing strategy is reinforced by the representations of tourists concerning Ladakh. This region generally appears, by virtue of the absence of extreme cultural and religious repression such as is commonly perceived in the case of Tibet, as a (Buddhist) religious Eden in the eyes of foreigners. Tourism contributes thus to a recasting of ethnic identities and inter-ethnic relations in Ladakh which does nothing to improve social cohesion – and which is also not thought of in those terms by the tourism industry or the government. At the same time, the formation of contemporary identities is certainly consolidated by the apprehension of the difference which the Ladakhis experience through tourism or, for example, Indian cinema. Tourism and Indian modernity, which seem to offer freedom, opportunity and mobility, are social ideals which the Ladakhis construct on a fictitious basis (that is, the tourists whom one inadequately knows, and television). They shape the outside world and the sense of self-identification, and bring into play individual and social values.

These are central elements in the construction of contemporary identities in Ladakh. The narratives on Ladakhi identity are taken up by the *amchi* elite and thus enter the medical field. The *amchi* form a specialized group confined to a given religion, which diminishes the problems arising from heterogeneity as known in Ladakh. Nevertheless, they do not feel themselves to be particularly united – quite the contrary (Pordié 2005) – and their identity is certainly polymorphous. On the other hand, the logics pertaining to (social and ethnic) identity in the particular case of IPRs are closely interlinked with the general phenomena in Ladakh.

Medicine and ethnic issues

The *amchi* emphasize the significance of their medicine in its cultural context. Their comments on pharmaceutical research and IPRs lead to a narrowing or transformation of the concept of culture. The culture to which the *amchi* allude is supposed to represent Ladakh, but it remains above all a Buddhist culture. The words of an *amchi* from the urban elite represent a clear example. On official occasions (government meetings, visits of foreigners, non-Ladakhis, donators and so on), this man extols the merits of his practice to disparage the potential intentions of 'bio-pirates'. He specifies that health coverage is mainly provided by the *amchi* in the rural area (about 90 per cent of the population live in the countryside), that this medicine is handed down from generation to generation and that it has a strong foundation in the villages. He describes the medicine as 'rooted in Ladakhi culture' and evokes its 'traditional' dimension.

This *amchi* puts forward aspects which he views as enhancing prestige by making a selection which enables him to distinguish both his medicine and the population to which he belongs from the rest of India. IPRs therefore help to cement the relationship between medicine and society. The medical arguments are given an ethnicizing dimension which, as in the case of regional political demands, lends a homogeneous (but Buddhist) image to Ladakh. The fundamental difference stems from the fact that the medicine is itself anchored in a Buddhist culture and that what is said in relation to it cannot be entirely detached from the latter. The *amchi* for this reason evince religion, but they do not deliberately express it in the case of IPRs. Nor do they attempt to deform the cultural or ethnic reality of Ladakh,[25] even though they ultimately arrive at homogenizing results equivalent to those obtained in the struggle for autonomy. This type of discourse pertaining to identity is fostered and reinforced in the political climate. The *amchi* evoke IPRs in a particular ethnic context and profit from this context to support their argument. The demands for protection and the social interactions which followed the 'crisis' in intellectual property in Ladakh have been ethnicized by the Ladakhi *amchi* and are not, as van Beek more generally shows (1998), a product of ethnicity. Intellectual property rights have enabled the crystallization of an *amchi* ethnic identity and have thereby become subject to hijacked uses. IPRs elucidate medicine as a marker of differentiation of a minority group in national society.

The claims concerning IPRs cast light on an interplay of relations between the local and national/global levels. This is an additional factor which, owing to the distance between the objects (the local medical community and international challenges), furthers the expunging of social and religious particularities in Ladakh, as well as the heterogeneity of the medical knowledge and practices which characterize the *amchi*. The international scope of issues pertaining to IPRs confers on the *amchi* a guise of identity which is useful to them because it presents the (virtual) image of a solidly linked, homogeneous group possessing a knowledge rich in meaning, which is necessary to justify their cause and to mobilize external passions and interests.

While *amchi* medicine is closely related to the local 'culture' and society, its possible exploitation by foreign interests (Indian or international) questions the rights of an entire community. IPRs can therefore serve as a support for claims concerning identity and political demands. Intellectual property rights pertain to an ideological discourse which can be easily superimposed on the contemporary political agenda in Ladakh. The statements of the leaders in the struggle to obtain Union Territory status, who argue their position by retaining elements of cultural, ethnic and bio-geographic orders, allow this comparison.[26] The two elected representatives of the newly constituted Ladakh Union Territory Front (LUTF), Namgyal Rigzin (N.R.) and Sonam Wangchuk (Pintoo Norboo, P.N.), commented on this subject (in Tashi 2002: 16–17):

> One of Ladakh's grievances, as a fallout of which Ladakhis are demanding UT [Union Territory] now, is that the power in the state failed to recognise Ladakh's regional identity.
>
> (N.R.)

> Ladakhis have all shared this opinion. . . because the problems that we share are not of caste, creed, colour, race or religion but the problems which arise from nature, which has been very harsh with the region . . . Nature has completely separated the districts of Leh and Kargil from [the] Kashmir valley as much as Kashmir from [the] Jammu region . . . This is an issue of common struggle against nature.
>
> (P.N.)

Sonam Wangchuk, from the Secmol educational association, specified in a newspaper article the reasons which, according to him, constitute the necessary basis for recognition of Union Territory status. He mentions three central points: geography, culture and history (Sonam 2002). This is echoed, to a great extent, by all protagonists of the claim for autonomy in Ladakh and is at times directly addressed, as when Thupstan Chhewang, then chief executive councillor of the LAHDC,[27] expressed his position towards the Kashmiris: 'Why should we be subjected to their cultural aggression?' (Sehgal 2002). The parallel with the discourse on intellectual property rights is striking, as the claims of each seek to keep out the 'evil foreigner'. Pharmaceutical research appears to be for the *amchi* what the Kashmiris are for the Ladakhis. These two motives, UT and IPRs, are however initially confined to different spaces (political and medical, respectively), but both concur in articulating nature, culture and politics.

In a context such as this, IPRs can be 'recuperated' to conduct or nourish 'nationalist [claims] on the cultural level', according to the terms of Michaud (1990), who characterizes thus the main Ladakhi NGOs. While activism for indigenous rights, generally implemented by NGOs, benefits from the support of public opinion, it also has the support of international instances of the highest standing, such as the World Health Organization (cf. WHO 2000, 2003). Remarks made by international organizations are taken up by the leaders in the fight against 'bio-piracy' and legitimate their activities, which can use the law as a screen to carry on nationalist political agendas. This case, which only exists in an embryonic stage in Ladakh and is not explicitly present on the regional political scene, is today a recognized social fact on the Indian subcontinent. The political range of IPRs is reinforced by their power to mobilize networks. They can convince traditionalist circles by presenting vernacular medicine as an integral part of culture, as well as those inclined towards modernism by representing medicine as a contemporary issue of regional, national and international policies.

Intellectual property rights and medical identity

While the elite *amchi* reinforce their social legitimacy through their discourse on intellectual property, they nevertheless do not obtain medical legitimacy. The corresponding logics are distinct, and although these logics may intersect this does not affirm the *amchi* medical legitimacy in the community. However, a more fertile terrain is found outside the community for displaying a medical identity and laying claim to its legitimacy. The arguments and social practices of the *amchi* are analysed with regard to the plasticity of their claimed identities, their apparent changing patterns and their actual social coherence. I retain for this purpose a selected number of evocative examples to uncover a series of respective push-and-pull strategies, experienced in relation to both biomedicine and āyurveda.

The *amchi* describe their medicine as highly devalued and disparaged. This they generally attribute to the emergence of biomedicine and new corresponding powers in the field of health, as well as to the new aspirations of their fellow citizens (Pordié 2000). This grievance is in part true, for the practitioners know the obvious difficulties which combine problems of monetary remuneration in the rural milieu with those of medical practice in a social climate privileging biomedical development. But the situation is not irreversible, and the *amchi* recognize that their practice is still to a certain extent socially and institutionally dynamic.[28] Their positioning vis-à-vis biomedicine relates essentially to medical identity. By asserting themselves in pharmaceutical research and in the exploitation of the 'biological heritage', the elite *amchi* demarcate themselves from the biomedical world.[29] In this respect, they emphasize the connection of their practice to the environment by employing an entire range of arguments, some of which are borrowed from works on Tibetan medicine for neophytes, which may be found on the market in the Ladakhi capital, and gleaned from tourists and local environmental activists.[30] IPRs therefore also reveal the encounter between the *amchi* and a more supportive West than that shown through bio-piracy. The image of the West as a pillager is confronted with that of the West which admires the local medicine and its environmental and cultural contexts. The *amchi* certainly do not have such a dichotomous view or understanding, but it is within these extremes that the social re-combinations of IPRs occur. The conjugation of such variants is neither a paradox nor a problem for the *amchi*, since they make use of both and turn them into a coherent social whole in which IPRs play a central role.

Through the appropriation of external rhetoric, *amchi* speak thus of 'natural' medicine, of the 'herbal' particularity of their medical practice, or of the absence of side-effects.[31] The *amchi* negotiate the authenticity and singularity of their medical identity by using a wide panoply of modern elements: IPRs, environmental conservation and so on. Their narratives pertaining to 'tradition' generally do not concern the past, but on the contrary express the present and the future (Tan 1999). Moreover, the *amchi* assertions reveal the following oppositions between their medicine and biomedicine: natural elements/industrial products, innocuousness/ toxicity and local cultural anchorage/importation from the West. They therefore denounce not only the 'violence' of biomedicine (Tan 1999; Zimmermann 1992), but also and above all the social violence of bio-prospecting. This recalls in substance the shortcomings of a dehumanized and dominating modern science, and is seen, as far as IPRs are concerned, as potentially harmful to the Ladakhis.

There are, however, paradoxes, notably when the *amchi* crystallize their discourse around medicinal plants and biomedicines potentially derived from them. The opposition of *amchi* medicine to biomedicine does not signify that medicinal plants are opposed to biomedicine, because they stand in a relationship of continuity, of which bio-prospecting constitutes the link. (Industrial) biomedicine is derived in this case from (natural) plants, which the *amchi* emphasize when arguing against pharmaceutical research or when specifying that 'most modern medicines come from plants'. But this continuity is perceived by the *amchi* as a break because it eludes their power, which is itself called into question by a violation or possible exploitation of their knowledge.

Medical identity, medicinal plants and IPRs are also conflated in the *amchi*'s demand for official legal recognition of their medical system in India. Although government *amchi* exist, and education programmes and infrastructures are funded and supported by the central government, *amchi* medicine itself is not officially and fully recognized in India. It is tolerated. The wish for legal recognition expressed by the *amchi*, classically described in the political approaches to identity (Tully 2000), applies here to medical identity. To be recognized by law, *amchi* medicine must be integrated into a unit of the Ministry of Health and Family Welfare: the Indian Systems of Medicine and Homoeopathy (ISM&H).[32] The *amchi*, by showing their adherence to national policies and their will to defend their intellectual property, hope to show leaders in Delhi that their scholarly medicine deserves the same status as an Indian system of medicine.

In this respect, a workshop was co-organized in July 2001 by the Ladakh Ecological and Development Group and the Ladakh Amchi Sabha, under the auspices of the Foundation for the Revitalisation of Local Health Traditions of Bangalore. The objective was to follow the recommendations of the Convention on Biological Diversity (CBD)[33] and the policies of the ISM – both considered as means of securing IPRs – such as providing practitioners with information and constituting data banks on medicinal plants (DISM 2001). The *amchi* drew up lists of plants without anyone appearing to really take seriously the difficulties and inconsistencies involved in the matter. Although the *amchi* lay claim to a 'scholarly tradition based on a written corpus', which would theoretically ensure a minimal standardization of knowledge, the practitioners' knowledge remains heterogeneous. Transmission is primarily oral and gives place to multiple interpretations of classical written works. Moreover, in Ladakh, the institutionalization of education and practice concerns only a very small minority of *amchi*. The intentions to systematize knowledge consequently lead to the closely related problematic of articulating heterogeneous indigenous knowledge in written form and to the difficulties, or indeed impossibilities, inherent in such projects (e.g. Ellen *et al.* 2000). The objective was therefore not so much to conduct a precise work without flaw as to demonstrate the local interest of the responsible *amchi* in national policies. This manoeuvre had a twofold goal: 1) integration in the ISM, which would represent for the *amchi* a significant social advancement in the official health care sector and a clear augmentation of material and structural support; and 2) affirmation of their own medical identity by supporting a unique pharmacopoeia in India.

Medical identity is therefore expressed particularly through plants, understood both as a distinguishing feature claimed by the *amchi* and as the centre of interest of a section of biomedical research constituted by bio-prospecting. Medicinal plants represent a relational space between the *amchi* and pharmaceutical research. Plants are necessary in the practice of the *amchi* and symbolize their knowledge of nature. Being concerned with the knowledge and practices of *amchi* medicine, pharmaceutical research promotes vernacular medical identity. Although religion would be a representative social characteristic of their group, the religious identity of the *amchi* seldom appears in the issues related to their medical identity in the context of intellectual property rights.[34] Religion may be occasionally taken into consideration, but it is immersed in the naturalism which arises from the argumentation of the *amchi* (environment, plants, biology). This naturalism thus fits more easily into the biomedical discourse of pharmaceutical research, a system they are opposed to. The collective medical identity expressed to the biomedical world tends, in the process, to assume shades of the latter.

A similar logic may be seen with regard to āyurveda, which also arises in the *amchi*'s contemporary narratives on IPRs, because this medicine is a major symbol of the Indian scholarly traditions and particularly illustrates the 'immemorial' medical knowledge of the subcontinent. The *amchi* attempt to distinguish themselves from āyurveda without, however, renouncing their affiliation. The singularity of the plant environment, the historical development and the cultural context of *amchi* medicine allow their distinction and thus justify the autonomy of the system. On the other hand, they retain certain theoretical characteristics and the historical foundations of their medicine to confirm their affiliation with āyurveda.[35] A text from the Health Department (2001: 3) supporting the demand for recognition and integration into the ISM observes:

> The fundamental concept of Sowa Rigpa Medicine [*sic*] is based on the theory of the five cosmo-physical energies earth, water, fire, air and space, and the three humours or primary energies called in Tibetan 'Nyspa' and in Sanskrit 'Dosha'. These three dosha are rlung – vayu, mKhrispa – pitta, and badkan – kapha, respectively, in the Ayurvedic concept.

The *amchi* avoid a lasting relegation to the status of *tribal medicine* and an overly close political assimilation with the medicine-of-the-Tibetans.[36] Proceeding in this manner, backing up their arguments attributed respectively to distinction and affiliation, the *amchi* share certain allegiances with the authorities of the ISM in order to better construct their differences.

The medical issues of identity expressed towards biomedicine and āyurveda reveal a 'chameleon-like medical identity' which assumes different shades according to the support on which it rests. This identity is certainly homogeneous in a given context, but it differs from context to context. The *amchi* draw elements of otherness from various medical systems and then include them in their own medical discourse. Medical identity is thus transformed according to the conjunction of circumstances by a partial and selective shift in the foreign paradigms. The overlapping in otherness appears in the case of IPRs as a strong argument of difference. This process is also to be found at the juncture of medical and social identities; it enables the reinforcement of the *amchi*'s ethnic and political claims.

An encounter between medical and ethnic identities: the Tibetan case

The outright separation of medical and ethnic identities such as I have described is obviously an expedient of presentation. Their boundaries are blurred, permeable and unstable; these mutually supportive 'identities' overlap and sometimes merge. The Ladakhi relationship to Tibetans, and more specifically to those living in India,[37] enables one to better understand this tangled state. The identity of medicine does not stand apart from that of its practitioners, and this, as said in Ladakh, has been the case since the tenth century:

> During the tenth century, the great translator and philosopher Rinchen Zangpo introduced this Tibetan system to Ladakh where he translated the text of Astanga Herdapa Vitta from Kashmir. Since then, the amchi medical system flourished in Ladakh. The local medical practitioners, under the initiative of the Kings of Ladakh, enriched their medical system by introducing new herbal and mineral drugs as well as medical texts . . . Nevertheless, Tibet has been the training centre of arts, culture and science, and the students from Ladakh used to avail this opportunity until Tibet has been occupied by the Chinese government. The relation inevitably broke down and the Ladakhi amchis began to preserve the guru-she system[38] from generation to generation. It is today an original Indian system of medicine. Today this system is recognised at a global international level [and it is] named as Tibetan medicine.
>
> (Health Department 2001: 2)

This quote is taken from the file addressed to the Indian prime minister in the summer of 2001, the objective of which was to request the integration of the medicine of the *amchi* in the ISM. It shows how the Ladakhi practitioners stand out in the existing forms of Tibetan medicines. They retain a number of historical particularities (the accuracy of which lies beyond the scope of this chapter) and thus argue for the autonomous development of Tibetan medicine in Ladakh. Identity is a historical construction, real or perceived, which is found again in an ideological, political, even cultural, and in cases also medical discourse. The medicine of the Ladakhi *amchi* has undergone a historical development distinct from the medicine in Tibet, the influence of which has clearly not declined. On the one hand, it would be socially and culturally unacceptable (and wrong historically) to reject the links with Tibet too quickly and, on the other hand, it makes it possible to benefit from the standing of the medicine-of-the-Tibetans. In this way Tibetan medicine has been 'enriched' by the introduction of a Ladakhi *materia medica* and of medical texts supposedly written in Ladakhi by Ladakhis. The environmental and medical particularities are accentuated to serve the identity of their practice and to firmly establish it as an indigenous Indian system. The double issue of identity is very clearly perceptible.

The Ladakhi *amchi*, however, know very well that their medicine *is* Tibetan medicine, theoretically at least. The differences between medicines (Ladakhi and Tibetan) follow the same logic as that shown in the case of biomedicine and āyurveda. They are alternately self-styled (local identities) or rejected (place to be gained in the 'Tibetan medicine' market) by the *amchi*, depending on the given objective. The origins of the knowledge of the *amchi* in Ladakh are known to all, but vary under the influence of socio-political, economic and identity issues. These manipulations express, for the *amchi* of Ladakh, their wish to acquire a recognized status in the field of Tibetan medicine. As said earlier, this expression of *Ladakhiness*[39] clearly appears in the naming of the practice, most often referred to as '*amchi* medicine', in order to distinguish it from the medicine-of-the-Tibetans.

The hijacked use of intellectual property serves as a screen for the existing social tensions between the communities of Ladakhi and Tibetan *amchi*. Let us take up once more the case of the Dutchwoman from the Plant Foundation who, as we know, was expelled from Ladakh for suspected bio-piracy. Her acceptance by the Ladakhi *amchi* to come and work illegally on medicinal plants in their region was mainly due to the letter which she brought with her. The letter, signed by her Tibetan master, justified the reasons for her presence and asked those concerned to facilitate her work. The master in question was none other than the late Trogawa Rinpoche, then a religious and *amchi* of renown, and founder (1992) and director of the Chagpori Institute of Darjeeling. The *amchi* of Ladakh considered the Venerable very highly both in medical and in religious terms. The acceptance of the foreigner reflected the logic of respect and sometimes of adoration witnessed among the Ladakhi towards Tibetan religious leaders. At the time of the expulsion, however, the origins of the presence of the Dutchwoman were no longer mentioned, because a public rejection of Trogawa Rinpoche and his project would have been unthinkable. There is a profound ambivalence in Ladakhi attitudes towards Tibet, but they tend publicly to be reverential, and this sets limits to what one is allowed to argue. The expulsion of the retired Dutchwoman exhibited *amchi* social power and was seen locally as refusing subservience to the will of the Tibetans. The situation generated a debate among leading *amchi*, some of them finding the sanction inappropriate and disrespectful. But what ultimately happened showed that bio-pirates have become a more important justification than the will of reincarnated lamas.

The relations between Ladakhis and Tibetans raise a new concern in the case of IPRs. The problems of intellectual property with regard to Tibetans are not evident, or even legitimate, when expressed by Ladakhis practising Tibetan medicine. This is perhaps the reason for which the discourse easily switches over to the field of environmental conservation, since IPRs and conservation are closely interrelated (Bodecker *et al.* 1997; Timmermans 2003). The Tibetans are notably accused of being among those mainly responsible for collecting wild plants in regions usually benefiting the Ladakhi *amchi* (in particular the Rhotang Pass, near Manali, and in Ladakh). Tenzin Choedrak, former personal *amchi* to the Dalai Lama, said in 1999: 'Upon my arrival [in India] the Tibetan doctors availed of less than eighty substances to make traditional remedies. I seriously started searching for raw materials which, for the most part, are sent from Tibet and from Ladakh' (interviewed by Tager 1999). In addition, a member of the Men-Tsee-Khang Cultural Centre (MCC), inaugurated in Leh in the first week of July 2003, told me in 2000: 'The Leh Men-Tsee-Khang is important because it is often too humid to dry the plants in Dharamsala. In Ladakh we can collect the plants and dry them easily.' The environmental degradation is obviously the result of multiple factors, and the Tibetans are certainly not the first and only cause (Pordié 2002). But the reason is regularly evoked by the *amchi* of Ladakh, although never explicitly to the concerned Tibetans, and sheds light on their problems vis-à-vis the latter. The recent construction of the MCC is perceived as major competition. The MCC is an immense building, which includes a clinic, a pharmacy and a museum, and future plans include the possibility of accommodating patients and courses for foreigners.[40] The Ladakhi *amchi* practising in Leh fear that their fellow citizens, as well as the tourists, will start to desert their clinics. One of them observed the progress of the work in 2000:

> What can I do? I am supposed to know what is happening here [he is one of the leading *amchi*] for *amchi* medicine but I even did not know about that centre. Tibetans can do whatever they want. They have money and support and a special status in India. They do much better than us. It is difficult to say I don't like them; I should not bother about this . . . [silence] But now there is a big competition . . . [laughter] When the Tibetan *sman rtsis khang* will come, then [laughter]. . . more competition! Then the Ladakhi *amchi* cannot sleep; they would either not be able to sleep or always sleep.

The Ladakhi *amchi* suffer in the confrontation with their Tibetan counterparts. Today, they are attempting to redefine their space. The tensions between the two communities are latent and emerge at particular moments. The construction of the centre encroaches at the same time upon the material, social and symbolic spaces of the Ladakhi *amchi*, who find themselves driven back to their subaltern position. They must therefore mobilize new registers, such as intellectual property, pharmaceutical research and environmental conservation, to establish more firmly their (medical and ethnic) identities and not, as they say, sleep for ever.

Conclusion

Intellectual property rights concerned with indigenous knowledge are expressed in the general framework of globalization. They represent a new element in the *amchi* medical system to which the concerned community provides a set of necessary responses. This localization of a global phenomenon sheds light on the logics which are involved in the contemporary construction of Tibetan medicine in Ladakh. Intellectual property rights are an evocative example for the study of the socio-political consequences of relations considered or legitimized as primarily medical.

Pharmaceutical research is an element of the culturally dominant biomedical authority, the dominion of which is beyond doubt.[41] Its relation with the medicine of the *amchi* ultimately benefits the latter. In fact, the 'medical authority' retains a power which it transfers to *amchi* medicine by showing its interest. Bio-prospecting acts as an agent in catalysing *amchi* power, notwithstanding local discourses which agree in demonstrating the contrary. In short, the symbolic power of biomedicine – through pharmaceutical research – enables an increase in the social and political power of *amchi* medicine and accords it medical legitimacy. According to one *amchi*:

> They [the bio-prospectors] are interested in our knowledge because it is rich and valuable. They start to understand this. . . but we have known it since long ago. Our people [the Ladakhi population] can tell. Our medicine works for many ailments; we do not always have success, like any medicine, but we certainly are not the worst [laughter].

The *amchi* exploit the prominence of foreign research institutions[42] to strengthen their positions, both in the field of health and on the level of society. As has been shown, the social use of IPRs makes it possible to modify the expression of this power and to transform the direct confrontation with biomedicine into derived confrontations with other medical systems.

The fact that knowledge can be a source of power is certainly not new, notably in ancient and contemporary Tibetan worlds. Money is to be made from knowledge, and economic affluence guarantees a privileged social status. Power is traditionally negotiated and defended; the case of IPRs clearly illustrates this point. But it seems that there is another phenomenon, for here an outside power (biomedicine) is being used, thereby adding credibility to local knowledge. This knowledge is then defended against biomedical power and socially negotiated in the Ladakhi context. This process reflects a transferral of forces manifested in different fields.

As Kuhn suggests (1994), the biomedical expansion that has been taking place in Ladakh since the 1970s has led to a domination of the traditional health systems. The *amchi*, as individuals of an increasingly acculturated society, do not evade these general social processes. The phenomena shown in this chapter are certainly located in the wider influential and authoritative role of biomedicine, but this cannot in itself be taken as a teleological conclusion sufficient to explain the actual changes.

Although specifically circumscribed, the reading that this chapter has offered is anthropologically indicative of a reconfiguration of the Ladakhi health system. It sheds light on new places and expressions of power among those who are considered to be dominated in the 'medical' field.[43] *Amchi* medicine exhibits a range of possibilities to actually benefit from the imposition of the national and international biomedical agenda in Ladakh. It articulates to a great extent its own politics around the element of domination to better domesticate it, as the case of IPRs clearly displayed. IPRs constitute an example in which the encounter between medical systems assumes an unexpected shape and reveals specific political and social locales extending far beyond their initial medical scope.

This text has shown three fundamental levels which are interlinked in context. The first level of analysis shows IPRs as a social object reserved for use within the group or on its immediate periphery; the second concerns the national and international claims in which the social expression of the group is homogenized to leave the field open to imagine and to express collective (medical and ethnic) identities; and the third combines the former two by making use of IPRs (through conservation) as social, medical and ethnic stratagems directed towards the Tibetan community in exile. The *amchi* concerned attempt in each case to limit the ascendancy of exogenous power over their world by reinforcing their individual or community power, by affirming or claiming their ethnicity and by adapting their medical identity, using its 'chameleon-like' character to better camouflage their interests. In all cases the changing performances of identities and power, whether located in social, 'ethnic' or medical registers, do not reflect the disparities and inconsistencies of the group, but rather cultivate and (re)define them. At the same time, this strategy, although it creates conflicts between the elite *amchi* and accentuates the difference between rural and urban practitioners, enables the medical system to be inscribed in the contemporary socio-political field. It thus brings the *amchi* into a closer hierarchical relationship with the contemporary agents of politics and modern science, and contributes to a greater differentiation of the social, political and therapeutic dimensions of their 'medical' space. More than personal power incarnated in the person of an *amchi*, it is first and foremost political power which is sought on a collective basis on local, regional and national levels. The reinforcement or the definition of other, economic and juridical, powers can also be an integral part of this approach, as Léonard has remarked (1981).

Intellectual property rights have a plural character in society, and the flexibility of that character makes it possible for them to be totally appropriated by the *amchi*. They are mobilized and socially negotiated in all the relations the group maintains within itself and outside. Thus IPRs illustrate the manner in which *amchi* medicine constructs itself on semantic, social, political and identity bases in an array of relations principally established between medicines, or rather 'medical worlds' (*amchi* medicine, biomedicine, āyurveda, Tibetan-medicine-of-the-Tibetans).[44] Intellectual property appears as an alibi with many facets, mobilized by diverse actors – *amchi*, politicians, tourists, NGOs – and purposefully employed to the advantage of social practices. One can approach IPRs as a sort of common language which people can translate as they wish. They become bearers of multiple meanings and can represent a justification for general social issues.

Notes

1 This is a category defined by the government of India which corresponds to 'ethnic minorities'. This socio-political construction differentiates, on a variety of levels, individuals belonging to this group from the rest of Indian society (see Xaxa 2003).

2 In Ladakh, these Tibetan medicine practitioners generally speak of their medicine as '*amchi* medicine'. See Chapter 1 for a discussion on the use of the generic term 'Tibetan medicine'. Among themselves, the Ladakhi *amchi* mainly use *gso ba rig pa*, a term which is also employed, albeit sparsely and recently, in English (Sowa Rigpa). This is subsequent to the recommendations aiming at homogeneity of denomination that were made by the Dalai Lama at the Indian National Conference of *Amchi* held in the summer of 2000 in Spiti, India. This was further elaborated and formalized by a Representative Committee formed in late 2003 under the aegis of the Himalayan Buddhist Cultural Association. This common denomination is used in the demand for full legal and institutional recognition by the government of India. The naming and its purpose have been ratified during the National Seminar 'Scope of Sowa-Rigpa (Science of Healing) Medical System and Medicinal Plants in Himalayan Region', held in Delhi in February 2004. The term 'Tibetan medicine' is only used with informative purpose by the *amchi*. I will use both '*amchi* medicine' and 'Tibetan medicine in Ladakh' in this chapter to designate the studied medical practice in the region.

3 He retired from this position in early 2003.

4 He was awarded a gold medal in 1987 by the State of Jammu and Kashmir in recognition of his service in the field of medicine. Dr S.T. Phuntsog is today Director of the Mahabodi Hospital in Ladakh.

5 Biomedicine is often referred to by the Ladakhis as allopathy in opposition to *amchi* medicine, although the term applies to both systems. The error is also found among scholars (cf. Kuhn 1994). See Pordié (2007: 10) for a short discussion of allopathy and its use in India.

6 Union Minister of State for Law, Chairman of the Standing Committee of Parliament on Law, Justice and Company Affairs, Chairman of the Expert Group on Patent Law, Central Council for Research on Ayurveda and Siddha (CCRAS) from the Ministry of Health and Family Welfare and so on.

7 The names used for persons are phonetically transcribed. I use elsewhere Wylie's system of transliteration. The names of the *amchi* are pseudonyms.

8 Although the 1994 petition had earlier stated that 'recently there have been several enquiries by individual foreigners from the industrially and economically developed countries with regard to the Amchi system of medicine', no proof of their intention was given.

9 According to my informants, the IPRs case in Ladakh involved well-known activists, such as Vandana Shiva or Helena Norberg-Hodge.

10 The nationality of the lawyer involved conjecture. He was recruited primarily because he was in the direct network of Nomad RSI and was willing to work on a voluntary basis. The fact that the lawyer came from Central America, where the question of indigenous rights is of particular significance, also made sense for the NGO.

11 The journal also has an English title carrying a different meaning: *Trans-Himalayan Amchi Medical Education Newsletter*. Its content, according to an evaluation I conducted with a number of *amchi* in Ladakh, has not been fully understood by the rural *amchi*, owing to its specialized, non-medical, nature.

12 One foreigner was said not to be very sociable; the other may have been targeted because she was never introduced officially, and not introduced for many months, to N.T. This

attitude upset him, since the foreigner would openly disregard his competence and thus paid no attention to his social status (the woman nevertheless told me later that she did not even know of the existence of the institution concerned).

13   The BJP, 'Party of the Indian People', was in power in India from 1998 to 2004. This is a political party advocating Hindu nationalism (cf. Hansen 1999; Jaffrelot 1996), which includes Buddhist radicals in Ladakh who came together initially in opposition to Muslims (van Beek 2004).

14   Although there are female *amchi*, I use the masculine pronoun because none of the women are yet involved in IPRs politics.

15   IPRs bring all types of social problems into the institutional scene. Individual *amchi* therefore require a rational-legal (here, institutional) form of social legitimation, in accordance with the Weberian tripartite classification (1959), to be able to gain or use power in the case of IPRs. When dissension occurs, if a particular individual should lack this type of legitimation he or she would not have the appropriate social instruments to respond to or resist the social pressure exerted by IPRs.

16   This geographical dimension of discourses on IPRs applies mainly to Leh district and to the Zangskar region of Kargil district, which correspond to the distribution of the Buddhist population in Ladakh and to the areas where *amchi* medicine is found.

17   These excursions may also be organized with foreign organizations.

18   This circular marked the renewal of activities pertaining to IPRs in 1999, catalysed by the presence of the Mexican lawyer, but also by a 'suspect' German student investigating edible plants. The circular was written 'under the direction of the President, other founders and Sr. members of LAS' and was intended for all clinics of Tibetan medicine, the District Magistrate, the Superintendent of Police, the Forest Officer, the Chief Medical Officer, the Amchi Medicine Research Unit and the Non-Timber Products Department of Forestry.

19   This is not to say that there is no customary form of ownership in Ladakh aiming to protect knowledge, but IPRs in their present form and scale, and the challenges they represent, are indeed a new element.

20   Notwithstanding the existence of major events in the political life of Ladakh in the 1830s and later, in the 1930s, I consider the period correlated to Indian independence as a factor triggering the constitution of one (or several) modern identity(-ies). I employ the term 'modern' identities so as to underscore the dynamism and fluidity in matters of identity and its historical evolution.

21   Communalism often evokes religion in the Indian context, although the word does not exclusively carry that meaning. 'In its common Indian usage the word "communalism" refers to a condition of suspicion, fear and hostility between members of different religious communities. In academic investigation, more often than not, the term is applied to organized political movement based on the proclaimed interests of a religious community' (Pandey 1990: 6).

22   The LAHDC has been active since 1996. It concerns the district of Leh, the majority of which is Buddhist – the chief executive councillor was, until recently, Thupstan Chhewang, who is none other than the former president of the LBA in 1989. The district of Kargil, the majority population of which is Muslim, has refused the offer until recently. The Ladakh Autonomous Hill Development Council Kargil was commissioned in July 2003. I do not consider here the struggle to obtain scheduled tribe status, which has also contributed to the formation of modern Ladakhi identity/(-ies).

23   This is not to say that this 'virtual' identity has no consistency. It has clear political repercussions and should therefore not be radically objectivized and relegated to the realm of illusion (Abélès 1997).

24   The strategies pertaining to *fictive* or *ideal* identities are often used in political contexts as instruments for political identification (Chebel 1998). Martijn van Beek (2000a, 2000b) has explored this matrix in great detail in Ladakh and goes beyond more commonly addressed issues of identity politics to show how it responds to an 'art of

representation', a fundamental condition of political action, which both transforms and jeopardizes the social reality. The author thus sheds light on particular practices of identification and social relations, and contributes to a revisiting of democratic theories.

25 Apart from this type of presentation, the *amchi* very readily include the Ladakhi Muslims in their discourse on culture if they are so questioned. They then list the similarity in language, writing, food habits, constraints linked to the health or geographical environment and so on. Statements they make in sustained discussions nevertheless tend to socially subordinate the Muslims. They refer to the minor role played by Muslims in the field of traditional health and their dependency on the *amchi* in the villages, should they be present.

26 Such arguments existed long before 2002 and tend to make the autonomy demand a non-communal (religious) issue. This also allows a reading of identities as supposedly 'natural' characteristics which are claimed to be collectively shared. It also sheds light on the ways in which identities unfold and become established in interacting with and imagining nature (see, for example, Roepstorff *et al.* 2003).

27 Thupstan Chhewang, also former president of the Ladakh Buddhist Association in 1989, later became the Ladakh Union Territory Front (LUTF) leader. He was then elected Member of the Parliament (MP) in May 2004. In autumn the same year, former members of the LUTF quitted this regional party to re-form the Congress so as to attain Union Territory status with support from their national party.

28 This is manifested through the creation of an autonomous department within the regional department of health, multiplication of activities, increase in the regional budget, increase in private clinics, existing demands from patients, existing development projects and so on.

29 The *amchi* are indeed aware of the existing relations between biomedicine and the pharmaceutical industry, as underscored by Csordas and Kleinman (1996).

30 A fair number of tourists in Ladakh, generally out of ecological romanticism, would mention the 'connection' the *amchi* supposedly have with the environment and the 'natural' dimension of their medicine. Many of them reject 'unfair bio-prospecting', since it is perceived as being in opposition to both the moral ideal the inhabitants are seen to incarnate (Bishop 1989; Lopez 1998) and their supposedly inherent ecological ethics (Huber 1997).

31 Classical Tibetan medical texts nevertheless mention the existence of side-effects. For example, the *rguyd bzhi* mentions in the Final Treatise (*Phyi-ma'i rgyud*) the 'perverse effects' of evacuative medicines and the means to master them (*log gnon*) (Meyer 1981: 184).

32 This unit has since then changed its name. The Department of Indian Systems of Medicine and Homoeopathy has been renamed the Department of Ayurveda, Yoga and Naturopathy, Unani, Siddha and Homoeopathy (AYUSH); *vide* notification issued by the Cabinet Secretariat on 11 November 2003. I will, however, retain the acronym ISM for the remainder of this chapter.

33 The CBD was signed at the UN Conference on Environment and Development (UNCED) held in Rio de Janeiro in 1992. This is the largest international legal agreement ever to have existed, having been signed by more than 175 countries in 2000. Articles 8(j), 15, 16 and 17 directly concern intellectual property (Dutfield 2000).

34 As we have seen earlier, religious identity appears more clearly in the ethnic issues surrounding IPRs, although not necessarily intentionally. It is, on the other hand, fully expressed elsewhere, notably in the political construction of local *amchi* associations (Pordié 2003).

35 See Meyer (1981) for details on the role of āyurveda in the historical construction of Tibetan medicine.

36 The latter two elements would make integration into the ISM more difficult. The Tibetans exiled in India have always refused the subsumption of their medicine under āyurveda. I must mention that recent developments on this matter may change the situation: the

integration of Tibetan medicine in the ISM was reconsidered in the summer of 2003 on the Tibetan side, motivated by economic interests (exemption of taxes on the sale of medicines and cosmetics in India). However, there is no consensus among the *amchi* of Ladakh on the form that this integration could take. While some *amchi* are not opposed to the integration of their medicine 'under' āyurveda, the great majority wish to preserve the very identity of their medicine and thus that it would be recognized as an independent system of medicine.

37 Rivalries with the Tibetan *amchi*, or at least the inferiority complex which characterizes the Ladakhi *amchi*, are expressed in a historical and cultural framework – Ladakh as a hierarchically inferior and reified Tibetan 'sub-culture' or 'satellite culture' (cf. Aziz 1987), geographic origin of Tibetan medicine and religious leaders. The mediation and the contemporary success of Tibetans on the international medical plane contribute a supplementary element.

38 This is how the Ladakhis term the teaching of medicine from master to apprentice: *guru-she* or *guru-shes*. It is certainly a contraction of the Sanskrit terms *guru* and *śiṣya* (master and disciple, respectively).

39 This type of neologism is used by various authors in the case of Tibet; like *Tibetanness*, it refers particularly to problems of identity.

40 This project aims at making capital out of the Tibetan medical market in Ladakh, benefiting notably from the popularity of Tibetan *amchi* among the tourists.

41 Acceptance of biomedical cultural authority is a widespread contemporary characteristic in traditional medicines. This phenomenon has involved classic Chinese medicine since the end of the nineteenth century (Croizier 1968) and was also shown in the case of Tibetan medicine (Janes 1999; Meyer 1986, 1993).

42 The relationship the *amchi* actually have with foreign research institutions is essentially a relationship of thought, that is, it seldom materializes in practice.

43 Albeit on a different register, Adams (2001) also shows that the appropriation of modernity by Tibetan medicine in Tibet does not mean its conditional surrender, but rather that it serves to strengthen some aspects of knowledge and practice.

44 The medical techniques are not of paramount concern, for the dynamics are, at least initially, located on other levels. The integration of biomedical techniques or practices in Tibetan medicine does not formally exist in Ladakh, as is the case elsewhere.

References

Abélès, M. (1997). La mise en représentation du politique. In M. Abélès and H.-P. Jeudy (eds), *Anthropologie du politique*, Paris: Armand Collin.

Adams, V. (2001). Particularizing Modernity: Tibetan Medical Theorizing of Women's Health in Lhasa, Tibet. In L. H. Connor and G. Samuel (eds), *Healing Powers and Modernity: Traditional Medicine, Shamanism and Science in Asian Societies*, Westport, CT: Bergin & Garvey.

Aggarwal, R. (2004). *Beyond Lines of Control: Performance and Politics on the Disputed Borders of Ladakh, India*, Durham, NC and London: Duke University Press.

Aubert, S. (2002). Protection juridique et éthique, la contribution des droits de propriété intellectuelle à l'ethnopharmacologie, *Ethnopharmacologia* 28: 74–87.

Aziz, B. (1987). Moving toward a Sociology of Tibet. In J. Willis (ed.), *Feminine Ground: Essays on Women and Tibet*, Ithaca, NY: Snow Lion Publications.

Balandier, G. (1980). *Le pouvoir sur scène*, Paris: Balland.

Baviskar, A. (2000). Claims to Knowledge, Claims to Control: Environmental Conflict in the Great Himalayan National Park, India. In R. Ellen, P. Parkes and A. Bicker (eds), *Indigenous Environmental Knowledge and its Transformations: Critical Anthropological Perspectives*, Amsterdam: Harwood Academic Publishers.

Bishop, P. (1989). *The Myth of Shangri-La: Tibet, Travel Writing, and the Western Creation of a Sacred Landscape*, Berkeley: University of California Press.

Bodecker, G., Bhat, K. K. S., Burley, J. and Vantomme, P. (eds) (1997). *Medicinal Plants for Forest Conservation and Health Care*, FAO Non-Wood Product Series, Vol. 11, Delhi: Daya.

Bray, J. (1991). Ladakhi History and Indian Nationhood, *South Asia Research* 11(2): 115–133.

Brush, S. B. (1999). Bioprospecting the Public Domain, *Cultural Anthropology* 14(4): 535–555.

Busch, L. (1995). Eight Reasons Why Patents Should Not Be Extended to Plants and Animals, *Biotechnology and Development Monitor* 24: 24.

Certeau, M. de (1980). *L'invention du quotidien*, 1. *Arts de faire*, Paris: Union générale d'éditions, coll. 10/18.

Challa, J. and Kalla, J. C. (1995). World Trade Agreement and Trade Related Aspects of Intellectual Property Rights: Relevance to Indian Agriculture, *Commonwealth Agricultural Digest*, Vol. 4, Farnham Royal: Commonwealth Agricultural Bureaux.

Chebel, M. (1998). *La formation de l'identité politique*, Paris: Petite Bibliothèque Payot.

Coombe, R. (1998). *The Cultural Life of Intellectual Properties: Authorship, Appropriation, and the Law*, New Brunswick, NJ: Routledge.

Croizier, R. (1968). *Traditional Medicine in Modern China*, Cambridge, MA: Harvard University Press.

Csordas, T. J. and Kleinman, A. (1996). The Therapeutic Process. In C. F. Sargent and T. M. Johnson (eds), *Medical Anthropology: Contemporary Theory and Method*, Westport, CT and London: Praeger.

Dhar, B. and Chaturvedi, C. (1998). Introducing Plant Breeders' Rights in India: A Critical Evaluation of the Proposed Legislation, *Journal of World Intellectual Property* 1(2): 245–262.

DISM (Department of Indian Systems of Medicine and Homoeopathy) (2001). *Draft National Policy on Indian System of Medicine*, New Delhi: DISM.

Dutfield, G. (1999). Protecting and Revitalising Traditional Ecological Knowledge: Intellectual Property Rights and Community Knowledge Databases in India. In M. Barkeley (ed.), *Intellectual Property Aspects of Ethnobiology*, London: Sweet & Maxwell.

Dutfield, G. (2000). *Intellectual Property Rights: Trade and Biodiversity*, London: IUCN Earthscan.

Ellen, R., Parkes, P. and Bicker, A. (eds) (2000). *Indigenous Environmental Knowledge and its Transformations: Critical Anthropological Perspectives*, Amsterdam: Harwood Academic Publishers.

Fassin, D. (1996). *L'espace politique de la santé: Essai de généalogie*, Paris: Presses Universitaires de France.

Hansen, T. B. (1999). *The Saffron Wave: Democracy and Hindu Nationalism in Modern India*, Princeton, NJ: Princeton University Press.

Health Department (2001). *Sowa Rigpa Tradition, Amchi Medical System: Demand for Registration under Indian System of Medicine*, 20 July, Leh: Health Department.

Huber, T. (1997). Green Tibetans: A Brief Social History. In F. J. Korom (ed.), *Tibetan Culture in the Diaspora: Proceedings of the Seventh Seminar of the International Association for Tibetan Studies (PIATS), Graz, June 18–24, 1995*, Österreichischen Akademie der Wissenschaften, Philosophisch-historische Klasse, Denkschriften, 262, Vol. 4, Vienna: Verlag der Österreichischen Akademie der Wissenschaften.

Jaffrelot, C. (1996). *The Hindu Nationalist Movement in Indian Politics*, New York: Columbia University Press.

Janes, C. (1999). The Health Transition, Global Modernity and the Crisis of Traditional Medicine: The Tibetan Case, *Social Science and Medicine* 48: 1803–1820.

Juma, C. (1999). *Intellectual Property Rights and Globalization: Implications for Developing Countries*, Science, Technology and Innovation Discussion Paper No. 4, Cambridge, MA: Center for International Development, Harvard University.

Kocken, J. and van Roozendaal, G. (1997). The Neem Tree Debate, *Biotechnology and Development Monitor* 30.

Kothari, A. (1999). Intellectual Property Rights and Biodiversity: Are India's Proposed Biodiversity Act and Plant Varieties Act Compatible?, Paper presented at the Workshop on Biodiversity Conservation and Intellectual Property Regime, RIS/Kalpavriksh/IUCN, New Delhi, 29–31 January.

Kuhn, S. A. (1994). Ladakh: A Pluralistic Medical System under Acculturation and Domination. In D. Sich and W. Gottschalk (eds), *Acculturation and Domination in Traditional Asian Medical Systems*, Stuttgart: F. Steiner Verlag.

Lanjouw, J. (1997). *The Introduction of Pharmaceutical Product Patents in India: 'Heartless Exploitation of the Poor and Suffering'?*, National Bureau of Economic Research Working Paper No. 6366, Los Angeles, CA: UCLA Department of Economics.

Léonard, J. (1981). *La médecine entre les savoirs et les pouvoirs*, Paris: Editions Aubier Montaigne.

Lopez, D. (1998). *Prisoners of Shangri-La: Tibetan Buddhism and the West*, Chicago, IL: University of Chicago Press.

Meyer, F. (1981 [2002]). *Le système médical tibétain, Gso-Ba Rig-Pa*, Paris: Presses du CNRS.

Meyer, F. (1986). Orient–Occident: un dialogue singulier, *Autrement* 85: 124–133.

Meyer, F. (1993). La médecine tibétaine: tradition ancienne et nouveaux enjeux. In O. Moulin (ed.), *Tibet, l'envers du décor*, Genève: Olizane.

Michaud, J. (1990). Mais entrez donc! Les entrepreneurs touristiques et le pouvoir au Ladakh (Inde), *Anthropologie et Sociétés* (14)3: 127–139.

Mills, M. (1999). Belief and the Priest, Religious Reform and Ethical Self-Determination in Buddhist Ladakh, *Scottish Journal of Religious Studies* 19(2): 167–185.

Namgyal, Sh. P. and Phuntsog, S. T. (1994). Intellectual Property Rights of the Amchi System of Medicine, Petition issued on behalf of the Ladakh Amchi Sabha, Leh.

Namgyal, Sh. P. and Phuntsog, S. T. (1995). Demand for Protection, Ladakh's Indigenous Medicine is under Threat from Large International Companies, *Ladags Melong*, Spring.

Pandey, G. (1990). *The Construction of Communalism in Colonial North India*, Delhi: Oxford University Press.

Pordié, L. (2000). Tibetan Medicine: The Dynamic of a Biocultural Object in a Context of Social Change, Paper presented at the International Academic Conference on Tibetan Medicine, University of Lhasa – CMAM, Lhasa, May.

Pordié, L. (2002). La pharmacopée comme expression de société: Une étude himalayenne. In J. Fleurentin, G. Mazars and J. M. Pelt (eds), *Des sources du savoir aux médicaments du futur*, Paris: Editions de l'IRD – SFE.

Pordié, L. (2003). *The Expression of Religion in Tibetan Medicine: Ideal Conceptions, Contemporary Practices and Political Use*, PPSS Series 29, Pondicherry: FIP.

Pordié, L. (2005). Claims for Intellectual Property and the Illusion of Conservation: A Brief Anthropological Unpacking of a 'Development' Failure. In Y. Aumeeruddy-Thomas, M. Karki, D. Parajuli and K. Gurung (eds), *Himalayan Medicinal and Aromatic Plants:*

Balancing Use and Conservation, Kathmandu: IDRC Canada, WWF Nepal, UNESCO/ WWF People and Plants Initiative.

Pordié, L. (2007). Ethnographies of 'Folk Healing', *Indian Anthropologist* 37(1), January: 1–12.

Roepstorff, A., Bubandt, N. and Kull, K. (eds) (2003). *Imagining Nature: Practices of Cosmology and Identity*, Aarhus: Aarhus University Press.

Sehgal, R. (2002). *Trifurcation Tangle* (interview with Thupstan Chhewang), *Times of India*, 20 August.

Sonam, W. (2002). Ladakhis Unite for UT Status, *Ladags Melong*, October.

Subramanian, A. (1999). India as User and Creator of Intellectual Property: The Challenges Post-Seattle, Paper presented at the Workshop on South Asia and the WTO, New Delhi, 20–21 December.

Swanson, T. (ed.) (1995). *Intellectual Property Rights and Biodiversity Conservation: An Interdiciplinary Analysis of the Value of Medicinal Plants*, Cambridge: Cambridge University Press.

Tager, D. K. (1999). Tendzin Tcheudrak vu de l'intérieur, *L'actualité des religions* 3.

Tan, L. M. (1999). *Good Medicine: Pharmaceuticals and the Construction of Power and Knowledge in the Philippines*, Amsterdam: Het Spinhuis.

Tashi, M. (2002). What Do the New MLAs Say?, *Ladags Melong*, October: 16–18.

Timmermans, K. (2003). Intellectual Property Rights and Traditional Medicine: Policy Dilemmas at the Interface, *Social Science and Medicine* 57: 745–756.

Tully, J. (2000). Une étude politique de l'identité. In W. Kymlicka and S. Mesure (eds), *Les identités culturelles*, Comprendre, 1, Paris: Presses Universitaires de France.

van Beek, M. (1998). True Patriots: Justifying Autonomy for Ladakh, *Himalayan Research Bulletin* 18(1): 35–45.

van Beek, M. (2000a). Beyond Identity Fetishism: 'Communal' Conflict in Ladakh and the Limits of Autonomy, *Cultural Anthropology* 15(4): 525–569.

van Beek, M. (2000b). Dissimulations: Representing Ladakhi 'Identity'. In H. Driessen and T. Otto (eds), *Perplexities of Identification: Anthropological Studies in Cultural Differentiation and the Use of Resources*, Aarhus: Aarhus University Press.

van Beek, M. (2001). Making a Difference? Reflections on Decentralization, Recognition, and Empowerment, Paper presented at the Conference on Global Developments in the 21st Century, Polson Institute of Global Studies, Cornell University, 21–22 September.

van Beek, M. (2004). Dangerous Liaisons: Hindu Nationalism and Buddhist Radicalism in Ladakh. In S. Limaye, M. Malik and R. Wirsing (eds), *Religious Radicalism and Security in South Asia*, Honolulu, HI: Asia-Pacific Center for Security Studies.

van Beek, M. and Bertelsen, B. K. (1997). No Present without Past: The 1989 Agitation in Ladakh. In T. Dodin and H. Räther (eds), *Recent Research on Ladakh*, Vol. 7, Ulm: Ulmerkulturanthropologishe Schriften.

Weber, M. (1959 [1919]). *Le savant et le politique*, Paris: Plon.

WHO (World Health Organization) (2000). *Announcement of the Inter-regional Workshop on Intellectual Property Rights in the Context of Traditional Medicine*, December, Bangkok: WHO.

WHO (2003). *Traditional Medicine*, Resolution of the World Health Assembly, WHA56.31, 28 May.

Xaxa, V. (2003). Tribes in India. In V. Das (ed.), *The Oxford Indian Companion to Sociology and Social Anthropology*, 2 vols, New Delhi: Oxford University Press.

Zimmermann, F. (1992). Gentle Purge: The Flower Power of Ayurveda. In C. Leslie and A. Young (eds), *Paths to Asian Medical Knowledge*, Berkeley: University of California Press.

7 Tibetan medicine and biodiversity management in Dolpo, Nepal

Negotiating local and global worldviews, knowledge and practices

Yildiz Aumeeruddy-Thomas and Yeshi C. Lama

The increasing importance being given to cultural knowledge in the context of global environmental management, and the commoditization of biodiversity and of certain forms of traditional environmental knowledge, raise important questions for ethnobiologists and ethnobotanists who mediate between local and international communities (Alexiades 2004). Within this context, we examine the flows of knowledge and information, as well as the redefinition of worldviews and practices in light of increased interactions between the local and international levels, using as a case study the WWF–UNESCO People and Plants project in Dolpo District, Nepal. This project aimed to develop applied ethnobotany, to explore local 'traditional/indigenous knowledge' of plant resources, and to work with local users to develop sustainable management systems.

Dolpo is one of the remotest districts of Nepal, located in the north-western area of the country and contiguous to the north with the Tibetan Plateau. We reflect upon how Tibetan medicine practitioners in Dolpo, known as *amchi*,[1] have entered the realm of international conservation, and the implications this has had for them, both individually and collectively. Lama's (2003) earlier discussion of the relationship between the *amchi* and the conservationists[2] places the two on a continuum between the local and the global. The current paper furthers this discussion by examining the ways in which Dolpo *amchi* have, at a particular point in global conservation history, entered into certain forms of partnership with conservationists and how the process of forming these partnerships has created new social dynamics. We frame our discussion around the concept of 'local/traditional knowledge' and explore how this concept, appropriated by the WWF–UNESCO People and Plants project, was reconstructed locally.

Much attention has been given to indigenous knowledge and practices in the discourse of conservation management over the last two decades. The central aim has been to find ways of bridging the gaps between scientific and local/traditional knowledge and practices (Ellen *et al.* 2000). Scientific knowledge is widely assumed to be disconnected from social and political spheres and to be essentially global, while indigenous knowledge is seen to be restricted to specific localities and socially constructed. Biodiversity conservation approaches are thus assumed to be scientific, while the approach and practices of the *amchi* are associated with local indigenous knowledge. However, it is becoming increasingly accepted that all knowledge, including scientific knowledge, is socially produced (Latour 1997) and that different knowledge systems represent 'a plethora of partial perspectives and situated practices among diverse social actors' (Leach and Fairhead 2002: 299).

We focus here on the forms of engagement between holders of different knowledge systems as they work towards a partially shared goal: the conservation and management of medicinal plants. Medicinal plant scarcity is indeed an issue faced by *amchi* throughout the Himalayas, owing to an increasing national and international demand for 'natural' medicines (Lama *et al.* 2001; Pordié 2002). Issues surrounding access to knowledge, and the contested rights to act upon it, emerge through this encounter between local dynamics and global agendas. Following earlier discussions by Lama (2003), we reflect on how the 'flexible selves' of different actors in development and conservation projects enable learning processes that bring together different types of knowledge and worldviews, thus reshaping social and political positions. We also discuss how traditional knowledge can transcend local and national frontiers to interact directly with international efforts for biodiversity conservation.

In examining relationships between *amchi*, conservationists and other social groups, we focus on the *amchi*'s knowledge of plants and their ecology, their symbolic understanding of plants and space, and the ways in which their knowledge interacts with that of the other actors through collaborative efforts. We examine how the work undertaken in Dolpo influenced the perception of medicinal plants and the transmission of knowledge from the *amchi* to other members of their community. We explore how the *amchi* saw in the project opportunities not only for improving local health and management of medicinal plants, but also for advancing their socio-political status, and the extent to which the conservationists accommodated their various agendas. The project made some aspects of the *amchi*'s knowledge known to the larger scientific community, resource managers and policy makers, both nationally and internationally and, in doing so, increased the visibility of the *amchi* as a group. We examine the means through which the project promoted a specific aspect of the *amchi*'s knowledge, the reasons for doing so and the implications of this.

From local indigenous knowledge to global heritage

The concept of 'local/traditional knowledge' is a social construct as well as an environmental tool. It is today strongly influenced by global environmental management discourse and norms, through the important position it has been afforded in the international arena (Cormier-Salem and Roussel 2002; Michon 2002). The very use of concepts such as 'local' enters in consonance with the importance attributed to indigenous knowledge by global environment decision makers (Agrawal 2002).

Studies of indigenous knowledge were originally rooted in social anthropology and ethnoscience, developed in the 1950s by the New Ethnologists such as Conklin (1957) and French ethnobiologists and anthropologists such as Haudricourt (1962) and Lévi-Strauss (1962). The ethnoscientists' work, using anthropology combined with naturalist approaches, contributed to systematizing the study of the relationships between local societies and their natural environments, as well as their underlying knowledge systems and socio-cultural dynamics. Linguistic methods were highly valued, in particular the analysis of the semantic categories used in classification processes. Beyond the simple cataloguing of the use of natural ·products such as medicinal plants – a current approach in colonial ethnobotanical works (Davis 1994) – the main aim was to put more emphasis on how knowledge and praxis, or technical knowledge, are linked to cosmology, religious beliefs, internal social cohesion, and relationships of power and authority within a given society. This approach helped in understanding more clearly how societies perceive, adapt and justify their actions in relation to the natural environment.

There is widespread theoretical consensus among scholars from many fields that finds the nature–culture dichotomy to be inadequate, thus rendering the purely biological dimension of nature, a concept that underpins the majority of classical biological research, non-operational. Contrary to the dichotomized view, many societies perceive the environment to be an integrated natural and cultural object, or a social construct (Descola 2002: 83). Furthermore, variations in nature conceptions are highly marked between different localized societies, and it has been argued that such variations 'might arise from particular practices of environmental interaction' sustained by particular social ideologies (Ellen 2002: 101). Such theoretical debates, supported by a large array of studies by anthropologists and ethnobiologists, show the intricate linkages between knowledge systems and practical management approaches and have, both directly and indirectly, raised the importance given internationally by academics and managers to 'local/ traditional knowledge'.

In the early 1970s and especially during the 1972 Stockholm summit, the United Nations Environment Programme (UNEP) began drawing the world's attention to the 'global environmental crisis'. Amongst the rhetoric surrounding the fate of the planet, local agricultural practices such as shifting cultivation, utilized by small farmers from third world countries, were portrayed as major contributors to deforestation and environmental degradation. Their knowledge and practices had faced decades, if not centuries, of dismissal as being 'indigenous', 'traditional' and damaging and had, ever since the development of the modern sciences, been labelled as 'backward'. The rhetoric generated by the world environmental crisis debate led many anthropologists and ethnobiologists to develop case studies and attempt to demonstrate the validity and internal coherence of indigenous peoples' resource management systems. Many found evidence of sound environmental bases to such systems (e.g. Posey and Balee 1989). An interdisciplinary approach was adopted, linking ecologists, anthropologists, economists and agronomists in attempts to better understand the overall relationships between different elements of anthroposystems or agro-ecosystems (e.g. Jollivet 1992).

During the early 1980s, a network of committed scholars began raising awareness of the importance of indigenous knowledge for environmental management. Strict conservation approaches, especially those that advocated the exclusion of local people from protected area management, were increasingly called into question (Colchester 1999; Descola 1999). Ethical questions were raised, as the exclusionary approach tended to have adverse affects on the livelihoods of the people who originally relied on the protected areas. These approaches were further criticized as exclusion was often found to have negative effects on the conservation efforts themselves. Thereafter, the idea of 'development' was included in many conservation approaches and the concept of 'integrated conservation and development projects' began to emerge. The roles of indigenous communities living in biodiversity-rich areas in shaping and preserving the overall landscape (Fairhead and Leach 1996; Balée 2000), or in shaping agro-diversity (Brush and Meng 1998), were highlighted. Thus the loss of cultural diversity became a major element of international concern, alongside more established fears about the loss of biological diversity. Organizations such as UNESCO developed an interest in the conservation of traditional knowledge, as illustrated by the mass of literature published on food habits (Hladik *et al.* 1993), land use dynamics and sacred sites (Ramakrishnan *et al.* 1998). This work portrays the intimate linkages between biological and social systems and emphasizes the utility of such knowledge and management systems for biodiversity conservation.

The first International Congress of Ethnobiology, held in Belem in 1988, and the International Society of Ethnobiology, founded at this occasion, developed a code of ethics, namely the Belem Declaration. This certainly contributed to raising local traditional knowledge to the rank of global heritage. It also paved the way for a diversity of claims by indigenous movements in relation to local/traditional knowledge. The Declaration states:

> We members of the International Society of Ethnobiology strongly urge action as follows. Henceforth:
>
> 1　A substantial proportion of development aid be devoted to efforts aimed at ethnobiological inventory, conservation and management programs;
> 2　Mechanisms be established by which indigenous specialists are recognised as proper authorities and are consulted in all programs affecting them, their resources and their environments;
> 　. . .
> 4　Procedures be developed to compensate native peoples for the utilisation of their knowledge and their biological resources;
> 5　Educational programs be implemented to alert the global community to the value of ethnobiological knowledge for human beings.
>
> 　　　　　　　　　　　　　　　(Extracts from the Belem Declaration)

The importance of the link between 'local/traditional knowledge' and 'nature conservation' emerged and was supported by many scholars (e.g. Warren *et al.*

1995), although a range of theoretical and practical problems remained concerning how these two epistemologically very different concepts could be effectively integrated. This led to a more generalized concept of 'traditional ecological knowledge' (TEK), which has been strongly instrumentalized for the purposes of natural resource management (Berkes *et al.* 2000; Berkes and Folke 2002).

In development circles there has also been a general shift in emphasis, at least rhetorically, from 'top-down' interventions to more participatory, or 'grassroots', approaches. Modernizing and scientific/technical approaches, based on the transfer of technology, have given way to a more populist discourse (Sillitoe *et al.* 2002), with a strong participatory focus that promotes local knowledge in problem identification. Olivier de Sardan defines populism in the development context as a:

> form of relationship between the intellectuals – associated to privileged classes and groups – and the people – that is, the dominated classes and groups – in which the intellectuals discover the people, have a feeling of pity towards them and/or marvel at their capacities, and intend to serve them and contribute to their well-being.
>
> (Olivier de Sardan 1995: 19)

This author further argues that such populism is consubstantial to development, as participatory approaches are based on a complex and fundamentally uneven set of relationships between those who make the rules, deciding who should participate and setting the agenda, and those who actually participate.

Nevertheless, the promotion of participatory approaches did lead to a major shift in environmental management, especially in the development of co-management systems. Such approaches gained momentum worldwide, but were particularly well accepted in India and Nepal (Hobley 1996; Aumeeruddy *et al.* 1999). The interaction between social and ecological dynamics and the role of interdisciplinary research were highlighted by proponents of the 'new ecology', who drew attention to the role of anthropogenic disturbances on the one hand and ecological stochasticity and resilience on the other as important factors in shaping the dynamics of ecosystems (Gunderson and Holling 2002). The ecosystem concept, previously seen as a linear system that tends towards a climax and a balanced state and where disturbances, especially human disturbances, have negative impacts for the ecosystem, is now highly controversial (O'Neill 2001).

The environmental crisis also led to new concepts, such as that of biodiversity, which was born in the 1980s (Wilson and Peter 1988) and whose limits are essentially blurred, being neither strictly biological nor social (Aubertin *et al.* 1998; Aubertin 2000). The concept of biodiversity is hybrid in nature, being simultaneously an economic object (strong emphasis given to genetic resources and benefit sharing in the Convention for Biological Diversity), a social object (it is closely associated to knowledge and practices) and a political object (the role local indigenous groups and nations may play in decisions regarding their biological resources). The Earth Summit held in Rio de Janeiro in 1992 produced both the Rio Declaration and the Convention for Biological Conservation, which strengthened the role of local indigenous knowledge in environmental management, especially in relation to biodiversity.

This overview of the evolution of the status of 'local/traditional knowledge' depicts the context in which UNESCO, within its Man and Biosphere programme, WWF and the Royal Botanical Garden at Kew established a new interdisciplinary programme, the People and Plants Initiative. The main aim of the People and Plants Initiative was to develop applied ethnobotany for conservation, and sustainable and equitable use, of plant resources. Local knowledge held a central position from the outset, as did the need to build bridges between traditional and scientific knowledge to achieve conservation with a strong people-centred approach (Martin 1995; Cunningham 2001; Aumeeruddy-Thomas and Pei 2003).

People and plants in Dolpo: preliminary interactions

Dolpo is an area culturally defined by its inhabitants' strong linkages to their land, the history of their migration from the ancient kingdom of Zhangzung in Western Tibet in the seventh or eighth century (Jest 1975; Snellgrove 1992) and a way of life based upon highland agro-pastoralism. Their seasonal migrations to Tibet, prior to the closure of the Tibetan border by China in 1959, and their ongoing visits to lowland valleys for trade and barter, have created a variety of social, economic and political linkages with different localities (Bauer 2004). Bauer's analysis of the socio-economic and political relationships between Dolpo and the plains areas of Nepal to the south and the Tibetan Changthang plateau to the north show that Dolpo is not as secluded as it has been sometimes portrayed (ibid.). A 'middle road' exists for Dolpo people, enabling them to relate to the 'outer' world despite their social marginalization in Nepal (Ramble 1997). Although an airstrip, between one and five days' walk from most villages, now links it to the outside world, the area remains one of the remotest in Nepal.

Dolpo is divided into two areas, known as Upper and Lower Dolpo. Access to the upper part was restricted to foreigners for security reasons until the late 1990s, when group trekking was introduced with the payment of hefty fees (Bauer 2004). Most of the formal administrative unit of Dolpa District was incorporated in Shey Phoksundo National Park in 1984. Beyond this administrative reality, local cultural and social representations also distinguish clearly between Upper and Lower Dolpo. The upper part is inhabited by Tibetan-speaking people, whereas the lower part comprises a mix of people of Tibetan origin, and a range of Tibeto-Burman ethnic groups, including Gurung and Magar, as well as groups who have migrated more recently from the Indo-Gangetic plains of southern Nepal. The two areas are thus culturally and ecologically distinct (Kind 2002; Aumeeruddy-Thomas *et al.* 2004). In the very harsh environment of Dolpo, social cohesion, as well as natural resources, plays a major role in local livelihoods. The natural resources, while being crucial locally, are also valued internationally both as commodities for the regional and international phyto-medical markets and for biodiversity, as Dolpo was identified as a place of global importance for biodiversity conservation (Wikramanayake *et al.* 2001).

Two surveys commissioned by WWF Nepal in Dolpo, one on the situation of *amchi* practice and the other on vegetation and the status of medicinal plants, had shown that there were significant links between the practice of the *amchi* and the conservation of medicinal plants (Gurung *et al.* 1996; Shrestha *et al.* 1998). Increased harvesting for trade by non-*amchi* commercial collectors was largely responsible for the depletion of certain species (Lama *et al.* 2001; Ghimire *et al.* 2004). The *amchi* also saw their medical practice declining, mainly because of economic difficulties.[3] They emphasized their lack of formal recognition by the government, which denied them the right to practise in local health posts despite the fact that these were largely empty owing to the lack of qualified staff willing to stay in such remote areas (Shrestha *et al.* 1998). As Dolpo was one of the most important areas for high-altitude medicinal plants in Nepal, WWF Nepal and the WWF–UNESCO People and Plants Initiative project team headed there in 1997.

The project team, comprising botanists and ecologists from Tribhuvan University in Kathmandu, an ethno-ecologist, an anthropologist and two expert *amchi*[4] from Mustang, reached Lake Phoksundo in Dolpo in June 1997. WWF Nepal's Northern Mountain Conservation Project (NMCP), a USAID-funded programme, was then operating in Dolpo as a partner of the Department of National Parks and Wildlife Conservation with the aim of strengthening community-based approaches in the park. A large gathering of people had been called for an initial field planning meeting of the People and Plants project. Many of the most prominent Dolpo *amchi* were present, as were the local and international NGOs operating in the area, and groups of women and young people from the adjoining villages who had recently been mobilized into Sister Groups and Eco Clubs.[5]

It is a common feature of 'new conservation' approaches to organize people into 'workable' groups, although this generally marks the members as somehow different from the rest of the community and may generate tensions. Such groups are given the opportunity to express their views in decisions and planning phases and in this case most were registered under the buffer zone user committee group. This committee was created specifically to represent the different interest groups living in the national park and surrounding zones.

It is in this culturally assorted context that Dolpo *amchi* were encouraged to express their views on the issues of scarcity and access to medicinal plants, individually as well as in an informally constituted group. The scientists put forward the essential paradigm of conservation, mainly through pointing out that some plants may become rare because of over-harvesting. Issues pertaining to the access to, and control over, plants by different social groups, and to the amounts of plants harvested, were introduced as vital factors underlying the concept of conservation.

It is notable that the Dolpo *amchi* remained relatively quiet following intro-ductory speeches by the Park warden, a representative of the WWF Nepal project in Dolpo, and representatives of international organizations. It was only following the speech of the young botanist Suresh Ghimire from Tribhuvan University in Kathmandu that the *amchi* reacted. The botanist voiced his concern about threats to medicinal plants species in the area, building his argument on his extensive knowledge of the botany and ecology of these species. The *amchi* then highlighted their own concerns about depletion and access, as the plants are essential elements of their practice. This shows that their initial encounter with scientific botanical knowledge highlighted certain areas of convergence concerning the concept of conservation and, at least to some extent, the reasons for plant depletion.

The *amchi*'s knowledge of medicinal species appealed to the project team, as it appeared to offer sound potential for setting up sustainable approaches to harvesting medicinal plants. Developing applied research that builds upon local ethnobotanical and ethno-ecological knowledge was indeed a key approach promoted by the People and Plants initiative. As a result of this new dynamic, which brought the *amchi* into interaction with the conservationists,[6] the *amchi* emphasized their knowledge and use of medicinal plants in meeting the health care needs of the local population.

However, their ability to practise medicine has been largely diminished by their material conditions, leaving them with little resources or time to devote to the study and practice of medicine. The *amchi* pointed to the recent degradation of their medical tradition, which was partly attributed to their invisibility and irrelevance to the policy makers in Kathmandu. Two major ideas germinated at this initial meeting: firstly, the forming of an association of Dolpo *amchi*; and, secondly, the building of a traditional health care centre. The association, which was actually formed two years later, represented an institutionalizing process by which the Dolpo *amchi* hoped to be able to strengthen their roles as health care providers and advocate their demands for support at the national level. These ideas may have been influenced by the *amchi* experts, who were themselves engaged in such actions elsewhere. While the sustainable use of medicinal and aromatic plants (MAPs) and the will to achieve national legitimacy and recognition for their medical system were key interests of the *amchi*, the conservationists were mainly interested in the former. The promotion of sustainable use of medicinal plants and of their management in and around Shey Phoksundo National Park was the conservationists' motto.[7]

At the occasion of this meeting another local group, the women, voiced their concerns, mainly in terms of access to knowledge related to the use of medicinal plants for primary health care. They pointed to their essential role in child care, as well as to their personal concerns surrounding what they termed as 'women's diseases', which were frequent in Dolpo and required more attention than they were being given by the male *amchi*. This advocacy role played by the Sister Groups, organized by the WWF Nepal project, show how a recently set-up project, through organizing people into formal and identifiable groups, has led the women to position themselves more formally in the health care sphere.[8]

Another group that attended this meeting comprised people from the southern buffer zone villages, largely representing the interests of the commercial collectors. They also expressed their interest in collaborating in the project, as they saw opportunities for obtaining support for the domestication of highly valuable medicinal plants, as well as the development of value addition processes. Although commercial collection represents a major threat to medicinal plants in Dolpo, the project chose to work in priority with the *amchi*. Several reasons led the team to make this apparently paradoxical choice: 1) people inhabiting the park were seen as immediate stakeholders and more directly affected by the establishment of the park; and 2) the immediate importance of medicinal plants conservation for the health care of the communities living inside the park and in its eastern buffer zone (Dho Tarap) seemed of higher priority. These proximate issues also appeared easier to address than those pertaining to commercial trade in the southern buffer zone, because of the complex role of market factors of which the team had little experience. The people inhabiting the park were seen as the logical 'stewards' of the natural resources, despite their lack of formal roles or decision-making power relating to resource management. The project team hoped that these groups would be able to recover their customary rights and to jointly manage their resources with the park managers – uniting against external poachers – to protect resources which were, at the same time, essential for their medical practice.

This approach aimed to favour cultural resources, include local people's knowledge and practices, and promote formal and informal institutions as means of guiding management practices in the protected area. This has been tried elsewhere, such as in the Kayan Mentarang conservation project in Kalimantan (Indonesia), and has been critically analysed by Eghenter and Sellato (2003). This project, entitled the Culture and Conservation Project, recommended a change of status from strict nature reserve to national park and proved that the communities' actual presence and strong cultural identity could contribute to minimizing the risk of encroachment by outside parties. This project also helped in the official recognition of traditional systems and regulation methods, as well as the role of local institutions in the management of the national park. One major and long-lasting effect of the project was the capacity building of the indigenous researchers, which helped local people to reflect on their own practices in relation to conservation. It also showed that traditional management could lead to over-exploitation in situations of competitiveness related to exogenous factors. The Dolpo People and Plants project, to a large extent, pursued very similar goals to the Kayan Mentarang project. Although some attempts had been made previously to integrate the cultural dimensions of conservation management pioneered in the Makalu Barun conservation area project (Ramble and Chapagain 1990), prior to the People and Plants project no such systematic approach, building upon local knowledge and practices, had been developed in the Himalayas.

In Shey Phoksundo National Park, existing policies do not allow resources to be used for commercial collection. The *amchi*, although not directly involved in commercial harvesting, expressed their wish that certain widely distributed and very common species of medicinal plants should be allowed for collection in the park, and not only for local medicinal purposes. The *amchi* felt that limited selling or bartering of such plants should also be allowed, to enable them to purchase the precious lowland medicinal plants that are crucial for their medical practice. This point was emphasized by an external technical analysis of the project (Leaman *et al.* 1999).

During the initial planning meeting, the *amchi* also called for more protection by the park authorities of the resources lying within the park. They highlighted the fact that, since the establishment of the national park, the *amchi* and their communities had lost any form of traditional control of their territory and thus the ability to protect the resources therein. Indeed, the establishment of the national park de facto subsumed all their customary rights, since the national park authorities are responsible for maintaining law and order within the park, according to the Forestry Act of 1993. Only the villages and agricultural lands lying within the park boundaries had been declared as buffer zones, while the high meadows that had been used for many centuries by the people, and on which a major part of their economy relies, had come under the jurisdiction of the park. People had been granted informal use rights for livelihood purposes, but no formal access rights to these areas had been offered. This is a vivid example of how state power dominates local authority systems, with little consideration of local social dynamics – a situation frequently encountered throughout the Himalayas (Saberwal 1996).

Therefore, people living inside the park relied entirely on the regulatory management system of the park to protect their cultural and natural resources against the commercial collectors, whom they considered to be ignorant and whose harvesting practices were perceived as having a depleting effect on the resources. Although cases elsewhere in the Himalayas, especially in Ladakh (Pordié 2002), show that *amchi* are engaged in different practices of collection linked to larger trade circuits, Dolpo *amchi* collect essentially for local health care use. Different studies undertaken by this project have demonstrated that their ethno-ecological knowledge has, to date, promoted harvesting practices that were sustainable (Ghimire *et al.* 2004, 2005).

A high priority was thus given for work with the *amchi*, who were perceived as having the highest level of ethnobotanical and ethno-ecological knowledge and assumed to be an important attribute for conservation. It was also assumed that the commercial collectors had a lower level of ethno-ecological knowledge. An analysis conducted later on, however, on variations in levels of knowledge between different medicinal plants users, showed that commercial collectors had relatively high and specific ethno-ecological knowledge regarding the plants that they collected for trade. This knowledge remained largely unused, because harvesting patterns are actually driven by very poorly organized market circuits (Ghimire *et al.* 2004). Rather than a case of lack of knowledge, problems were arising from knowledge that was not being put into practice, compounded by a range of economic factors. Although more time and resources were spent to work with the Tibetan communities living inside the park, the project rectified this initial oversight by including some work with external commercial collectors in 2001, four years after its inception. A major component of this work concerned setting up domestication and cultivation trials with the collectors.

Navigating across different knowledge systems

The *amchi* of Shey Phoksundo National Park and its surrounding areas practise Tibetan medicine, a regionally shared knowledge system based on the scholarly Tibetan medical texts, with the addition of local empirical knowledge. Our studies in Dolpo confirmed that the *materia medica* used in Dolpo was partly based on species only found in Nepal, which differ from those highlighted in contemporary medical texts such as the Trungpe Dimey Shelgi Melong (*'khrungs dpe dri med shel gyi me long*).

The relationship between the *amchi* and the conservationists was forged largely owing to the increased trade in medicinal plants from Dolpo and the importance of these plants for the practice of the *amchi*. The global concern for biodiversity conservation has some partial connections with these local realities, conceptually, symbolically and materially, while being on the other hand partly incommensurable. How then does the global agenda of conservation and sustainable use of medicinal plants play out in the day-to-day lives of the *amchi* in Nepal? To answer this question we must identify the specific pathways by which these different realities meet and explore the exchanges and transformations that ensue from these encounters.

The work of the People and Plants project involved close interactions with the *amchi* in different ways and under a variety of conditions. Many discussions took place during meetings, whereby the Dolpo *amchi*, as a group, expressed their opinions about plant scarcity, uses, and harvesting patterns, and engaged in species prioritization exercises for inclusion in a book on *amchi* knowledge and medicinal plants (see Lama *et al.* 2001). The team, made up of both the authors, an ecologist, a botanist, park game scouts and a few expert *amchi*, worked with individual *amchi* in identifying medicinal plants in the alpine meadows and searching through local medical texts to figure out the properties and effects of key medicinal plants and their botanical identification.

The focus, beyond the simple identification of medicinal plant species, was on the interpretation of semantic categories and on seeking to understand how the *amchi* classify plants and how they understand their life cycles, design land units and elements of landscapes. The major aim was to learn from *amchi* knowledge and to discuss and cross-examine this knowledge in view of the reference system that arises from 'scientific knowledge'. This work entailed discussions with individual *amchi* on their specific knowledge about medicinal plants, as well as discussions with larger groups of *amchi*, which served to establish the level of homogeneity in plant classification amongst the Dolpo *amchi*. Work focused, for example, on identifying the categories by which the *amchi* organize the plant world. Two or three of the *amchi* who worked directly with the research team dug out terminologies not in current usage, but which corresponded to certain botanical concepts, such as how to define a plant family. Results of this exchange are given in the box.

The box does not show complete correspondence between botanical and *amchi* classifications. For example, the differentiation of herbs and grasses into seven categories and the differentiation of trees into two major categories (trees with and without thorns) are forms of classification that are not found in the botanical classificatory system. In conducting this analysis, it became obvious that many of these terms are the closest equivalents that the *amchi* could find for the purpose of sharing their knowledge with the botanists. The botanists, having developed a strong practical working relationship with the *amchi* in the field, were able to distinguish

Ethnobotanical rank categories in amchi botanical classification

In life form, *shing* (woody plants) are further classified into four categories, namely *shing sdong* (large trees), *nag sdong* (small trees or large shrubs), *'khri shing* (climbers) and *'db ma* (shrubs), whereas *sngo ldum* (herbaceous plants) are further classified into *sngo ldum* (herbs) and *rtswa* (grass).

Below life form ranks, there are two intermediate ranks, based on flower and fruiting characters. In intermediate 1, all the *shing sdong* (which contains various species of trees) are further divided into two categories based on whether the plant flowers or not: *me tog can gyi shing sdong* (plant with flower) and *me tog med p'i shing sdong* (plant without any distinct flower). Similarly in intermediate 1, all the *sngo ldum* (herbs and grass) are directly classified into seven categories based on the morphology of fruits, roots and flower. These seven categories of *sngo ldum* are *gng bu can* (plants with bean-like fruits), *'brs bu can* (plants with ovoid fruits), *tsug* (plants with mustard-like fruits), *rtsa ba* (plants with small roots), *rtaa ba che ba* (plants with large roots), *me tog can* (plants with distinct flower) and *me tog med pa* (plants without flower or with indistinct flower). All the lower plants (fungi, lichens, hepatics, mosses and ferns) are grouped in *sngo ldum* under *me tog med pa*.

In intermediate 2, all the trees which flower, *me tog can gyi shing sdong*, are further divided into two on the basis of presence or absence of thorn. Thus, the thorny trees are divided into *tshar ma can gi shing* (*tshar ma* – thorn), and non-thorny trees are grouped into *tshar ma med p'i shing*.

Below the two intermediates, there is another rank locally referred to as *rigs*. However, the word *rigs* is used only in some cases. It is a theoretical concept that *amchi* use when asked to comment in relation to the integration of different groups of plants into a higher level of hierarchy. It represents a small grouping of several groups of plants bearing a similar generic term (generics) that are considered to be similar in either habit, plant morphology, use, property, etc.

(Source: Lama *et al.* 2001)

within this discourse between what was approximation for the sake of promoting understanding and what was actually the current discourse used by the *amchi*. This was particularly necessary regarding the ways of distinguishing one species from another. During long discussions with larger groups of *amchi*, it was generally acknowledged that the terminologies were correct, although some of the *amchi* seemed puzzled because some of the terminologies, although useful for interacting with the research team, were rarely used among themselves.

In scholarly research, the ethnobotanist aims to understand and record the meanings of local semantic categories, with no other objective than to establish the coherence of the classification system. In this case of applied research, *amchi*, scientists and conservationists engaged in an exchange of knowledge, for the purpose of gaining social and political recognition for the former, and for the purpose of conservation for the latter. Their different forms of knowledge were thus in an ongoing state of engagement and negotiation, following similar processes to those detailed by Leach and Fairhead (2002). Partial perspectives and situated practices play a major role in the expression of knowledge, which is itself a mirror reflecting the engagements between the researcher and the local 'informants'. This form of analysis, which has been extensively used in academic ethnoscientific research, can thus be used in applied research. How social and biological scientists position themselves in such situations raises a number of ethical and political issues because, although they are involved in research, they are also social mediators between local groups and larger national and international forums (Orlove and Brush 1996: 330; Eghenter and Sellato 2003: 17).

This classification exercise illustrates how the *amchi* adopted certain aspects of the system used by the botanist, thus offering an example of the local interpretation of scientific classifications. Ordering and classifying are known to refer to worldviews and to ways of conceptualizing nature, as well as to arise from particular practices (Friedberg 1992). In this case, the partial expression of the *amchi*'s knowledge and the effort made to integrate the scientists' classificatory approach was a way for the *amchi* to navigate and negotiate between two worldviews.

Vernacular classifications are also known to be multilayered, with much overlapping between purely naturalist approaches and other forms of symbolic or utilitarian classification processes, which are not necessarily made explicit in vernacular nomenclature. Thus, other forms of classifications used by the *amchi*, such as ordering medicinal plant resources according to their medical properties and uses, were downplayed in the course of interactions with scientists and conservation managers, whose main purpose was the sustainable management of resources. For example, the three fruits of *Terminalia chebula*, *Terminalia bellerica* and *Phyllanthus emblica* referred to as 'the three fruits' (*'brs bu gsum*, *'brs bu*), which are crucial to *amchi* medicine, and the six species including *Elletaria cardamomum*, *Syzigium aromaticum*, *Myristica fragrans* and *Carthamus tictorius* referred to as the *bzng po drug* (literally the 'six good', meaning six good plants highly appreciated for medicine, but also in religious rituals as offerings) are equivalent to panacea types in *amchi* medicine. However, they were barely mentioned at all in the classifications discussed with the botanist. All medicinal plants and materials for making medicine are said to have six tastes: sweet (*mngar*), sour (*skyur*), salty (*lan tshwa*), pungent/acrid (*tsha ba*), bitter (*kha ba*) and astringent (*bska ba*). In addition to the six tastes, medicines have three post-digestive tastes (*zhi rjes*) and eight potencies (*nus pa*): heavy (*lci*), light (*yang*), oily (*snum*), coarse (*rtsub*), cool (*sil*), hot (*tsha*), blunt (*rtul*) and sharp (*rno ba*). Examples of medicinal plants having a sweet taste were given by the *amchi* during the course of discussions relating to their medical practices, while such classifications were never referred to in the context of situated practices relating to management.

The analysis of this knowledge proved very useful in establishing how best to define the objects around which the project revolved, i.e. the medicinal plants. It also provided a framework for discussing plant life cycles and habitats, as well as collection practices, parts of plants collected, seasons of collection, and choice of best habitats for collection, as understood by the *amchi* on the one hand and the ecologist on the other. This framework was also used in a joint exercise between the *amchi*, the game scouts and the project botanist/ecologist, which focused on two species of major importance both for local use and for trade. This exercise was conducted in high-pasture areas in Pungmo, with the *amchi* involved in the design of the ecological experiment (e.g. the sampling of sites) and in the simulation of their selective harvesting practices, as well as in the ecological monitoring processes, which used the different stages of plant life cycles to follow up on the fate of medicinal plant populations (cf. Ghimire *et al.* 2005).[9] Such stages were used by both the local team and the scientific team, on the basis of a consensual understanding.

Apart from the use of this collaborative framework, the exercise derives entirely from classical approaches in ecology, through the monitoring of densities, frequencies and abundances. Further to this experiment, which obviously incorporated the two types of knowledge, the *amchi* were asked to simulate *in situ* their very selective approach to harvesting, which is based upon the selection of mature life stages and those plants seen as most vigorous and potent from a medical perspective. They were instructed to simulate their own approach to collection, i.e. collection of about 10 per cent of the plant population, and then to increase this level to 75 per cent to enable the measurement of the population's reaction to different levels of harvesting. In other words, this exercise aimed to establish whether *amchi* collection practices are sustainable, as well as to determine the highest level of pressure that could be sustainably applied (Ghimire *et al.* 2005). These exercises illustrate how the knowledge of the *amchi* was integrated with that of the scientists in the course of what are referred to as 'practising relationships'. It is also an example of how what is generally thought of as local knowledge can transcend the local level, through its integration in broader scientific experiments that may have a demonstration value at a larger level.

Understanding management systems in a particular locality also implies understanding how people manage the space where medicinal plants grow. Studies of local toponomy in a high-pasture area in Pungmo showed that the landscape is ordered, and therefore appropriated in everyday life, on the basis of morphological characteristics such as vegetation types or specific plant species (e.g. *spng rtsi do bo*), real and symbolic animals either visiting or related symbolically to ecological zones (e.g. *skyung ka thang*; *skyung ka* is a mythical bird in Tibetan cosmology), and types of forbs and grass quality, as well as spirits known to inhabit the landscape (Aumeeruddy-Thomas *et al.* 2004). In addition to naming the landscape, ritual and religious practices, such as annual pilgrimages and festivals, are celebrated to pay tribute to local deities, such as *lha*, *gzhi bdag* and *klu*, and to request permission to use the area, practices which are common in many other communities of Tibetan origin (see Ramble 1997). The analysis of how people related to the high-pasture area during the different circumambulations of the Yulha Chulsa[10] pilgrimage in Pungmo highlights the gap between the scientist's naturalist vision, which generally considers morphology, relief and sometimes vegetation, and the local relationship to the landscape, which does not draw a stark divide between natural and supra-natural elements. However, as the project essentially aimed at understanding the cultural dimension of local management practices, it moved beyond strict scientific understandings of the landscape to incorporate supra-natural elements in different exercises. These included resource mapping, during which the *amchi* located the distribution of medicinal plants, including mythical as well as naturalist elements.

The greatest resistance encountered in terms of sharing knowledge (which was generally done quite openly) was in the discussions on the use of substitutes for species that are rare and endangered. Such species face depletion because of their limited distribution, their high extraction for trade, their difficult regeneration owing to the parts used, and their high number of users. In earlier times, when access to the Terai was more laborious, the *amchi* used local species as substitutes for important lowland species such as *Terminalia*. While the *amchi* disclosed several species for which substitutes were currently being used, this subject found less enthusiasm and interest than others. Although some learned *amchi* advocate using substitutes for problematic species and many *amchi* claimed to be doing so, others, including one of the expert *amchi*, felt that the use of substitutes would degrade the quality of their medicines. It is interesting to note here the differences of opinion amongst *amchi* themselves on this topic. At the national-level *amchi* workshops, however, the *amchi* came up with a list of substitutes that were acknowledged to be effective for use by the authoritative Chagpori (*Lcags po ri*) Institute at Darjeeling. During his visit to Nepal, one of the Institute representatives enumerated a list of plants that should be used as substitutes to avoid over-exploitation of the original species. In theory, medicinal substances may be substituted for one another if their taste (*ro*) and potency (*nus-pa*) are similar to the original ingredient. However, the project held back in the push for substitution, as it was felt that the impetus came largely from a narrow vision of species focused on conservation.

Another instance of 'practising relationships' relates to the engagement of the services of the 'expert *amchi*' from the neighbouring district of Mustang in the initial years of the project. Reflecting upon this practice of importing expertise and its unspoken impact upon the Dolpo *amchi*, in later phases the project started to rely more upon a local expert, who was unanimously declared as the most knowledgeable *amchi* by the other Dolpo *amchi*. Such a move no doubt enhanced the confidence of those *amchi* who had experienced less exposure to the mainstream of events and processes that concerned them and impacted upon them. The local expert *amchi* was directly involved in determining local priorities and preparing agendas and programmes for *amchi* workshops, and was in regular consultation with the various *amchi* associations. Furthermore, he had to be in constant communication with the Nepali-speaking project personnel, who were from outside Dolpo. Through dialogue, however slow and laborious, the Dolpo *amchi* must learn to speak a new language and engage more closely with development and conservation concepts in order to promote their tradition. The switch from external experts to a local expert *amchi* thus provided greater opportunities to the Dolpo *amchi* to increase their visibility and participation in wider development processes.

Practising relationships are, however, rarely smooth or clear and often entail a fair degree of misunderstanding and negotiation. Following requests from the *amchi* for medical texts to further their pursuit of knowledge and training, especially among younger *amchi*, the project team procured some key materials, including modern Tibetan medical texts. However, there were concerns about some texts, which were considered by the external evaluators of the project to be eroding or downplaying the knowledge of the local *amchi*. These texts included the *'khrungs dpe dri med shel gyi me long*, a classical Tibetan text book illustrated with a large number of botanical plates. This book has been widely adopted by the Dolpo *amchi*, who lengthily commented on its content, especially on the recipes and identification of plants. In certain cases, the plants differed from the Dolpo species they used. External evaluators, however, were concerned that such texts, seen as external to Dolpo, may act as a type of authoritative standardized knowledge base which could transform the Dolpo *amchi*'s own knowledge. However, the project considered that there was no need to cut Dolpo *amchi* from information sources, since they had themselves expressed their interest in having access to medical texts that they did not possess.

Such concerns, although relevant, were not viewed as major by the project team, as specificities of *amchi* knowledge are unlikely to disappear if they are relevant to the *amchi* themselves. Furthermore, in the quest for government recognition, there have been moves by the Himalayan Amchi Association towards the standardization of knowledge (through developing a standard curriculum to present to the government). In the last few years, the Himalayan Amchi Association has introduced training on medical theory taught by *amchi* graduates from a medical school in Darjeeling, India, courses which most of the Dolpo *amchi* attended.

Changing social relationships

A community-based model for the management of medicinal plants and for the promotion of *amchi* practice in Dolpo emerged as a major objective of the project after the first year of general surveys that were conducted throughout the region. One community, that of Pungmo in Lower Dolpo, chose to construct a Traditional Health Care Centre (THCC) through their Village Development Committee – a decision that was strongly supported by the project team. This situation created some tensions between the Upper and Lower Dolpo *amchi*, with the former believing that they had been left out of the whole planning process. They strongly voiced their interest in having the THCC in Upper Dolpo rather than Lower Dolpo. This tension finally led to the Upper Dolpo *amchi* achieving, at a later stage of the project and on their own initiative, the establishment of a second clinic in Dho Tarap, as well as forming the Upper Dolpo *amchi* association, which was supported by the project only after its formation.

The People and Plants project saw the first clinic, in Lower Dolpo, both as an opportunity to develop a monitoring centre for the conservation of medicinal plants inside the park and as a way to provide quality health care services and promote *amchi* knowledge. Negotiations took place with the *amchi* to ensure that the conservation and sustainable use of medicinal plants would be a major objective of the centre, in addition to the health care and promotion role, which were the primary concerns for the *amchi*. Before the THCC was inaugurated in June 2000, an exercise aimed at identifying species to be used at the clinic and to identify the potentially vulnerable species was developed. The concept of 'vulnerable species' was not well understood by the *amchi* at the outset. However, over the course of the exercise they came to understand more clearly the purpose of this prioritizing exercise, which was based on their own knowledge of plant distribution, abundance, parts used and amounts needed by the clinic (Tripathi and Schmitt 2001). Thus a list of potentially vulnerable species was established, on the basis of the criteria outlined above, but also considering the potential external demand. These priority species were to be closely monitored by a Medicinal Plants Management Committee that, although not yet recognized by the national park, was formed on a voluntary basis and comprised young people from Phoksundo villages. This group had been proposed previously, in the management plan of the national park, to serve as a link between the THCC and the park for the monitoring of medicinal plants.

This approach has not yet proved to be a workable one, however, as the *amchi* generally prefer to collect the plants themselves. Any assistance they might require is generally organized informally, on the basis of mutual confidence and the *amchi*'s appreciation of the harvesters' knowledge. Women have thus been identified in Pungmo village as the main providers of medicinal plants to the *amchi*, because of the long periods they spend in the highland pastures during summer while taking care of the herds. While the *amchi* did not reject entirely the forming of the Medicinal Plants Management Committee, it became obvious that, without continuous support from the project, the committee would not function. However, the committee did continue to collect plants for the clinic and record the amounts collected for each species, which allows for some degree of assessment of the impact of collection for the clinic.

The Lower Dolpo THCC inauguration was a subject of pride both for the *amchi* and for the local communities. It also was an occasion for representatives from the district administration offices to extend their wishes to further support the *amchi* in their new endeavour. Religious chanting and prayers in the clinic central room by the groups of Upper Dolpo and Lower Dolpo *amchi* is one of the activities that helped in establishing linkages between the Dolpo *amchi* as a group. Other activities included the plantation of selected medicinal plants species in the THCC garden.

Domestication of Himalayan medicinal plants is a subject of high interest among the *amchi*. All of them had individually attempted some experiments in their home gardens, but most efforts had been directed towards *in situ* planting, where it was felt that the species would retain their medical potency. Besides plantation trials, all *amchi* had brought about ten of the most used species of medicinal plants for the purposes of identification. These dried samples were used for verifying their identification by going through botanical flora and Tibetan medical texts, and the samples were displayed in the clinic, with both Tibetan medical terms and botanical names. One expert *amchi*, who was previously involved in domestication trials in Mustang, had been actively exchanging experiences, seeds and planting materials with the Dolpo *amchi*.

The project also encouraged the planting of medicinal plants in the THCC garden for demonstration purposes, but the *amchi* were not convinced by this as they thought that the plants would not thrive in the conditions around the centre. That they still went ahead with the garden was a sign that they were willing to engage and share experiences with the project. Moreover, it shows the symbolic importance of this practice vis-à-vis all the people who visited the garden during the inauguration.

The THCC inauguration was an important occasion for social representation for the *amchi* of Dolpo, both Lower and Upper. It asserted their identity as a group, despite their internal tensions, and in this respect was shown to be quite successful. The *amchi*'s reach to patients had now increased from the local communities to the members of the district administration, national park staff, army personnel, occasional tourists and even passing insurgents. However, the social consequences of this new institution are still difficult to assess. A major issue lies in the fact that the *amchi* were no longer seen as village *amchi*, but as clinic *amchi* living outside their villages in a place that, although more or less equidistant from the different villages using the clinic, was nonetheless somehow disconnected from village life. Their new status and positioning at the clinic appeared to be in contradiction to their village-based social role, and this issue certainly needs further anthropological research for all the implications to be unpacked.

Negotiations and transformations

A 'globalizing' world means that even the most remote corners of the world are now accessible to environmental policies and management approaches, and residents must often adhere to, or negotiate with, preset terms and conditions of interaction. The conservationist, the ethno-ecologist, the botanist and the anthropologist are only a small part of the (mostly well-intentioned) influx of people who arrive in the mountain village with their own worldviews and sets of values, aiming to do 'good' both for themselves and for the local community. But following their departure, what remains? What aspects of their way of life have the local population been empowered, coerced or seduced into transforming? Very often, it turns out to be those aspects of indigenous and traditional activities which are contrary to the notions of science and modernity and hence 'in need of change'. Conservation knowledge, like other forms of 'governmentality', through its strategies and action plans, impacts upon local people, how they secure a livelihood, practise medicine, graze livestock, collect medicinal plants and so forth.

Research on *amchi* knowledge and practices have opened up the space, both literal and metaphorical, for collaboration with the *amchi*. Even if it is only certain aspects of their knowledge that are valorized by the conservationist, the *amchi* have benefited from the overall visibility in the local and trans-local arenas. The *amchi* of Nepal have been able to reframe their status and identity in the national arena, just as 'indigenous' and 'traditional' peoples elsewhere in the world have, through deployment of these labels, been able 'to reframe their disadvantageous relationship vis-à-vis the nation-states that encompass them' (Kearney 1995: 560).

The formation of *amchi* associations, at the district and national levels, has made the relationship between the *amchi* and the conservationist more visible. At the local level, the *amchi* associations are key actors through which the project implements its activities. The Dho Amchi Association, for example, took on the key responsibility for the construction of an *amchi* health care centre as well as the organization of local-level workshops to discuss *amchi* activities. At the national level, the Himalayan Amchi Association (HAA), formed in 1998, has continued its activities of seeking government recognition for its medical tradition. Examining the relationship between the *amchi* and the conservationist requires looking beyond the context of medicinal plant conservation and local health care development to embrace issues of identity and cultural survival and to maintaining 'a particular social existence' amidst processes of nationalism, nation building, democratization and ongoing conflict in Nepal.

Association with the project offered the marginalized *amchi* an opportunity to legitimate their own knowledge in the eyes of their community and the nation. As Sillitoe points out, 'the privileging of some knowledge [over others] will extend a degree of power to those who hold that knowledge; alternatively making it widely known may undermine the position of its holders' (Sillitoe 1998: 233). On the other hand, the conservationists, with their attractive packages of training, capacity-building schemes and publications, have perhaps raised expectations beyond what can actually be offered, for example the expected construction of THCCs in every village where there are *amchi*. The establishment of the THCC as an imported social institution will no doubt have long-term consequences in the way education is imparted in the future, and in the *amchi*'s relationship to patients.

Needless to say, any relationship involves negotiations, transformations and a good deal of moulding of those involved. We now turn to the complex agents mediating the relationships between the local and the global, the 'flexibility' of their selves, and the contradictions inherent in these relationships, which are often based on asymmetrical relations of power, perceptions and interests. Given the changing socio-cultural, political and environmental circumstances in the region, what seems to be required is a 'flexibility' and a willingness to transform, if necessary, received wisdoms, be they the 'textual certainties' of the *amchi* or the endangered status lists of the conservationists.

Mediating between different knowledge, worldviews and interests is fraught with difficulties. The agent in the context of trans-local processes in Nepal, such as development or biodiversity conservation, is similarly placed in a position whereby she or he is constantly negotiating between the different agendas and personas that come into play. To say the least, it is not an easy task. The juxtaposition of the *amchi* and the conservationist across the divide between the local and the global does not posit an essential identity or stability. Such a positioning is more a temporary identification that constitutes and reforms the subject, so as to enable that subject to act. There is nothing essentially 'local' about the *amchi* as he travels with his yak miles across the Himalayan passes to purchase food supplies on the Tibetan Plateau, or to Kathmandu to attend the national workshop of *amchi* organized by the Himalayan Amchi Association, or the training by the Remote Area Development Committee of the Ministry of Local Development, or to Lhasa under the auspices of WWF to meet with the *amchi* at the *sman rtsis khang*, or to the international conference of Tibetan medicine in Washington, DC, seeking new donors. Similarly, to think of the conservationist as 'global' is also to see only one aspect of a complex role: conservationists working with the *amchi* in Dolpo defy categorization as 'global' because they operate at the national, district, village and sub-village levels.

Neither the knowledge of the *amchi* nor that of the conservationist is a closed, static system, but is open to reinterpretation and adaptation, based on the ever-changing social, political and economic environment. For the *amchi*, the practice of experimentation with new medicinal ingredients (plants and minerals) for use as substitutes for endangered species of plants and animals is a challenge of the late twentieth century, caused by the over-harvesting of these species which have now been 'red-listed'. Although the causes of the over-harvesting and poaching are often very distant from the *amchi* themselves – aggravated by the increasing commercialization of herbal medicine, or the opportunistic poaching of rhinoceros in a period of political turmoil – the impact upon the *amchi* lies in their reduced ability to produce medicines according to the formulas that they have long been using.

Thus, although it is a neologism when the *amchi* use the term '*sung-kyob*' (conservation, roughly translated) when they talk about medicinal plant conservation, it is also not something entirely new. The *amchi* have in fact been involved in 'conservation' practices, such as harvesting only the amounts needed for preparation of medicine, collecting from different sites each year, and waiting until after the seeds are dispersed to uproot the tuber, for centuries before they came into contact with the conservationists (Shrestha *et al.* 1998; Ghimire *et al.* 1999). However, it is clear that the more sustained the encounter between the *amchi* and the conservationists, the stronger the emphasis the former puts on plant conservation and the more central it becomes as a distinct concept in their day-to-day lives.

Conclusion

The main postulate of the People and Plants Initiative considers local vernacular knowledge and practices as important components of environmental management. Developing such an approach implies an encounter between different worldviews, knowledge systems and practices and thus carries various epistemological and social implications. A variety of these issue areas have been examined in this chapter. We have stressed the fact that the different parties involved in this encounter between the local and the global had partially shared concerns for a common subject – the conservation of medicinal plants – although the paradigm of conservation, as understood by the conservationists, was new to the *amchi*. While the concerns of the different parties were not fully symmetrical or integrated, they did engage in some common actions, such as the Traditional Health Care Centre and the ecological experiments that built upon local ethno-ecological knowledge.

In spite of the fact that the knowledge and worldviews of the different parties were only partially commensurable and that there were divergent agendas,[11] the identities of certain actors facilitated a largely positive encounter. *Amchi* have important, highly localized and embedded roles, yet are also recognized as actors within a trans-Himalayan medical system that transcends local Dolpo practices. These identities may be connected with Lama's discussion about 'flexible selves' (Lama 2003), where the *amchi* uses his capacity, just as the inhabitants of Dolpo generally do (Bauer 2004), to develop new ways to deal with the 'Other', in this case the conservation managers, the national Ayurvedic doctors and the representatives of international organizations. It can be seen as an experiential learning process between the different actors concerned and a rich form of 'practising relationship' during which divergent agendas may appear to converge.

Processes of learning are important aspects of this encounter. The fact that local knowledge has entered international arenas through debate hinges on the particular thought processes and directions of the different actors present (Dumoulin 2003). As far as the botanist, ecologist and ethno-ecologist were concerned, the local knowledge of the *amchi*, integrated into their ecological research, provided a new outlook to their work, uniting naturalist, social and cultural dimensions. In the context of the global environmental crisis, ecology as a science is moving rapidly towards understanding mankind as an integrated part of ecosystems (O'Neill 2001). The nature/culture dichotomy, in which scientific knowledge explicitly excludes mankind in its attempts to understand so-called natural and biological dynamics, is now either blurred or rejected. Every scientist must now accept the general 'constant' that each and every part of 'nature' is significantly influenced by human activities, be that influence interpreted as positive, negative or neutral.

Some authors, such as Agrawal (2002), have criticized the 'scientifization' of ethno-ecological knowledge, suggesting that facile generalization about this knowledge, and its scientific validation through experiments, in many ways extracts the knowledge from its local cultural specificity. Although this argument carries strength, it appears to the authors that such questions are very much dependent upon how this 'scientifization' process takes place. Here, issues of participation, and of how participation is effectively played out, are of central relevance. More than participation in decisions, which is a familiar issue in development projects that build on indigenous knowledge (Sillitoe *et al.* 2002), processes of learning themselves have arisen from analysis of the People and Plants project as a key issue area. This has been inadequately discussed to date and would certainly benefit from more theoretical and practical attention in the future.

Notes

1 See Chapter 1, note 4.
2 Lama (2003: 3) uses the term 'conservationist' for all personnel belonging to a conservation project. In this paper, we differentiate between the various members of the project: the scientists (ecologists, sociologists or anthropologists), who are scholars

holding scientific knowledge, and the conservation managers, who develop management approaches that are assumed to have a scientific basis.

3 See, for an example drawn from other areas, Pordié (2002).

4 These were termed 'expert *amchi*' because they were involved in supporting the development and recognition of *amchi* practices at both the national and the international level. Both were also practising *amchi*, recognized for their extensive knowledge and skills.

5 Although it was difficult to fully understand the social structure and membership selection criteria of these groups, it was evident that the representatives at the meeting were either socially prominent people or those who, for different reasons, were able to speak out. One such group, the Medicinal Plants Management Committee, was formed during the course of the project. The process of group formation consisted of an open village meeting and a general discussion, during which members were selected. People became members either because of their capacity to be good brokers between the village and extra-local organizations or because of their high level of knowledge relating to medicinal plants. Many already represented the village at the Village Development Committee, the major administrative unit relating to village life.

6 It was in fact a team composed of scientists and managers coming from different cultural backgrounds and representing both national and international agencies.

7 Large volumes of MAPs are being extracted for trade from this area (see Lama *et al.* 2001).

8 See Gururani (2002) for an account of the increasing emphasis being given to gender issues in environmental management generally, and Gurung *et al.* (1999) for details of women's medicinal knowledge in Dolpo.

9 An example of a perennial herb's life cycle, which includes the different stages of the cycle as perceived by the *amchi* and which was used during the ecological monitoring process, is given in Ghimire and Aumeeruddy-Thomas (2005).

10 Yulha Chulsa is a major pilgrimage celebrated in the high pasture of Kunasa of the village of Pungmo, the main aim of which is to celebrate the protecting deities of this particular high pasture (Aumeeruddy-Thomas *et al.* 2004: 119). 'The "local god" (*yul lha*), often also referred to as the village god, or god of the land, [presides] over the well-being of a village community' (Kind 2002: 21).

11 These agendas include sustainable resource management (conservationists), social and political visibility and the promotion of a collective national identity (*amchi*), domestication and value addition (commercial collectors), and increased access to training and education (women).

References

Agrawal, A. (2002) Indigenous Knowledge and the Politics of Classification, *International Social Science Journal* 173: 287–297.

Alexiades, M. N. (2004). Ethnobiology and Globalization: Science and Ethics at the Turn of the Century. In T. J. S. Carlson and L. Maffi (eds), *Ethnobotany and the Conservation of Biocultural Diversity: Advances in Economic Botany*, Vol. 15, New York: New York Botanical Garden Press.

Aubertin, C. (2000). L'ascension fulgurante d'un concept flou, *La Recherche* 333: 12–17.

Aubertin, C., Boisvert, V. and Vivien, F.-D. (1998). La construction sociale de la question de la biodiversité, *Nature, Sciences, Sociétés* 6(1): 7–19.

Aumeeruddy, Y., Saigal, S., Kapoor, N. and Cunningham, A. B. (1999). *Joint Management in the Making: Reflections and Experiences*, People and Plants Working Papers Series 7, Paris: UNESCO.

Aumeeruddy-Thomas, Y. and Pei, S. (2003). *Applied Ethnobotany: Case Studies from the Himalayan Region*, People and Plants Working Paper Series 12, Paris: UNESCO.

Aumeeruddy-Thomas, Y., Lama, Y. C. and Ghimire, S. K. (2004). Medicinal Plants within the Context of Pastoral Life in the Village of Pungmo, Dolpo, Nepal. In C. Richard and K. Hoffmann (eds), *Strategic Innovations for Improving Pastoral Livelihoods in the Hindi-Kush Himalayan Highlands*, Vol. II, *Technical Papers*, Kathmandu: ICIMOD.

Balée, W. (2000). Qui a planté les décors de l'Amazonie?, *La Recherche* 333: 18–23.

Bauer, M. K. (2004). *High Frontiers: Dolpo and the Changing World of Himalayan Pastoralists*, New York: Columbia University Press.

Berkes, F. and Folke, C. (2002). Back to the Future: Ecosystem Dynamics and Local Knowledge. In L. H. Gunderson and C. S. Holling (eds), *Panarchy: Understanding Transformations in Human and Natural Systems*, Washington, DC: Island Press.

Berkes, F., Colding, J. and Folke, C. (2000). Rediscovery of Traditional Ecological Knowledge as Adaptive Management, *Ecological Applications* 10: 1251–1262.

Brush, S. B. and Meng, E. (1998). Farmers' Valuation and Conservation of Crop Genetic Resources, *Genetic Resources and Crop Evolution* 45: 139–150.

Colchester, M. (1999) Parcs ou Peuples?, *Ethnies*, Documents, 24–25 (*Nature Sauvage, Nature Sauvée? Ecologie et peuples autochtones*): 159–193.

Conklin, H. C. (1957). *A Report of an Integral System of Shifting Cultivation in the Philippines*, FAO Forestry Development Paper 12, Rome: FAO, p. 209.

Cormier-Salem, M.-C. and Roussel, B. (2002). Patrimoines et savoirs naturalistes locaux. In J.-Y. Martin (ed.), *Développement Durable? Doctrines, pratiques, évaluations*, Paris: Editions IRD.

Cunningham, A. B. (2001). *Applied Ethnobotany: People, Wild Plant Use and Conservation*, London: Earthscan.

Davis, W. (1994). Towards a New Synthesis in Ethnobotany. In M. Rios and B. Pedersen (eds), *Las plastas y el hombre: Memorias del primer simposio ecuatoriano de etnobotánica y botánica económica*, Quito: Ediciones Abya-Yala, Pontificia universidad católica del Ecuador.

Descola, P. (1999). Diversité biologique, diversité culturelle, *Ethnies*, Documents, 24–25 (*Nature Sauvage, Nature Sauvée? Ecologie et peuples autochtones*): 213–235.

Descola, P. (2002). Constructing Nature, Symbolic Ecology and Social Practice. In P. Descola and G. Palsson (eds), *Nature and Society: Anthropological Perspectives*, London: Routledge.

Dumoulin, D. (2003). Local Knowledge in the Hands of Transnational NGO Networks: A Mexican Viewpoint, *International Social Science Journal* 178: 593–605.

Eghenter, C. and Sellato, B. (2003). Introduction. In B. Eghenter, B. Sellato and G. S. Devung (eds), *Social Science Research and Conservation Management in the Interior of Borneo: Unravelling Past and Present Interactions of People and Forests*, Bogor: CIFOR, WWF Indonesia, UNESCO, Ford Foundation.

Ellen, R. (2002). The Cognitive Geometry of Nature: A Contextual Approach. In P. Descola and G. Palsson (eds), *Nature and Society: Anthropological Perspectives*, London: Routledge.

Ellen, R., Parkes, P. and Bicker, A. (eds) (2000). *Indigenous Environmental Knowledge and its Transformations: Critical Anthropological Perspectives*. London: Routledge.

Fairhead, J. and Leach, M. (1996). Enriching the Landscape: Social History and the Management of Transition Ecology in the Forest–Savanna Mosaic of the Republic of Guinea. In J. I. Guyer and P. Richards (eds), *The Social Shaping of Biodiversity, Africa* 66(1): 14–35.

Friedberg, C. (1992). Représentations, classifications: comment l'homme pense ses rapports au milieu naturel. In M. Jollivet (ed.), *Sciences de la nature, Science de la société: Les passeurs de frontières*, Paris: Editions du CNRS.

Ghimire, S. K. and Aumeeruddy-Thomas, Y. (2005). Approach to In Situ Conservation of Threatened Himalayan Medicinal Plants: A Case Study from Shey-Phoksundo National Park, Dolpo, Nepal. In Y. Aumeeruddy-Thomas, M. Karki, K. Gurung and D. Parajuli (eds), *Himalayan Aromatic and Medicinal Plants: Balancing Use and Conservation*, Kathmandu: IDRC, Canada, WWF–UNESCO, PPI, WWF Nepal Programme.

Ghimire, S. K., McKey, D. and Aumeeruddy-Thomas, Y. (2004). Heterogeneity in Ethno-ecological Knowledge and Management of Medicinal Plants in the Himalayas of Nepal: Implications for Conservation, *Ecology and Society* 9(3): 6 (http://www.ecology andsociety.org/vol9/iss3/art6).

Ghimire, S. K., McKey, D. and Aumeeruddy-Thomas, Y. (2005). Conservation of Himalayan Medicinal Plants: Harvesting Patterns and Ecology of Two Threatened Species, *Nardostachys grandiflora* DC. and *Neopicrorhiza scrophulariiflora* (Pennell) Hong, *Biological Conservation* 124: 463–475.

Ghimire, S. K., Parajuli, D. B., Gurung, T. N., Lama, Y. C. and Aumeeruddy-Thomas, Y. (eds) (1999). *Conservation of Plant Resources, Community Development, Training in Applied Ethnobotany at Shey Phoksundo National Park and its Buffer-Zone, Dolpa*, WWF Nepal Programme Report Series No. 38, Kathmandu: WWF Nepal Programme.

Gunderson, L. H. and Holling, C. S. (eds) (2002). *Panarchy: Understanding Transformations in Human and Natural Systems*, Washington, DC: Island Press.

Gurung, T. N., Lama, Y. C. and Aumeeruddy-Thomas, Y. (1999). Improving Local Health Care in Phoksundo VDC. In S. K. Ghimire, D. B. Parajuli, T. N. Gurung, Y. C. Lama and Y. Aumeeruddy-Thomas (eds), *Conservation of Plant Resources, Community Development, Training in Applied Ethnobotany at Shey Phoksundo National Park and its Buffer-Zone, Dolpa*, WWF Nepal Programme Report Series No. 38, Kathmandu: WWF Nepal Programme.

Gurung, T. N., Lama, G. G., Shrestha, K. K. and Craig, S. (1996). *Medicinal Plants and Traditional Doctors in Shey Phoksundo National Park and Other Areas of the Dolpa District*, WWF Nepal Programme Report Series No. 26, Kathmandu: WWF Nepal Programme.

Gururani, S. (2002) Construction of the Third World Women's Knowledge in the Development Discourse, *International Social Science Journal* 173: 313–323.

Haudricourt, G. (1962). Domestication des animaux, culture des plantes, traitement d'autrui, *L'Homme* 2(1): 40–50.

Hladik, C. M., Hladik, A., Linares, O. F., Pagezy, H., Semple, A. and Hadley, M. (eds) (1993). *Tropical Forests, People and Food: Biocultural Interactions and Applications to Development*, Man and Biosphere Series, London: Parthenon Publishing.

Hobley, M. (1996). *Participatory Forestry: The Process of Change in India and Nepal*, ODI Rural Development Forestry Study Guide, London: ODI.

Jest, C. (1975). *Dolpo, communautés de langue tibétaine du Népal*, Paris: Editions du CNRS.

Jollivet, M. (ed.) (1992). *Sciences de la nature, Science de la société: Les passeurs de frontières*, Paris: Editions du CNRS.

Kearney, M. (1995). The Local and the Global: The Anthropology of Globalization and Transnationalism, *Annual Review of Anthropology* 24: 547–565.

Kind, M. (2002). *Mendrup: A Bonpo Ritual for the Benefit of All Living Beings and for the Empowerment of Medicine Performed in Tsho, Dolpo*, Kathmandu: WWF Nepal Programme.

Lama, Y. C. (2003). The Amchi and the Conservationist: Practising Relationships in the Nepal Himalaya, MA thesis in Social Anthropology, School of Oriental and African Studies, University of London.

Lama, Y. C., Ghimire, S. K. and Aumeeruddy-Thomas, Y. (2001). *Medicinal Plants of Dolpo: Amchis' Knowledge and Conservation*, Kathmandu: WWF Nepal Programme.

Latour, B. (1997). *Nous n'avons jamais été modernes: Essai d'anthropologie symétrique*, Paris: La Découverte.

Leach, M. and Fairhead, J. (2002). Manners of Contestation: 'Citizen Science' and 'Indigenous Knowledge' in West Africa and the Caribbean, *International Social Science Journal* 173: 299–311.

Leaman, D. J., Malla, S. B. and Fatima, N. (1999). Report of a Mid-Term Evaluation of the People and Plants Initiative WWF/UNESCO/Kew, Himalayas Regional Programme, WWF Project No. 9Z0556.

Lévi-Strauss, C. (1962). *La pensée sauvage*, Paris: Plon.

Martin, G. J. (1995). *Ethnobotany: A People and Plants Conservation Manual*, London: Chapman & Hall.

Michon, G. (2002). Du discours global aux pratiques locales, ou comment les conventions sur l'environnement affectent la gestion de la forêt tropicale. In J.-Y. Martin (ed.), *Développement Durable? Doctrines, pratiques, evaluations*, Paris: Editions IRD.

Olivier de Sardan, J.-P. (1995). *Anthropologie et développement: Essai en socio-anthropologie du changement social*, Marseille, Paris: APAD-Karthala.

O'Neill, R. V. (2001). Is It Time to Bury the Ecosystem Concept?, *Ecology* 82(12): 3275–3284.

Orlove, B. S. and Brush, S. (1996). Anthropology and the Conservation of Biodiversity, *Annual Review of Anthropology* 25: 329–352.

Pordié, L. (2002). La pharmacopée comme expression de société: Une étude himalayenne. In J. Fleurentin, J.-M. Pelt and G. Mazars (eds), *Des sources du savoir aux médicaments du futur*, Paris: IRD-SFE.

Posey, D. and Balee, A. (eds) (1989). *Natural Resources Management in Indigenous and Folk Societies of Amazonia*, Advances in Economic Botany No. 7, New York: New York Botanical Garden.

Ramakrishnan, P. S., Saxena, K. G. and Chandrashekara, U. M. (eds) (1998). *Conserving the Sacred for Biodiversity Management*, New Hampshire: Science Publishers.

Ramble, C. (1997). Tibetan Pride of Place: Or, Why Nepal's Bhotiyas Are Not an Ethnic Group. In D. Gellner and J. W. Pfaff-Czarnecka (eds), *Nationalism and Ethnicity in a Hindu Kingdom*, Amsterdam: Harwood Academic Publishers.

Ramble, C. and Chapagain, C. P. (1990) *Preliminary Notes on the Cultural Dimension of Conservation*, Kathmandu: National Parks and Wildlife Conservation Office.

Saberwal, V. (1996). Pastoral Politics: Gaddi Grazing, Degradation, and Biodiversity Conservation in Himachal Pradesh, India, *Conservation Biology* 10(3): 741–749.

Shrestha, K. K., Ghimire, S. K., Gurung, T. N., Lama, Y. C. and Aumeeruddy, Y. (1998). *Conservation of Plant Resources, Community Development, Training in Applied Ethnobotany at Shey Phoksundo National Park and its Buffer-Zone, Dolpa*, WWF Nepal Programme Report Series No. 33, Kathmandu: WWF Nepal Programme.

Sillitoe, P. (1998). The Development of Indigenous Knowledge: A New Applied Anthropology, *Current Anthropology* 39(2): 223–252.

Sillitoe, P., Bicker, A. and Pottier, J. (eds) (2002). *Participating in Development: Approaches to Indigenous Knowledge*, London: Routledge.

Snellgrove, D. (1992 [1967]). *Four Lamas of Dolpo: Tibetan Biographies*, Kathmandu: Himalayan Book Series.

Tripathi, G. R. and Schmitt, S. (2001). Rapid Vulnerability Assessment of Medicinal Plants. In S. K. Ghimire, Y. C. Lama, G. R. Tripathi, S. Schmitt and Y. Aumeeruddy-Thomas (eds), *Conservation of Plant Resources, Community Development, Training in Applied Ethnobotany at Shey Phoksundo National Park and its Buffer-Zone, Dolpa*, WWF Nepal Programme Report Series No. 41, Kathmandu: WWF Nepal Programme.

Warren, D. M., Slikkerveer, L. J. and Brokensha, D. (eds) (1995). *The Cultural Dimension of Development: Indigenous Knowledge Systems*, London: Intermediate Technology Publications.

Wikramanayake, E. D., Carpentert, C., Strand, H. and McKnight, M. (2001). *Ecoregion-Based Conservation in the Eastern Himalaya: Identifying Important Areas for Biodiversity Conservation*, Kathmandu: WWF and ICIMOD.

Wilson, E. O. and Peter, F. M. (eds) (1988) *Biodiversity*, Washington, DC: National Academy Press.

Part III

Tibetan medicine and the West

8 The integration of Tibetan medicine in the United Kingdom

The clinics of the Tara Institute of Medicine

Colin Millard

This research took place in the clinics of the Tara Institute of Tibetan Medicine, which is part of Tara Rokpa Edinburgh, an organization set up by Akong Rinpoche, a Tibetan lama who along with Chogyam Trungpa Rinpoche founded Kagyu Samye Ling Tibetan Centre at Eskdalemuir in Scotland in 1967. Tara Rokpa Edinburgh is concerned with the healing arts and has two main areas of activity: Tara Rokpa Therapy, a form of psychotherapy, developed by Akong Rinpoche and several psychotherapists, which combines techniques of Western psychotherapy with the methods of Buddhism; and the Tara Institute of Tibetan Medicine. Concerning Tibetan medicine, Tara Rokpa Edinburgh has two goals: to support Tibetan medicine in Tibet and to establish Tibetan medicine in the West. The Tara Institute of Tibetan Medicine aims to establish Tibetan medical clinics where patients are able to consult with highly trained Tibetan doctors and to provide a training programme in Tibetan medicine.

The Tara Institute's training programme began in 1993 when the Tara College of Tibetan Medicine was established, and a teaching programme was developed under the guidance of Khenpo Troru Tsenam, directing physician and professor of medicine at the Central Institute, Lhasa. Since that time two groups of health care professionals have undertaken in-depth introductory courses in Tibetan medicine. At the present time the college is not running any programmes and the main focus of the Tara Institute's activity is the Tibetan medical clinics. The Tara Institute runs clinics with visiting doctors from Tibet, once a week in Edinburgh and once a month in London, Glasgow and Dundee and at the Kagyu Samye Ling Tibetan Centre.[1]

This chapter explores some of the complex issues related to the integration of Tibetan medicine in the West, particularly as they relate to these clinics. Just as biomedical knowledge and practice vary within one society (Hahn and Gaines 1985), and at an international level (Lock 1980), the idea that there is a monolithic uniform 'traditional' Tibetan medicine must be brought into question. The discussion in this chapter on the adaptation of Tibetan medicine in this particular Western context contributes to the heterogeneity of the Tibetan medical field and it analyses the degree of flexibility of Tibetan medicine.[2] From issues that have arisen during the establishment of these clinics, and from my observations working in them,[3] there are four main forms of adaptation that need to be considered. These are: adaptations to meet legal requirements; adaptations to fit a Western socio-economic and political context; adaptations in ideology; and adaptations to what might be called a Western disease ecology. I will answer two fundamental questions pertaining to contemporary Tibetan medicine: What are the elements of Tibetan medical practice that have been most easily adapted to the clinical context in the UK? And which are the elements that have had to be transformed or left out?

The argument will be set within the theoretical grounding concerning the transformative effects on social behaviour and knowledge of what has been variously called the modern bureaucratic state (Berger *et al.* 1973), the commodity mode of production (Taussig 1980) or modernity (Giddens 1991). Such an environment consists of social mechanism that lead to disease being reified as an isolated entity and reduced to breakdowns in biological systems in the human body.

A further issue that will be considered is existing relationships of power and the hegemony of biomedicine in the health care arena. Generally speaking, biomedical knowledge is not relativized like other medical traditions. Most often it is not thought about as one medical tradition amongst others, but as *the* medical tradition, which others may complement if they meet existing legal requirements.

Tibetan medicine and European and UK law

In this section I will make some observations about changing legislation in the UK and Europe that has direct relevance for the practice of Tibetan medicine in European countries. These observations are partly based on my experience of how these regulations had affected Tibetan medical practice in the Tara clinics and partly on documents that are available on the websites of the Medicines and Healthcare Products Regulatory Agency, the European Herbal Practitioners Association[4] and the Department of Health. For those who want to know more, a wealth of information can be found from these sources. Legislation on herbal medicines and complementary and alternative medicines has been in a constant state of flux in the past decade, and what follows is only a snapshot of the situation as it stands at present; some progress has been made, but the debates remain unresolved and are ongoing.

The way that Tibetan medical practice in the Tara clinics has been affected by legislation relates to two areas: therapy modifications and statutory self-regulation. Tibetan medicine uses a range of external and internal therapies. In the Tara clinics the only external therapies that were used were moxibustion, hot applications and massage. The present doctor[5] who practises in the clinics, Dr Lobsang Dhonden, has also been trained in acupuncture, but during the period of this research he did not use it.[6] Two of Tibetan medicine's traditional therapies, venesection and cauterization, are not used. However, this can be taken as only a minor modification, as during the two years I spent at the clinic in Dhorpatan I never observed venesection, and cauterization was only rarely performed.

By far the largest therapeutic method used in Dhorpatan and in the Tara clinics was the administering of medicines. It is in this area that Tibetan medical practice in the Tara clinics has undergone its greatest modification. European law on medicines goes back to the 1965 Directive 65/65 EEC. This directive gives a very broad definition of what a medicine is and requires that all medicines on the market in European member states have a licence or, in other words, are granted 'market authorization'. Over the years this Directive has gone through various revisions, culminating in the Directive 2001/83/EC; throughout this process the licensing position remained essentially the same. The procedure presents a number of intractable problems for herbal medicine. First, licences are not given to medicinal plants but to single chemical substances, and these bioactive constituents of plants are not easy to identify. Second, herbs as natural substances cannot practically be patented; this presents problems in terms of potential profitability if a company is to invest the large amounts of money needed to acquire a licence. Finally, there is the problem that the trials and evaluations which need to be undertaken for the licensing procedure to prove the efficacy and safety of the plant are very costly.

Most member states found their own solutions to the problems of the original Directive, such as classifying herbal medicines as food supplements (in the US they are classed as 'dietary supplements') or by using country-specific legislation. The law on the use of herbal medicines in the UK is covered by sections 12 and 56 of the 1968 Medicines Act. Section 12(1) relates to prescribing herbal medicines through consultation, and section 12(2) relates to over-the-counter sales. Herbal medicines are exempt from requiring a licence provided that: they are manufactured or assembled in the herbalist premises and are given after a consultation (section 12(1)); or they have not been produced by any means other than drying, crushing or comminuting, they are sold with a title indicating only the constituent plant or plants, and no recommendations are given as to their use (section 12(2)).

These exemptions have meant that up to now herbal medicine in the UK has been subject to very little control. The Act contains no regulations concerning the quality control of herbal medicine, and no definition is given of what constitutes a herbal practitioner; consequently anyone, no matter what their knowledge or experience, could legally give herbal medicines. Those in favour of statutory regulation see the setting up of a statutory register as a way of overcoming these shortcomings.

One of the rules of exemption in the 1965 Act is that a herbal medicine should not contain non-herbal active ingredients. Tibetan medicine has a vast pharmacopoeia. One of the most famous Tibetan pharmacopoeias is Dilmar Geshe Tenzin's *The Pure Crystal Orb and Crystal Rosary* composed in 1717, which lists 2,294 medicinal ingredients. Most of these ingredients are derived from plants, but a significant proportion consists of mineral and animal products. Here therefore was a huge problem for the Tara Institute, as none of the large number of Tibetan medicinal compounds which contain minerals or animal products can be legally used in the UK. This problem was partly overcome when Akong Rinpoche found a little-known pharmacopoeia of the nineteenth-century Tibetan lama and scholar Mipham Jamyang Gyatso (1846–1912). This pharmacopoeia lists a large number of plant-based medicinal compounds, the logic being that it is possible to substitute animal or mineral ingredients with a plant ingredient having the same medicinal properties. At present all the medicines that are used in the clinics in the UK are manufactured from the Mipham formulary in a Tibetan medical hospital at Shilling

(Xinning) in East Tibet. Dr Dhonden told me that one of the most important differences between his practice here and his practice in Tibet and India is the restricted pharmacopoeia. This is a constant source of frustration for him. Whilst discussing this with me, he half jokingly said, 'Sometimes it is the law that is unlawful.'

But this was not the only difficulty. In the UK it is the function of the Medicines and Healthcare Products Regulatory Agency (MHPRA), an executive agency of the Department of Health, to regulate the use of medicines and health care products. The MHPRA publishes a list of toxic plants which are restricted under separate legislation; some of these plants can be obtained as medicines by prescription only from registered doctors or dentists, and others are restricted to pharmacists (MCA 2001, 2002). The Tara Institute had thus to first identify any of these plants in the Mipham pharmacopoeia and advise the Tibetan doctor in Shilling to replace the restricted plant with another plant having the same medicinal characteristics, according to Tibetan pharmacology.

For some time now European law on herbal medicine has been under revision. From 2002 onwards various amendments were made to the 2001 Directive, leading eventually to the publication of the Directive on Traditional Herbal Medicinal Products (DTHMP) 2004/24/EC, which makes it easier to acquire licences for herbal medicines. It is important to make clear here the exact focus of this Directive. As we have seen in the 1968 Medicines Act, legislation on herbal medicines has followed two routes: regulations on herbal medicines that can be sold over the counter, and regulations on herbal medicines that can be given after a consultation. The DTHMP is only concerned with the selling of herbal medicines over the counter, and for such medicines it stipulates that a licence is required. The new ruling which it brings in is that licences can be acquired for herbal medicines in the European Union without having to conduct the usual clinical trials and biomedical evaluations; instead for herbal medicines evidence must be provided of safe traditional use. Exactly what this evidence amounts to is that herbal medicines originating within the European Union must provide proof of thirty years' continuous safe use in Europe up to the date of the inception of the DTHMP ruling; for products originating outside the European Union this is reduced to fifteen years in Europe plus fifteen years outside. This ruling of the Directive has been criticized for the restriction it imposes on herbal medicines originating from countries outside the European Union; for instance, Tibetan medicine has only just begun to establish itself in European countries.

The DTHMP was implemented in the UK in 2005. All herbal medicines that are now currently sold over the counter under section 12(2) will now need to be registered and evidence provided of safe traditional use. The registration scheme includes a transition period that ends on 30 April 2011. Unlike under section 12(2) of the 1968 Medicines Act it will now be possible to put the ingredients of the medicine on the label and give instructions regarding its use. The government's intention is that after the transitional period section 12(2) will be replaced by the DTHMP. Once a herbal medicine has been registered, manufacturers, wholesalers and importers will all need licences to produce or retail it. In order to acquire a manufacturer's licence it will be necessary to demonstrate recognized standards of good manufacturing practice and undergo two-yearly inspections by MHRA staff at the manufacturer's premises.

As I have mentioned, the DTHMP is only concerned with medicines that are sold over the counter. Medicines that are given after a consultation are still regulated by section 12(1) of the 1968 Medicines Act. The first major step to revising this regulation was the publication in November 2000 of the House of Lords Sixth Report of the Science and Technology Committee on Complementary and Alternative Medicines, the first ever inquiry of a Parliamentary Select Committee into this subject (House of Lords 2000). Based on evidence gathered over a period of eighteen months, the report makes various recommendations to the government.

The report begins by grouping all complementary and alternative medicine (CAM) therapies into one of three groups. Group one consists of five therapies which the report states have already built up some evidence base, have individual diagnostic procedures, and are the most organized and the closest to achieving statutory regulation. Two of these five, osteopathy and chiropractic, are already regulated; the other three are herbal medicine, acupuncture and homoeopathy. In group two it places a range of therapies that do not incorporate diagnostic procedures and are often used in conjunction with conventional medicine. In this category it lists therapies such as: Alexander technique, aromatherapy, reflexology and Bach flower remedies. Group three consists of therapies with little evidence base that are based on notions which in the opinion of the report 'diverge from the scientific principles of conventional medicine'. Group three therapies are divided into two groups: one which comprises therapies such as iridology, radionics, dowsing and crystal therapy; and a second group where the report places traditional medical systems such as Ayurveda and Chinese medicine, and though it is not mentioned by name Tibetan medicine would most likely fit into this category as one of Asia's great medical traditions.

In summary, the report recommends that: more detailed qualitative information be gathered on CAM; that, where claims are made of therapeutic efficacy, these claims be validated; that the diagnostic procedures should also be evaluated and shown to be reliable and reproducible; and that evidence be provided on the safety, cost-effectiveness, and mechanisms of action of therapies. The question as to how these evaluations can be made is problematic and will be discussed in more detail below.

The report also recommends that each therapeutic profession unify itself under one voluntary regulatory body. It will then be the function of this body to set professional standards, such as providing a code of conduct, a disciplinary procedure and a complaints procedure. It should also set the standards of training and provide supervision of the training and accreditation. Once the professional structure is in place the therapy can then apply for statutory self-regulation under the 1999 Health Act. The report considers statutory regulation appropriate, if a therapy fulfils three conditions: that harm may arise from poor practice; that a voluntary regulatory system is in place; and that a valid evidence base has been gathered. The report considers that herbal medicine and acupuncture satisfy these conditions, and therefore it supports their attempts to achieve statutory regulation.

The government's response published in March 2001 generally agrees with these recommendations (Department of Health 2001). The document begins by suggesting a modification to the report's threefold classification of CAM therapies. For the purposes of self-regulation it suggests moving group three therapies that include herbal remedies, such as Chinese medicine and Ayurveda, to be subsumed within the group one herbal medicine category; this is where Tibetan medicine is now positioned. Following from this, the Department of Health, in collaboration with the Prince of Wales's Foundation for Integrated Health and the European Herbal Practitioners Association, established a Herbal Medicines Regulatory Working Group whose remit was to provide recommendations on the regulation of herbal medicine and on possible reform of section 12(1) of the Medicines Act. The group presented its recommendations in a report published in 2003, *Recommendations on the Regulation of Herbal Practitioners in the UK*.

The report recommends that, in order to maintain unified standards amongst the various herbal medicine traditions, a core curriculum should be established that will be shared by all training programmes in herbal medicine to satisfy the requirements of statutory self-regulation. The core curriculum that is presented in the report consists of nine modules: human science, nutrition, clinical sciences, plant chemistry and pharmacology, pharmacognosy and dispensing, practitioner development and ethics, practitioner research, a module specific to each herbal tradition, and clinical practice. It is quite clear from these titles that what the training will provide is a thorough grounding in biomedical science. It is left to the eighth module to provide the student with an understanding of the specific herbal tradition. This module, which has come to be known as the 'eighth element', has already been formulated for Tibetan medicine, Western herbal medicine, Chinese medicine and Ayurvedic medicine.[7]

The eighth element for Tibetan medicine was developed by the Tara Institute of Tibetan Medicine, in discussion with Dr Dhonden and various other Tibetan doctors. This was not without some considerable difficulty. In the past the formal training of Tibetan doctors sometimes lasted as long as twelve years. In contemporary Tibetan medical schools in Tibet, and in exile communities in India, it takes five years for students to complete the theoretical part of their studies.

The time that is allotted for the eighth element is 1,150 hours of tuition, which is considerably less than any of the traditional curriculums. As the total hours of the core curriculum as it stands at the moment is 2,560, this means that students will be spending more time learning biomedically orientated material than the subject matter of their chosen medical tradition. The core curriculum is not fixed; it is meant to give only an indication of what should be done, but at this stage it is unlikely that any substantial modifications will be made.

What statutory self-regulation amounts to for Tibetan medicine is that it will be regulated along with other herbal medicine traditions (at present Chinese, Ayurvedic and Western herbal medicine) under one piece of legislation. One possible advantage of statutory regulation is that it may pave the way for registered practitioners to use plants that are currently restricted, and some mineral and animal products. Discussions between the government and interested parties have been going on for some years now as to the form this legislation will take. In 2006 the Department of Health established a steering group with the aim of progressing this legislation.

Meeting the socio-economic and political context

Biomedicine's exclusive focus on disease entities and the concomitant neglect of the psychological and social dimensions of disease are a product of wider social and economic mechanisms. Tibetan medicine, on the other hand, allots a fundamental role to the psycho-social dimensions of disease, which are sometimes overemphasized, particularly as a response to the international demand of the herbal medicines market (Samuel 2001). The commodity mode of production creates the situation where disease becomes a dehistoricized, desocialized fact of nature (Taussig 1980). Diseases that are the products of social and political relationships are presented as problems of isolated individual bodies, therefore eluding the three realms of meaning, social, psychological and biophysical, in which they occur (Dunn 1976). In this view, disease representations are part of capitalist ideology; they are mystifications that obscure an underlying socio-political reality (Comaroff 1982; Taussig 1980). As Keesing puts it, cultures 'constitute ideologies, disguising human and economic realities . . . cultures are webs of mystification as well as significance' (1987: 161).

In the Tara clinics, following along with Tibetan medical notions of the interrelationships between the body, mind and natural environment, diseases are not thought to be problems of isolated individual bodies. Dr Dhonden gives due consideration to everything the patient has to say whether it relates to symptoms or to the patient's social circumstance. Furthermore he is fully aware of the relationship between the patient's psychological state and the patient's physiological condition. The clinical interactions in the next section clearly demonstrate this.

Quite frequently Dr Dhonden enquires about how the patient's condition is affected by seasonal changes, a question I often heard him ask his patients (see 'Patient 4', p. 201). Another question I often heard Dr Dhonden ask was about the patient's psychological state. Initially he used to phrase this 'How are your emotions?', but following discussion on this he now asks about the patient's mood (see 'Patient 3', p. 200).

Often patients would spend considerable time explaining about their relationships or about difficult past events, and about stress factors in their lives. Some patients also recounted their dreams, which they thought might relate to their condition. One 'schizophrenic' patient brought along a detailed journal to the clinic every month where she had recorded many of her psychotic experiences. She took on average about 30 minutes at the beginning of each session to recount all the dreams, sensations, thoughts, feelings and hallucinations that she had recorded in the journal. The doctor would always listen patiently. Certainly some of the cultural factors that were present in the patients' narratives must have eluded him. However, he could always gather enough information on the social and psychological factors to understand how they were contributing to the patient's humoral condition.

The Tara Institute relies to a large extent on payments made by patients coming to its clinics. It can be argued that it has been 'disembedded' from its original context of social interactions and forced into the mould of the capitalist economy (Giddens 1991). The patients at the Tara clinics thus have two identities: on one hand they are sick people seeking a cure, and on the other they are patients buying a service or consumers purchasing a product. The Tara clinics entail an adaptation in the economic relationship between the doctor and the patient.[8] However, this does not seem to have affected Tibetan notions of disease, and the wider picture of disease causation is still taken into consideration, as the examples in the following section show. The patients pay for the consultation and their medicines, so in a sense medicine in the clinics is a commodity, but this has very little effect on the relationship between the doctor and his patients. There is always plenty of time for patients to discuss all matters relating to their condition and whatever other questions they might have on their mind. The clinic is a relaxed and friendly environment. The following clinical interactions give a flavour of this.

Inherent to the Western socio-economic and political context, the modern bureaucratic state, are certain institutional forces and relationships of power that have a strong coercive affect on the form that Tibetan medicine can take. These institutional forces involve attributes such as a propensity to proper procedure and to rules and regulation which are predictable. There is also the strong imperative to orderliness; everything must be defined in such a way that it can be placed within a certain jurisdiction (Berger *et al.* 1973). Related to this orderliness is a taxonomic propensity. 'Bureaucracy is not only orderly but orderly in an imperialistic mode. There is a bureaucratic demiurge who views the universe as dumb chaos waiting to be brought into the redeeming order of bureaucratic administration' (ibid.: 50). There is a 'componentiality' whereby phenomena are classified and placed in categorical boxes, in order that they can be further subdivided or recombined to form greater wholes. This taxonomic style filters through into other areas of social life, biomedicine being no exception.

Another important coercive force impinging on Tibetan medicine in the West is existing relationships of power. Friedson (1970) has shown how by using legal and political means biomedicine gained professional dominance over competing traditions. This process still applies to the way Tibetan medicine is currently shaped in the UK. Up to now it has been regulated and organized according to the culture and institutions of biomedicine. This not only has consequences for the social organization of the tradition, but also leads to transformations in its theories and practices to make them consistent with those of biomedicine.[9] The regulations on herbal medicines and the process of statutory self-regulation in the UK have come about through such institutional forces and relationships of power.[10] They are dominated by a biomedical ethos. The proposed core curriculum in herbal medicine which herbal practitioners will have to pass in order to achieve statutory regulation includes, as we have seen, a substantial component of biomedical science. The regulatory process also requires the building up of an evidence base on the safety and efficacy of Tibetan medicine therapies, the reliability of its diagnostic methods and the cost-effectiveness of its treatments. Needless to say, the standards whereby this evidence base will be evaluated are those of biomedicine.

Clinical interactions: an ethnographic account

In this section I will present a number of clinical interactions that I recorded whilst working in the Tara clinics. The purpose of this is to illustrate the issues that are presented in this chapter and to give a feeling of what Tibetan medical consultation involves in the West. In what follows I have tried to be as faithful as possible to what actually happened; the turns of phrase I have used are in most cases those of the patients. I have given more details for the patient's first session and provided a brief summary of subsequent sessions.

Most of the patients who came to the clinic were over the age of 20; patients from all different age groups above this came. There were roughly equal numbers of male and female patients. As four of the five clinics are situated in centres of Tibetan Buddhism it follows that some of the patients had an interest in Buddhism and Tibetan culture. However, most of the patients came to the clinic because they had heard about it from a friend or had seen some publicity. When patients arrive at the clinic the procedure follows a set pattern. New patients are given a booklet which contains some basic details about Tibetan medicine, in particular the kinds of medications that are used. They then fill in a form giving personal details for the clinic records. After this they explain to the doctor the nature of their condition. The doctor told me that, following the Tibetan medical text, Tibetan medical diagnosis has aspects that relate to listening, looking and feeling. The doctor listens to what the patient has to say about his or her condition, and looks for any indicators of illness on the patient's body, such as discoloration of the skin or eyes and the appearance of the tongue. The doctor may also get important information about the condition of the patient's body by the appearance of his or her urine. The feeling aspect relates primarily to pulse diagnosis, but also to searching the body for unusual features or areas of pain.

The doctor listens to the patient and asks questions to refine his understanding. He then takes the pulse and asks further questions. At this point a conversation ensues between the doctor and the patient whereby the doctor explains to a certain extent the conclusion of his diagnosis. He may then give advice about helpful behaviour and diet. Usually the patient is given three medicinal compounds in the form of powders, to be taken with breakfast, lunch and the evening meal. These medicines are posted to the patient. Depending on the nature of the disorder, Dr Dhonden sometimes uses external therapies such as massage or moxibustion. Often the doctor advises the patient to come back after one month in order that he can carry out another diagnosis and assess how the patient has responded to the treatment. The booklet that is given to the patient contains a section where the patient can write down how his or her condition has changed in each of the ensuing weeks before the next appointment.

Because the medicines are manufactured in the pharmacy at Shilling in east Tibet and have to be imported to the UK, it is sometimes difficult to maintain supplies. During the research period the doctor had around ninety medicinal compounds at his disposal. Most of these compounds came in the form of powders, usually to be taken with water or occasionally to be prepared as a decoction. According to the Tibetan medical text there are ten types of medicinal compounds: decoctions, powders, pills, pastes, butters, ashes, concentrates, beers, herbal preparations and precious medicines. I witnessed the use of all these forms of medicine in the clinic in Dhorpatan, but at the Tara clinics medicinal powders and pills were used most often.

Patient 1

This patient was a 50-year-old man. At the time of the research he had been to see the doctor once a month for five months and his treatment was ongoing. As he had been working as an ambulance man for twenty years he was very well versed in biomedical techniques and terminology. On his first visit he explained that he had a bowel disorder. He had been to see a specialist doctor at the hospital and had been told that he was suffering from Crohn's disease, or ulcerated colitis. He told Dr Dhonden that his condition is also related to irritable bowel syndrome. He had been given anti-inflammatory steroids to build up the damaged tissue. The specialist at the hospital had mentioned the possibility of surgery, but first a biopsy needed to be done. He had told the specialist that he was coming to see a Tibetan doctor. The doctor was curious to be kept informed about the Tibetan medical treatment.

At this point Dr Dhonden took the patient's pulse. Whilst taking the pulse he asked two questions. First he asked the patient whether he had back or joint aches. The patient replied no, but he sometimes suffered from sciatica. Next, he asked the patient to explain what he experienced when he went to the toilet. The patient said that his stool had been very soft, with mucus and blood. When he started taking the steroids about a month before, initially the medicines had greatly improved his condition, but now the blood had come back. Dr Dhonden gave the patient three medicines to be taken with breakfast, lunch and the evening meal. He told him to continue to take the Western medication, but not to take it at the same time as the Tibetan medicine. Afterwards, he explained to me that he was treating the disorder with medicines used for a *tren* (*skran*) in the colon. This Tibetan word covers a range of growths and tumours.

One month after, on his second visit to see Dr Dhonden, the patient explained that his condition was slightly better. During the first two weeks he had been constipated; then he went on holiday and the constipation had stopped. He had taken the steroid again, which had stopped the bleeding for a while but then it had continued. He said that on the whole in the first two weeks his condition had improved, but in the following two weeks it had regressed. He said that in the third week he felt nauseous, but attributed this to a virus he had contracted from his ambulance work. He also added that the nature of his work meant that he ate irregularly, and he thought this might be part of the problem.

The doctor took his pulse, during which time he asked the patient if he had any sensation of acid coming up from his stomach. The patient replied no. He thought the pulse was a little improved and he gave the same three medicines. He explained that sometimes Tibetan medicine can bring about results quickly, but on the whole it acts gently and depending on the nature of the disorder it can take some time to bring about positive tangible results.

In the following three months the same sequence was repeated in the clinics. In the third month the patient reported that his condition had improved but now he was feeling an uncomfortable sensation of pressure in his lower back. He was also uncertain about which medicine was working as he was taking both Western and Tibetan medicine. In the fourth month his condition had again improved and he had cut down his intake of the steroid; at this point Dr Dhonden changed his morning medicine. In the fifth month the patient said that he was now much better, and the specialist had told him that surgery was not necessary. Dr Dhonden told him that his pulse was now healthy, and that he would give him only two medicines.

The patient was very happy with the way his condition had improved. He was still taking the Tibetan medicine and the steroid, but was now feeling well. He thought that it was the Tibetan medicine that had prevented him from needing surgery.

Patient 2

This patient was a 45-year-old woman. At the time of the research she had been to see the doctor once a month for four months and her treatment was ongoing. She explained that she had suffered from ME for twelve years, but this was now much better. Her main problem now was a range of conditions: for some time she had been slightly constipated and had recurring flatulence; she had eczema on her feet that became worse when the weather was hot; for ten years she had suffered from bad arthritis in her lower vertebrae; and she had low energy. The doctor took her pulse during which time he asked whether she had problems with her period. She replied no, but she had problems with her bladder. Then the doctor asked her if she had any problems with her knees or her joints. She said that she did have a little pain in her joints. The doctor gave her three medicines to be taken at breakfast, lunch and dinner. He also said that she should avoid spicy food, alcohol and potatoes.

The following month she explained that she had caught a virus, one cold after another. She was feeling at a very low ebb. Her constipation and flatulence had improved a little. The doctor took her pulse and afterwards he asked several questions. He asked the patient about her sleep. She said it had been mixed; sometimes she had awoken in the middle of the night and couldn't go back to sleep. She added that in the last month she had slept well on a few nights, which was better than before. The doctor then asked her about her eczema. She said this was a little better and that her arthritis had improved. The doctor said the medicines were working well but she would need to take them longer. The patient wanted to know how long, to which the doctor replied that this was uncertain, but maybe three months.

In the following two months her arthritis and eczema had improved to the extent that the doctor stopped giving her medicines for these disorders. Her sleeping pattern had also greatly improved. Though the constipation and flatulence had improved, they still continued to be a problem. The patient at one point in her assessment attributed this problem to parasites, but later she changed her view to a viral or bacterial infection. During the last visit the doctor said that her pulse was much more balanced.

Patient 3

This patient was a 30-year-old man. He had seen the doctor once a month for three months. The first time he visited Dr Dhonden I was not present; at this time he had told the doctor that he had a skin problem and small ulcers in his mouth. He had received three medicines. On the second visit he was very happy because the mouth ulcers had gone. He then went on to say that in the last month he had been very busy, and he had 'got a bit hyped'; also he felt confused and had not slept very well. When he exerted himself he felt hot inside. At that time he had the sniffles. He explained that he had had glandular fever when he was young.

The doctor took his pulse and asked how his skin problem was. The patient replied that it was still a problem. He said that it was like dermatitis. He had used cortisone cream for one year but had stopped. Dr Dhonden asked him if he had any digestive problems, to which he replied that he sometimes had diarrhoea, but now it was not so bad. He continued that the problem is that he has so much work, sometimes up to eighteen hours a day; he does not have the time to eat three regular meals. Dr Dhonden asked about his mood. The patient said that generally it is fine but when he is under stress he feels that the tension accumulates in his stomach.

Dr Dhonden gave him the same three medicines. He said that, as the mouth ulcer problem was now under control, a further month of the same medicine should stop this from coming back; then after he would give him medicines for his skin condition. He told the patient to avoid sweet foods. He gave chocolate as an example. This dismayed the patient as he had a particular penchant for chocolate.

The following month the patient explained that he had been more or less all right. He had 'forgotten' to take the medicines for a week and had got two mouth ulcers, but on resuming the medicine they had gone. He said that he had been very busy and he had had no time to think about anything. He said that he had been sleeping well, though he still had 'low energy'. He felt that cutting back on sugar had helped. Whilst taking the patient's pulse Dr Dhonden asked him whether he had any digestion problems. The patient replied that in the previous week he had argued a lot at work, and all the pent-up emotion had accumulated in his stomach; this had caused him to have diarrhoea. Dr Dhonden said that he would give the same morning and lunch medicines, the purpose of which was to stop the patient's mouth ulcers, and bring about mental balance and calmness, and that he would change the evening medicine to one which would focus on his stomach and digestive problem.

Patient 4

This patient was a 30-year-old woman. This was her first consultation with Dr Dhonden. She said that she had many problems. First she explained that she had recently been diagnosed as having an underactive thyroid condition. She was taking thyroxin, which had stabilized her. She was suffering from pain in her body, particularly in her left shoulder. Mentally she wasn't feeling very well; she was feeling very stressed and tired. She also mentioned that she had been getting dark blemishes and rashes on her chin and forehead. She said that this is the sort of thing that women get after childbirth, but it had been a long time since the birth of her child.

Dr Dhonden took her pulse and asked her if she had any problems with her stomach. She replied that she often had wind and burps. He then asked if she had noticed any seasonal changes in her condition, to which she replied no. As with the previous patients, Dr Dhonden gave her three medicines. The patient asked him what he thought about her problem. He told her that she had a weak constitution. Her digestion was weak and this was disrupting the functioning of her body. The three humours in her body were not balanced. A brief explanation was then given about the three humours. She asked if this was the cause of her muscular pain. Dr Dhonden thought it was. He said that the imbalance can sometimes affect the nerves, which can lead to muscular pain. He added that he was giving her medicines to balance her humours.

Patient 5

This patient was a 25-year-old woman. She had seen the doctor once a month for two months. She explained that she had been suffering from ME for over a year. She had difficult mobility and had been tired for the last fourteen months. The doctor took her pulse and asked her a series of questions. First he asked whether she had any problems with her stomach. She replied no. Then he asked if she had problems with her joints, and again she answered no. Then he asked about her period, which she said was fine. He asked her if she had backache, to which she responded that she did sometimes. Finally he asked about her sleeping. She said that she was sleeping too much, at least ten hours a day. Dr Dhonden then gave her three medicines. He explained that these medicines were to increase her energy and to bring balance into the wind (*rlung*) humour, which he had diagnosed to be in a disturbed condition. On her following visit she remarked that her strength and stamina had increased.

Adaptations to Western medical ideology

Having outlined what happens in the clinic I will now proceed to discuss issues that relate primarily to communication and the possibilities of translation between different medical ideologies. In the following section I will move on to discuss issues related to treatment evaluations. Tibetan medicine and biomedicine hold apparently incommensurable views on the body, mind and disease.[11] The personal views of practitioners and patients aside, biomedicine is a secular discipline. Tibetan medicine on the other hand is intimately related to Buddhist philosophy. In Dhorpatan it was possible to categorize diseases into two sorts related to their cause. Disease caused by behavioural patterns, seasonal changes or the presence of factors with characteristics that disturb one or more of the humours is amenable to the standard forms of treatment. Disease that is caused by harmful spirits, and this was quite common in the valley, requires ritual intervention. In the Tara clinics, this aspect of Tibetan medicine is not used, and the Buddhist elements of Tibetan medicine are usually only discussed if a patient requests it. The reason for this is not that there is a policy to present Tibetan medicine as a rational secular medical science. It is rather that most of the patients who come to the clinics are not conversant with Tibetan Buddhism, and Tibetan medicine can be practised without reference to it. Most of the patients who came to the Tara clinics knew very little, if anything at all, about Tibetan medicine. On the other hand all the patients were conversant in varying degrees with the notions and categories of biomedicine. Obeyesekere (1976) has noted that generally during consultations, whatever the type of medicine being practised, the patient wants to feel that he or she has successfully communicated his or her problem to the doctor. Generally, the biomedical consultation has been criticized for not achieving this. The two main criticisms pertain to the brevity of the consultation (Waitzkin and Stoekle 1976) and to the fact that not enough importance is given to psychological and social issues relevant to the patient (Frank 2002; Roter *et al.* 1988). In the Tara clinics the duration of the consultation or neglect of psychological and social factors is not an issue. The consultation is allowed to take a natural course; there is no attempt to finish within a given time; usually it takes about twenty minutes. Communication between the doctor and his patients is however a more opaque subject.

Tambiah (1990), in a discussion of multiple orderings of reality in anthropology, points to the work of the French historian Lucien Febvre (1878–1956). In Febvre's (1982) famous book *The Problem of Unbelief in the Sixteenth Century*, he presents the view that, in sixteenth-century France, anti-Christian thinking was impossible. In a discussion of the kind of thinking that was possible at this time, he gives a list of adjectives such as 'absolute', 'relative', 'abstract', 'concrete' and 'intentional'. To this he adds the nouns 'causality', 'concept', 'analyses', 'syntheses', 'deduction', 'induction', 'coordination', 'classification' and 'system'. He ascribes the absence of these words to a deficiency in thought. Hobsbawm points to the same idea when he says 'words are witnesses which often speak louder than documents' (1962: 13). Words such as 'industry', 'factory', 'capitalism', 'scientist' and 'crisis', along with many others, were all either invented or gained new meanings during the period 1789–1848, the period of the French Revolution and the British Industrial Revolution. Then what of the words 'cystitis', 'menopause', 'ulcerated colitis', 'myalgic encephalopathy' (ME), 'arthritis', 'eczema', 'diabetes', 'blood pressure', 'bowel stricture', 'underactive thyroid', 'stroke', 'giardia', 'stress', 'anxiety', 'depression', 'urinary tract infection', 'Crohn's disease', 'AIDS', 'schizophrenia', 'pernicious anaemia', 'endometriosis', 'prolapse', 'fibroid', 'motor neuron disorder', 'infection', 'cancer', 'virus', 'hormone' and 'immune system'? All these words were used in the Tara clinics during the period of this research.

In my task as translator for the doctor, often it was impossible to find an exact equivalent Tibetan term, and I had to resort to describing the biomedical idea that these words signify in a roundabout way. My background is in anthropology; I have no formal training in biomedicine. However, it was not necessary, for the purposes of his diagnosis, that the doctor fully understood the intricate technical details of a given biomedical classification. After I had conveyed to him some idea of the meaning of a biomedical term, the doctor would often come up with an approximate Tibetan notion. For example, 'cysts', 'abscesses' and 'boils' all come under the Tibetan term *nyen bur* (*gnyan 'bur*); 'cancer' is *tren* (*skran*) or *dre né* ('*bras nad*); 'allergy' is *mi thrö pa* (*mi 'khrod pa*); 'hormone' is *bu nön* (*bu snon*) or *ser min bu* (*gser rmin bu*); 'germs', 'viruses' and 'bacteria' all come under the term *sin bu* (*srin 'bu*); 'infection' is *gö né* ('*gos nad*); and for 'immune system' Dr Dhonden gave a Tibetan phrase which denotes '28,000 *sinbu* situated in the body', which protect it from disease (*lus la gnas p'i srin 'bu nyi khri brgyad stong*).

Some authors, such as Meyer, have commented on the tendency amongst Tibetans to modernize the Tibetan medical system by using biomedical terms. He is critical of Rechung Rinpoche (1973) for his use of the biomedical terms 'lupus', 'typhoid' and 'germs' (Meyer 1981: 39), Yeshi Dhonden's (1986: 96) translation of *rim tshé* (*rims tshad*) as 'infectious disease', and Lobsang Dolma Khangkar's (1986: 166) translation of *sinbu* as 'bacteria' (Meyer 1990: 239). I am not saying here that Tibetan medicine has an equivalent concept to the biomedical notions of 'hormone', 'virus' or 'immune system'; I wish only to indicate the problems that exist in translating the concepts of one medical system into the concepts of another (see Adams and Li, Chapter 5). The main text of Tibetan medicine is known as the Gyushi, (*Rgyud bzhi*).[12] This text consists of four volumes, most of which has been translated now except for the third volume, which deals with Tibetan nosology; this is because of the complex task of trying to match up Tibetan disease categories with those of biomedicine, which is generally problematic except, as Meyer suggests (1995b: 13), in cases where elementary symptoms make the association obvious.

However, there still remains the problem of divergent understandings in the nature of disease. The biomedical model views disease as a pathological entity, whereas Tibetan medicine involves a more process-orientated model (Lambert 1988; Nichter 1992). According to Tibetan medical notions disease develops through three progressive stages: formation, accumulation and manifestation (Meyer 1981; Barmark 1991). A similar notion is found in Chinese medicine where serious organic disorders are thought to be preceded by a series of functional disorders; if they are recognized in time they can be prevented from reaching the organic stage (Porkert 1976). The process model of disease is also found in Ayurvedic medicine. Lambert (1988) found in her study of local discourses on sickness and the body in rural Rajasthan that disease was considered to have a natural course and the villagers were less concerned with aetiology than they were with the disease's progression and outcome. Therapies concentrated not so much on cure as ritual techniques to encourage the natural course of the sickness. One such therapeutic ritual is known as *jhara*, 'sweeping', and involves downward sweeping motions made with margosa leaves or peacock feathers. This attitude to disease she refers to as a 'prognostic orientation'. She refers to Zimmermann (1978), who has argued that this way of approaching disease is very much the form adopted by Ayurvedic practice and this has been overlooked by orientations deriving from the biomedical model.

I should add here that it would be wrong to think that the process orientation of Tibetan medicine means that it does not have a notion of disease entities; many can be found in the third volume of the medical text. Disease is still related to a pathological condition in the humours, but the outcome of this can manifest as an organic disorder or a fixed set of symptoms. Paul Unschuld's (1993) comments on representations of Chinese medicine in Western literature are of relevance here. These representations focus exclusively on flows of 'energy', the five phases and *yin* and *yang* correspondences; yet from his readings of the Chinese medical texts there is in fact a well-worked-out concept of a disease entity.

Though modern Western literature might dwell more on the mystical side of Tibetan and Chinese medicine representing physiology in terms of flows of 'energy' in the body, this notion did not often occur in the Tara clinics. The three humours were not described as three 'energies' in the body; rather they where described as groups of psychological and physiological processes. Because they consist of material, dynamic and psychological components, at the Tara Institute they are referred to as 'bio-dynamic agents'. As we can see in the above clinical interactions, Dr Dhonden often uses the English word 'energy', but he uses this in the sense of vitality. The Tantric texts of Tibetan Buddhism speak of a subtle anatomy which is permeated by a vast network of channels. The mind in these texts is related to 'winds' or 'subtle energies' that flow through these channels. A yoga practitioner learns to manipulate these 'winds' to gain spiritual insight. Some of these winds are related to physiological functions and are mentioned in the Gyushi (Meyer 1995b: 127). When he talks about subtle 'energies' in the body he uses either the English word 'wind' or the Tibetan word *lung* (*rlung*). It is only in Patient 5 that 'energy' is used in the sense of subtle force, and this derives from the patient's own familiarity with yoga and martial arts.

Obeyesekere has pointed out that a major problem for Western medicine in Sri Lanka is that the doctors and the peasant patients in his study speak in 'mutually incomprehensible idioms' (1976: 225). Western medicine is effective but it is not rational. We are told that this problem does not exist between the peasants and Ayurvedic practitioners, whose explanations 'flow logically from a shared body of assumptions' (1976: 225). It may well be that for the sake of his argument here Obeyesekere has overstressed his case. The problem of incomprehensible idioms is not only applicable to cross-cultural medical encounters; research has shown that in biomedical consultations general practitioners sometimes use terminology that is incomprehensible to their patients (Hadlow and Pitts 1991), and the same could well be true for Ayurvedic practitioners and their patients. However, the epistemological question remains. Could it be that in the Tara clinics Dr Dhonden and his patients speak in incomprehensible idioms and that Tibetan medicine is effective but not rational to his patients?

Many of the patients, prior to coming to see Dr Dhonden, had consulted with their GP and sometimes practitioners of other forms of therapies. Quite often they had tried a biomedical treatment with no success. A great number of the patients had chronic disorders. Sometimes a patient (see Patients 1, 2 and 4 above), whilst describing his or her condition, would use biomedical terms, such as 'Crohn's disease' and 'ulcerated colitis' in Patient 1, 'ME' in Patient 2, and 'underactive thyroid' in Patient 4. But often the patients did not explain their illness using biomedical categories; the patient would present to the doctor a range of symptoms, as in Patient 3. Sometimes patients presented their own views on the cause, which they attributed to such agencies as 'bugs', 'parasites', 'viruses' and 'stress', as with Patient 2.

It was also quite common, as again we can see from the above clinical interactions, that patients have concurrent multiple disorders. Tibetan medicine's focus on the functioning of the system as a whole allows it to accommodate such multiple disorder syndromes with some success, as with Patient 2. These disorders are understood not in terms of static disease entities but in terms of humoral disharmonies. Dr Dhonden adapted his treatment to fluctuations in the patient's humoral condition throughout the course of the disorder. Treatments involved medicines, and advice on behaviour and diet. Dr Dhonden often explained to his patients that Tibetan medicine is a gentle therapy which works slowly and may take some months to fully attend to the cause of the disorder.

The issue of unintelligible idioms was seldom a problem in the Tara clinics. If patients requested an explanation of their condition in Tibetan medical terms, every attempt was made to give this in a simple and lucid manner, as was the case with Patient 4. Patients often asked Dr Dhonden what he thought was the cause of their condition or what he had perceived from their pulse. Sometimes he would use a Tibetan disease category, but most often he would relate their disorder to some humoral imbalance. Sometimes this was explained in terms of a general humoral imbalance and sometimes in terms of a problem with a specific humour, such as for Patient 5.

As we can see from the clinical interactions, the patients were not fixed into one idiom of understanding their own condition. Young (1982) has pointed out that patients often hold different epistemological accounts of their illness at the same time. For example, Patient 1 was fully conversant with the biomedical conceptions and treatment of his condition whilst at the same time being completely open to Dr Dhonden's views and methods. Some of Dr Dhonden's long-standing patients had internalized aspects of Tibetan medical theory and in their descriptions of their symptoms would include statements like 'my *lung* is not balanced'. Therefore, to answer the question as to whether in the Tara clinics Tibetan medicine is effective but not rational to its patients, it is often one reasonable explanation amongst a host of possible others.

Treatment evaluations

As we saw earlier in discussing the recommendations made in the Select Committee report, the process of statutory regulation in the United Kingdom involves the building up of an evidence base on: therapeutic efficacy beyond the placebo effect; the reliability and reproducibility of diagnostic methods; the safety and cost-effectiveness of the treatments; and the mechanisms of therapeutic action. One of the principal aims of the Tara Institute of Tibetan Medicine is to carry out this kind of research in the Tara clinics, but, with limited resources, evaluating therapeutic efficacy is no easy matter.

Anderson (1992), in a review of research methodologies for evaluating the efficacy of treatment, discusses four possible approaches. First, there is laboratory research, which involves biochemical analyses of changes in physiological functions, the use of animals, and chemical analysis on medicines to isolate therapeutically active components. Second, there is the case study. Case studies involve documenting the therapeutic effects of single isolated patients. They are useful in what they suggest about therapeutic efficacy, but it is not possible to extrapolate from case studies conclusive data on the effects of specific therapies. For example, in the case of Patient 1 (p. 198), the patient thought that Tibetan medicine had helped his condition, but such self-evaluations provide no substantial evidence that the positive result in these cases was not due to the placebo effect.

Third, there is the blinded randomized controlled trial (RCT). In biomedicine this is the so-called 'gold standard' for establishing therapeutic efficacy. This involves randomly dividing a group of people suffering from the same disorder into two groups: a treatment group and a control group. The treatment group is given the treatment that is to be evaluated; the control group is either given another form of treatment, a placebo that is indistinguishable from the real treatment, or is not given any form of treatment. Controlled trials that give the most valid evaluations of treatment efficacy are those that have been blinded. In single blinded trials the researcher assessing treatment efficacy should not know whether the patient is part of the treatment group or the control group. In double blind trials the patients are also not aware to which group they belong.

The fourth approach Anderson lists is the longitudinal observational study. This involves observing a group of patients with the same disorder undergoing the same therapy over a long period of time. Ideally patients taking part in the longitudinal study should be randomly selected and stratified according to criteria such as age, sex, ethnic group, social class and so on. In order to ensure validity of the data, the sample group should also be large.

At the present time research in the Tara clinics involves collecting data about the patients, including background information about the patient, how the patient describes his or her condition, the doctor's questions, forms of diagnosis and therapies, the patient's questions and comments and the doctor's responses, and gathering information about how the patient responds to the treatment. During the period of this research I have documented numerous case studies, some of which I have presented above. A number of longitudinal studies are also under way.

However, this type of evaluation, if it is to be undertaken in the way that Anderson prescribes, is problematic. The first problem is logistical. At the moment there are only relatively small numbers of patients attending the Tara clinics suffering from the same disorder. The second problem is relevant to all the research methods that Anderson lists, with the possible exception of case studies: that is, they involve an implicit biomedical notion of disease.

As we saw earlier, the Tibetan medical model of disease is largely process orientated. The success of the longitudinal study, as Anderson describes it, requires certain conditions: that one disease entity is present throughout the study and that a single therapeutic response is used to treat it. Nichter (1992) has pointed out that this kind of disease entity orientation in research is well suited to pharmaceutical companies whose aim is to develop new drugs.

In the Tara clinics Dr Dhonden often adapted the patient's medicines according to how he assessed that their condition had changed, and this could happen two or three times during the course of the disorder. Nichter observed the same perspective on treatment amongst Ayurvedic practitioners in India. He concludes that treatments are often adapted to the patient's humoral condition rather than an abiding disease entity. This is demonstrated in a longitudinal study that he carried out in order to assess the efficacy of an Ayurvedic therapy for diabetes. His idea was to measure the blood sugar level of a number of patients while they were undergoing treatment and then after eight weeks to stop the treatment and examine the effects this had on the blood sugar levels. The Ayurvedic practitioner was happy for Nichter to conduct the tests, as he was interested in the blood sugar levels himself, but:

> he found it wrongheaded to reason that after suspending treatment the body would return to the state it had been before, complete with the original disease. This assumed the same set of conditions that caused the illness persisted, that the medicine alone was affecting symptoms, and that a disease entity persisted as a definitive form.
>
> (Nichter 1992: 228)

Nichter points to Trawick's remarks in the same volume, which are equally applicable to Tibetan medicine:

> Just as diagnosis and treatment may vary from moment to moment in Ayurveda, so may the disease itself. Disease is not an isolated entity, it is a disturbance in the pattern of the system as a whole. And when symptoms of an illness abate, it is generally not said that the illness is gone, rather it is said that the disease has changed.
>
> (Trawick 1992: 228)

As I mentioned earlier, all disorders in Tibetan medicine are related to pathological conditions in the functions of the three humours. In the Tara clinics, with many patients there was no abiding disease entity; the disease was understood in terms of dysfunctions in the humoral system; this could change, and Dr Dhonden would adapt his therapy accordingly. Such patients would not fit the requirements of longitudinal studies that require a single disease entity and a single remedy in a large sample group. On one occasion a patient came to see Dr Dhonden with cancer who was about to undertake a course of chemotherapy. The patient had asked the specialist in the hospital if it was fine to take Tibetan medicine at the same time as the chemotherapy. The specialist thought that there should be no problem but wanted to see a list of the plants. Dr Dhonden gave the patient a list of the plants in the medicinal compounds but told her to tell the specialist that this was the medicine that was relevant to her condition at that particular moment and, as her condition progressed, the medicine would have to be changed.

Adams (2002) has drawn attention to the same problem for RCTs when they are applied to therapies of other medical traditions. They are adapted to the biomedical therapeutic approach which involves a medicine containing one or very few ingredients, and the medicine used remaining constant throughout the course of the treatment. Another problem is that biomedical researchers and Tibetan doctors may assess the same empirical evidence differently. Where a biomedical assessment using technical measures of treatment outcomes such as scans of organ systems, or blood tests, might indicate a negative result, the Tibetan doctor may get information that contradicts this from the pulse or urine diagnosis. Adams also draws attention to the contradiction in the scientific approach to assessing treatments' efficacy. Built into the scientific method is a notion of equal access and objectivity, yet the measurement of the therapeutic efficacy of Tibetan medicine is only considered valid if it accords with the standards of the biomedical model. Tibetan medicine is not considered in its own terms. There is more at stake here than medical knowledge. The process involves relations of power which define what is legitimate and what should be outlawed, what knowledge is deemed valid and what should be kept out of the arena, and this all hinges on issues related to margins of profit.

However, as I mentioned earlier, certain types of disorder in Tibetan medicine, though understood in humoral terms, have the characteristics of disease entities, and where this is the case RCTs may be used. Successful RCTs have been carried out showing the benefit of Tibetan medicine for intermittent claudication (blockages in the leg arteries) (Drabaek *et al.* 1993; Smulksi and Wojcicki 1994)[13] and arthritis (Ryan 1997). Although at the moment research in the Tara clinics mainly consists of case studies and longitudinal observational studies, and despite the many pitfalls we have seen, it is hoped that in the future this will be expanded to include RCTs and laboratory research. The aim of the laboratory research will be to provide chemical identification of plant bioactive components and to identify suitable 'fingerprint' components for quality assurance purposes. It will not be assumed that therapeutic action is the consequence of isolated chemical components. Research has shown that therapeutic action in certain cases is not due to single bioactive components but to the synergistic action of multiple organic substances present in the medicine (Cassella *et al.* 2002). The Tara Institute hopes that laboratory tests will also be made to monitor the patient's physiological responses to the treatment, such as major organ and immune cell functions, in order that biomedically valid evidence will be gathered on the safety of Tibetan medicine.

Conclusion

In the introduction to this paper the questions were posed as to the elements of Tibetan medical practice that have made an easy transition to the UK context and those that have had most difficulty. What is it that can be concluded at this stage from the Tara clinics about the affects of the various social and political forces on Tibetan medicine in the Tara clinics in the UK? I am reminded here about the determinative role that Horton (1982) and Goody and Watt (1963) ascribe to the advent of writing in transforming traditional modes of thought to the modern scientific mode of thought. This argument was refuted by Parry (1985), whose work amongst Brahman ritual specialists in Benares showed that the advent of literacy in a once oral tradition had not transformed the features of the original Brahmanical tradition; on the contrary, literacy had been used to reinforce these traditional features. There are indications that the forces that are bearing down on Tibetan medicine in the Tara clinics could, in a similar way, rather than transform Tibetan medicine into something vaguely resembling biomedicine, be used to reinforce the traditional features of the Tibetan medical system.

The reason why there has been so much government interest in CAM is not because of a pure interest in medical knowledge, but rather because people are turning to these traditions in great numbers. The irony is that nobody can deny the power that biomedicine has to cure many forms of disease, yet at the same time people are becoming increasingly dissatisfied with its institutions, knowledge and therapies, and are looking for alternatives. Statutory regulation has come about because of this growth in the popularity of CAM. Those in favour of statutory regulation see it as a positive measure which will maintain good standards of practice and ensure the safety of the medicines used. On the other hand people who are against statutory regulation view it as an unnecessary form of control, one which sanctions alternative therapies whilst in the same motion subordinating them to the structures of biomedicine by using its framework as the standard by which they are judged. The outcome of this could be that in time the theory and practice of Tibetan medicine in the UK will be transformed in a way that makes them more closely resemble those of biomedicine, such as an emphasis on disease entities rather than a process orientation, and the neglect of social, psychological and environmental causative factors.

People turn to alternative forms of medicine such as Tibetan medicine because of the negative image that is associated with biomedicine, that it is impersonal, its treatments sometimes involve negative side-effects, and it is not holistic in approach; in other words it does not take into consideration the functioning of the body and mind as an interrelated whole. The patients in the clinical interactions presented in the paper show that Tibetan medicine's focus on the interrelationship of the systems within the body give it a framework whereby it is able to understand and treat patients who come with chronic disorders or a range of symptoms but with no single disease entity. As more patients turn to Tibetan medicine because they favour its 'holistic' approach this will act as a strong force to support and sustain this view.

We have seen that the process of statutory regulation involves the building up of an evidence base on therapeutic efficacy and the validity of diagnostic procedures. As the situation stands, Tibetan medicine is not to be evaluated according to its own criteria, but according to the standards of biomedicine. The problem here is that biomedical methods of assessment are adapted to a biomedical model of disease. But this might not always work to the disadvantage of Tibetan medicine. It is possible that a randomized controlled trial could show a given Tibetan medicine to be efficacious. It may also be that in the future it will be possible to do a scientific assessment of Tibetan medical pulse diagnosis and show it to be valid. On many occasions in my research both in Dhorpatan and in the Tara clinics I witnessed the Tibetan doctors making very accurate diagnosis through the pulse reading. If this was scientifically validated it would support the Tibetan medical notion that the condition of most of the major internal organs is reflected in the pulse. The point I am making here is that it may be that a biomedical assessment of a Tibetan medical diagnosis or treatment will produce evidence that will bring into question the accepted biomedical model and lead us to a greater understanding of the nature of health and disease.

Notes

1 The Edinburgh clinic is situated in a complementary therapy and counselling centre. The London, Glasgow and Dundee clinics are located in branch centres of Kagyu Samye Ling.

2 I will draw at certain moments, as a comparative category, on fieldwork that I conducted between 1996 and 1998 in a Tibetan medical school and clinic in the valley of Dhorpatan in West Nepal (Millard 2002). Following on from the above argument, Tibetan medicine in Dhorpatan should not be thought of as the traditional form of Tibetan medicine; rather the contrast is between two localized forms of Tibetan medicine. In addition, I have presented five clinical interactions which illustrate issues raised during the discussion.

3 In October 1993 I was employed as clinical facilitator in the Tara clinics. My main role was to serve as translator for the Tibetan doctor. By the time I began my work the doctor could already speak quite good English, and my translating duties consisted of explaining to him the meaning of terms and phrases that he did not understand. Where necessary I also had to explain Tibetan medical concepts to the patient.

4 The European Herbal Practitioners Association (EHPA) was founded in 1994 to represent the interests of the various herbal traditions practising in Europe. It has representative members from the associations of different herbal medicine traditions. To become a full member of the EHPA an association must satisfy certain conditions: it must be a register of qualified herbal practitioners, and it must have thirty or more members. If an association cannot meet these criteria it can become an associate member, which is the present status of the Tara Institute within the British Association of Traditional Tibetan Medicine.

5 The word that is used in Tibetan to signify a trained Tibetan medical practitioner is *amchi* (*am chi*) or *menpa* (*sman pa*) (see Chapter 1). I do not use this title in this text because Lobsang Dhonden is generally referred to as 'Dr Dhonden' by his friends, acquaintances and patients. It is a possibility that the process of statutory regulation will entail the prohibition of the use of the title 'doctor' applied to statutory regulated herbal medicine practitioners.

6 He began his studies in Tibetan medicine at the age of 10 with his uncle Chime Dhundul at Sera monastery in Tibet. He went on to study Tibetan medicine at the Lhasa Medical

and Astrological College and received his degree in 1990. After working for some time in the hospital in Lhasa, he came to the Tibetan Medical and Astrological Institute in Dharamsala, India, where after working for several years at its branch clinics in Ladakh and Orissa he was awarded the *menrampa* (*sman rams pa*) degree. Dr Dhonden explained that, on graduating from the Tibetan medical school in Lhasa, the student is awarded with the lower degree, *du ra pa wa* (*sdus ra pa ba*), or a higher degree, *kachupa* (*dka' bcu pa*). After practitioners pass an exam after eight years of practice, the degree of *menrampa* is awarded to them; this is the shortened form of *menpa bum ram pa* (*sman pa 'bum rams pa*).

7   The 'eighth element' for each of Tibetan medicine, Ayurvedic medicine, Chinese medicine and Western herbal medicine is given as an appendix to the report.

8   In Dhorpatan, the patients had to pay for medicines. Usually this was a nominal cash payment, but sometimes it was a payment in kind, such as a few eggs or some potatoes. As the clinic was sponsored by the Snow Lion Foundation based in Kathmandu, it did not rely entirely on money coming from patients to support it. The Dhorpatan clinic, in contradistinction to the Tara clinics, is an integral part of the local community where everyone knows the doctor. Medicine is not seen as a commodity; it is a public service. However, Tibetan medicine is not always integrated in the community in this way; nowadays it also exists as a commodity in private clinics in India, Nepal and Tibet.

9   This process has been shown elsewhere in the case of Asian medicines, in both industrialized and non-industrialized countries (Janes 1995; Leslie 1980; Lock 1990).

10 Although in a different context, Janes (1995) gives examples of how Tibetan medicine was affected by socio-economic forces in Tibet after it was formally resanctioned by the Chinese authorities in 1980. In his view what has taken place is a transformation in medical theory which downplays the Buddhist elements of Tibetan medicine, moves away from considering the wider social, psychological and environmental factors of disorders, and tends towards approaching medicine as a cataloguing system of disease entities and treatments.

11 Tibetan medicine and biomedicine are expressions of two contrary modes of knowledge, what I have referred to respectively as synthetic and analytic modes of knowledge (Millard 2002). See also, for a detailed discussion of the Tibetan medical system, Meyer (1981, 1990, 1995a, 1995b).

12 This is the main medical text for Tibetan Buddhists. There is however an almost identical text that is used by the Tibetan Bön religion called the *Bumshi* (*'bum bzhi*). I have written about the history and subject matter of these two texts (Millard 2002).

13 To be precise, the drug Padma 28, which was used in these trials, is not a traditional Tibetan medicinal compound, but a medicine that has been developed by the Swiss company Padma AG from Tibetan medicine formulas.

References

Adams, V. (2002). Randomized Controlled Crime: Postcolonial Sciences in Alternative Medicine Research, *Social Studies of Science* (Special Issue: *Postcolonial Technoscience*) 32(5–6): 559–690.

Anderson, R. (1992). The Efficacy of Ethnomedicine: Research Methods in Trouble. In M. Nichter (ed.), *Anthropological Approaches to the Study of Ethnomedicine*, Tucson, AZ: Gordon and Breach Science Publishers.

Barmark, J. (1991). Tibetan Buddhist Medicine from the Perspective of the Anthropology of Knowledge, *Tibetan Medicine* 13: 3–37.

Berger, P.L., Berger, B. and Kellner, H. (1973). *The Homeless Mind*, London: Random House.

Cassella, S., Cassella, J. and Smith, I. (2002). Synergistic Antifungal Activity of Tea Tree (Melaleuca Alternifolia) and Lavender (Lavandula Angustifolia) Essential Oils against Dermatophyte Infection, *International Journal of Aromatherapy* 12: 2–15.

Comaroff, J. (1982). Medicine: Symbol and Ideology. In P. Wright and A. Treacher (eds), *The Problem of Medical Knowledge*, Edinburgh: Edinburgh University Press.

Department of Health (2001). Government Response to the House of Lords Select Committee on Science and Technology's Report on Complementary and Alternative Medicine, http://www.archive.official-documents.co.uk/document/cm51/5124/5124.pdf.

Dhonden, Y. (1986). *Health through Balance: An Introduction to Tibetan Medicine*, Ithaca, NY: Snow Lion Publications.

Drabaek, H., Mehlsen, J., Himmelstrup, H. and Winther, K. (1993). A Botanical Compound – PADMA 28 – Increases Walking Distance in Stable Intermittent Claudication, *Angiology* 44(11): 863–867.

Dunn, F. L. (1976). Traditional Asian Medicine and Cosmopolitan Medicine as Adaptive Systems. In C. Leslie (ed.), *Asian Medical Systems*. Berkeley: University of California Press.

Febvre, L. (1982). *The Problem of Unbelief in the Sixteenth Century: The Religion of Rabelais*, trans. Beatrice Gottlieb, Cambridge, MA: Harvard University Press.

Frank, R. (2002). Homeopath and Patient: A Dyad of Harmony?, *Social Science and Medicine* 55: 1285–1296.

Friedson, E. (1970). *Profession of Medicine: A Study of the Sociology of Applied Knowledge*, New York: Dodd, Mead and Co.

Giddens, A. (1991). *The Consequences of Modernity*, Oxford: Polity Press.

Goody, J. and Watt, I. (1963). The Consequences of Literacy, *Comparative Studies in Society and History* 5: 304–345.

Hadlow, J. and Pitts, M. (1991). The Understanding of Common Health Terms by Doctors, Nurses and Patients, *Social Science and Medicine* 32: 193–196.

Hahn, R. A. and Gaines, A. (eds) (1985). *Physicians of Western Medicine*, Dordrecht: D. Reidel Publishing Co.

Herbal Medicines Regulatory Working Group (2003). *Recommendations on the Regulation of Herbal Practitioners in the UK*, London: Prince of Wales's Foundation for Integrated Health.

Hobsbawm, E. J. (1962). *The Age of Revolution*, London: Weidenfeld & Nicolson.

Horton, R. (1982). Tradition and Modernity Revisited. In M. Hollis and S. Lukes (eds), *Rationality and Relativism*, Oxford: Basil Blackwell.

House of Lords (2000). *Select Committee on Science and Technology: Sixth Report on Complementary and Alternative Medicine*, http://www.parliament.the-stationeryoffice. co.uk/pa/ld199900/ldselect/ldsctech/123/12301.htm.

Janes, C. R. (1995). The Transformations of Tibetan Medicine, *Medical Anthropology Quarterly* 9: 6–39.

Keesing, R. M. (1987). Models, 'Folk' and 'Cultural': Paradigms Regained? In D. Holland and N. Quinn (eds), *Cultural Models in Language and Thought*, Cambridge: Cambridge University Press.

Khangkar, L. D. (1986). *Lectures on Tibetan Medicine*, Dharamsala: Library of Tibetan Works and Archives.

Lambert, H. (1988). The Cultural Logic of Indian Medicine: Prognosis and Etiology in Rajasthani Popular Therapeutics, *Social Science and Medicine* 34: 1069–1076.

Leslie, C. (1980). Medical Pluralism in World Perspective, *Social Science and Medicine* 14B: 191–195.

Lock, M. (1980). *East Asian Medicine in Urban Japan: Varieties of Medical Experience*, Berkeley: University of California Press.

Lock, M. (1990). Rationalization of Japanese Herbal Medicine: The Hegemony of Orchestrated Pluralism, *Human Organisation* 49: 41–47.

MCA (2001). Traditional Ethnic Medicines: Public Health and Compliance with Medicine Law, http://www.mca.gov.uk/.

MCA (2002). Safety of Herbal Medicine Products, http://www.mca.gov.uk/.

Meyer, F. (1981). *Gso-Ba Rig-pa: Le système médical tibétain*, Paris: Editions du CNRS.

Meyer, F. (1990). Théorie et pratique de l'examen des pouls dans un chapitre du Rgyud bzhi. In T. Skorupski (ed.), *Indo-Tibetan Studies: Papers in Honour and Appreciation of Professor David L. Snellgrove's Contribution to Indo-Tibetan Studies*, Buddhica Britannica Series Continua II, Tring: Institute of Buddhist Studies.

Meyer, F. (1995a). Introduction. In J. V. Alphen and A. Aris (eds), *Oriental Medicine*, London: Serindia Publications.

Meyer, F. (1995b). Theory and Practice of Tibetan Medicine. In J. V. Alphen and A. Aris (eds), *Oriental Medicine*, London: Serindia Publications.

Millard, C. (2002). Learning Processes in a Tibetan Medical School, Unpublished Ph.D. thesis, University of Edinburgh.

Nichter, M. (1992). Ethnomedicine: Diverse Trends, Common Linkages. In M. Nichter (ed.), *Anthropological Approaches to the Study of Ethnomedicine*, Tucson: AZ: Gordon and Breach Science Publishers.

Obeyesekere, G. (1976). The Impact of Ayurvedic Ideas on the Culture and the Individual in Sri Lanka. In C. Leslie (ed.), *Asian Medical Systems*, Berkeley: University of California Press.

Parry, J. (1985). The Brahmanical Tradition and the Technology of the Intellect. In J. Overing (ed.), *Reason and Morality*, London: Tavistock Publications.

Porkert, M. (1976). The Intellectual and Social Impulses behind the Evolution of Traditional Chinese Medicine. In C. Leslie (ed.), *Asian Medical Systems*, Berkeley: University of California Press.

Rechung, R. (1973). *Tibetan Medicine*, London: Wellcome Institute of the History of Medicine.

Roter, D. L., Hall, J. K. and Katz, N. R. (1988). Patient–Physician Communication: A Descriptive Review of the Literature, *Patient Education and Counselling* 12: 99–119.

Ryan, M. (1997). Efficacy of the Tibetan Treatment for Arthritis, *Social Science and Medicine* 44: 535–539.

Samuel, G. (2001). Tibetan Medicine in Contemporary India: Theory and Practice. In L. Connor and G. Samuel (eds), *Healing Powers and Modernity: Traditional Medicine, Shamanism and Science in Asian Societies*, Westport, CT: Bergin & Garvey.

Smulksi, H. and Wojcicki, J. (1994). Placebo-Controlled Double-Blind Study to Investigate the Efficacy of the Tibetan Plant Preparation PADMA 28 in the Treatment of Intermittent Claudication, *Forschende Komplementärmedizin* 1: 18–26.

Tambiah, S. J. (1990). *Magic, Science, Religion, and the Scope of Rationality*, Cambridge: Cambridge University Press.

Taussig, M. (1980). Reification and the Consciousness of the Patient, *Social Science and Medicine* 14B: 3–13.

Trawick, M. (1992). An Ayurvedic Theory of Cancer. In M. Nichter (ed.), *Anthropological Approaches to the Study of Ethnomedicine*, Tucson, AZ: Gordon and Breach Science Publishers.

Unschuld, P. (1993). Epistemological Issues and Changing Legitimation: Traditional Chinese Medicine in the Twentieth Century. In C. Leslie and A. Young (eds), *Paths to Asian Medical Knowledge*, Berkeley: University of California Press.

Waitzkin, H. and Stoekle, J. D. (1976). Information Control and the Micropolitics of Health Care: Summary of an Ongoing Research Project, *Social Science and Medicine* 10: 263–276.

Young, A. (1982). The Anthropologies of Illness and Sickness, *Annual Review of Anthropology* 11: 257–285.

Zimmermann, F. (1978). From Classic Text to Learned Practice: Methodological Remarks on the Study of Indian Medicine, *Social Science and Medicine* 12B: 97–103.

9 Tibetan medicine revisited in the West

Notes on the integrative efforts and transformative processes occurring in Massachusetts, USA

Ivette Vargas

There is ample evidence attesting to the evolving interest in Tibetan medicine in the US: the ongoing influx of Tibetan refugees into the US and Europe; the gradual opening of doors for Westerners to study in Tibetan medical institutions; favorable Western responses toward Tibetan physicians and practices; university programs studying Tibetan medical texts; Tibetan medical practices being established in the West; and numerous international conferences on Tibetan medicine. Curiosity over Tibetan medicine's origins, and its distinctive theoretical framework and treatments are appealing to American concerns about finding new models for healing. But what exactly is appealing about Tibetan medicine in the American context? What happens to Tibetan medicine when studied, applied, and dissected by a Western audience? These questions draw our attention to the complexity of studying, "integrating," and applying (whether whole or piecemeal) a foreign medical culture in a new socio-cultural setting.

In an attempt to find answers to these questions, a focused case study was thus conducted on Tibetan healing in one state of the US, namely Massachusetts. The aim was to explore the local impact of the Tibetan medical tradition and from that to catch a glimpse of its wider significance in the North American landscape.[1] In this chapter, I offer preliminary explorations of these issues, for I mainly provide descriptive data on specific institutions and individuals. This, however, set the ethnographical milieu in which further study may be conducted. The case study was based on fieldwork, which included interviews and observations in medical and educational institutions, and on library research. Tibetan medicine was found to have made an impact in several fields: the field of religion, the commoditization of Asian medicines, and the biomedical realm, although impacts have not been restricted to these fields and are not always present in all fields at the same time. The findings reflect diverse concerns and assumptions about the parameters of Tibetan medicine – should it be limited to an "objective" traditional medical institution with its own bounded theories and practices (with or without religious overtones)? Or should it be broadened into a healing system that encompasses the religious and/or spiritual, the *amchi*, the medium, and the Tibetan monk?

Among the diverse information collected during the research, certain key individuals and institutions clearly stood out among the rest. Not only were these long-standing representatives of Tibetan medicine (either in its broad or in its specific conception) or students of the system in the American context, but they also drew upon their own cultural resources in their understandings and applications of Tibetan medicine. In this chapter, attention is drawn to the perception of Tibetan medicine in the US through the eyes of these actors who have engaged with it as long-term scholars, practitioners, and/or physicians. Diverse voices within the Western context are presented, revealing how Tibetan medicine is increasingly shaping, and being shaped by, the American medico-cultural landscape.

Making Tibetan medicine religious

Perhaps one of the most explicit examples of Tibetan medicine's impact in the US concerns the activities of those non-profit organizations that explicitly link Tibetan medicine with religion. This association is certainly made in order to attract the public and is rendered easy because the differentiation between the two sectors is generally opaque to most people interested by Tibetan medicine and Tibetan Buddhism.[2] Through hosting Tibetan *amchi* and providing educational resources and public workshops on Tibetan medicine, religion and meditation, one such organization, namely the Shang Shung Institute, highlights the Buddhist foundations of Tibetan medicine, which has attracted Westerners for a number of years.

The Shang Shung Institute is based in Conway, Massachusetts, and was established in 1994. It has had a significant impact locally and is becoming increasingly influential on a wider scale. Malcolm Smith, board member of the Institute, Jacqueline Jens, program director/treasurer of the Institute (at the time of interview) and manager of resident *amchi*, and resident *amchi* Phuntsog Wangmo have revealed the grand efforts of a dedicated staff and religious practitioners. The Institute is a branch of the Shang Shung Institute in America, a non-profit, tax-exempt organization (publicized as being without political or religious aims), dedicated to the study of Tibetan medicine. As Malcolm Smith pointed out, this Institute is "not for cultural preservation as such" but it attempts to "integrate traditional medicine into modern society."[3]

The Shang Shung Institute was begun by, and is sustained through the efforts of, Namkhai Norbu Rinpoche,[4] a well-respected religious dignitary and *Rdzog chen* teacher. Originally from *Sde dge*, Tibet, he fled to Sikkim in the late 1950s. With the aid of the prominent Italian Tibetologist Giuseppe Tucci, he began a teaching career in Italy and since 1964 has been professor at the Instituto Orientale at the University of Naples. Here he investigated literary texts from the *Bon po* tradition in an attempt to reconstruct the history of Tibet. In 1963, Norbu Rinpoche hosted the first International Convention on Tibetan Medicine in Venice, Italy, and since then he has informally conducted teaching retreats around the world. From these activities arose an organization called the Rdzog Chen Community, based in Conway, Massachusetts. The Rdzog Chen Community provides the spiritual guidance for the Shang Shung Institute, while the latter advertises itself as an educational medical organization and resource center.

The Institute provides a comprehensive three-year Tibetan medical program with a two-year practicum, including an astrology program and "massage" courses open to the public. It is currently redesigning its program and hopes to expand to a four-year program and start a clinic that would be separate from the training institute. Alongside Tibetan medical training such as *bsku mnye*, adapted and presented as "massage,"[5] there are sessions conducted by the Rdzog Chen Community on a variety of Tibetan practices, other Buddhist and non-Buddhist meditation techniques, and yoga.

The impact of this Institute and its members on the Western medical community in Massachusetts is steadily developing. According to Malcolm Smith, there has been interest from the general public, Western physicians, scholars in Tibetan studies, and others. However, for the moment the Institute mostly attracts traditional Chinese medicine (TCM) practitioners, who seek to learn more about Tibetan medicine and its techniques of diagnosis, such as pulse and urine analysis, and external treatment practices like moxibustion.

One of the first resident *amchi* at the Institute was Thubten Phuntsog, who is professor of Tibetan medicine at the Central University of Nationalities in Beijing and the Institute of Tibetan Studies in Sichuan Province, China. He is the author of numerous books on Tibetan history, grammar, astrology, and medicine, as well as running a Tibetan medicine practice in New York City. During his years of residence at the Institute, between 1998 and 2001, he launched the three-year foundation in Tibetan medicine course.

In late 2001, *amchi* Phuntsog Wangmo became resident at the Institute and director of the Tibetan medical program. She was educated at the Lhasa Medical College and studied under Tibet's foremost doctors, Khenpo Troru Tsenam and Gyaltsen, who are credited with the revival of Tibetan medicine within Tibet under the Chinese (cf. Holmes 1995). According to her translator, Jacqueline Gens, Phuntsog Wangmo also spent a number of years studying in Dharamsala, India, and trained under the Dalai Lama's personal physician, Tenzin Choedrak. She also directed ASIA, a non-profit organization founded by Chogyal Namkhai Rinpoche, through which hospitals and training centers were built in Eastern Tibet and Western China. Prior to 1996, she was on the faculty of the Shang Shung Institute in Italy.

The Institute, especially with its links to the famed rinpoche, is greatly raising the profile of Tibetan medicine in American life through the training of Westerners in Tibetan medicine by actual Tibetan *amchi*. The Institute provides a resource center on Tibetan medicine and religion, and acts as a center for translation projects.[6] Although there are Western physicians and a considerable number of TCM practitioners attracted to the Institute in order to learn about Tibetan medicine, a large draw seems also to be coming from those already sympathetic to Tibetan religion as practitioners and/or scholars. The Buddhist aspects of Tibetan medical theories and practices are heavily emphasized, especially in the activities conducted by the Rdzog Chen Institute and by those who participate in the workshops. The link between Sangye Menla (the Buddha Master of Medicine) and efficacy in Tibetan medicine is highlighted and is reinforced by some *amchi*, who note, for example, that "traditionally Tibetan medicine only works with the permission of the Medicine Buddha."[7]

What then is the result of the religion–medicine linkage highlighted by this prominent organization in the American context? Although it is as yet too early to tell, the emphasis on the Buddhist consonance of Tibetan medicine tends to direct it towards some form of "spiritual" healing, in some ways evocative of what are widely referred to as "New Age" practices. This is, somewhat paradoxically, accompanied by arguments that assert the scientific character of Tibetan medicine (medical theories, the biological and physiological effects of medicinal substances, etc.).[8]

Adapting and commoditizing Tibetan medicine

Tibetan medicine is, without doubt, an increasingly globalized medical practice. In today's Tibet Autonomous Region in the People's Republic of China, cultural and capitalist pressures are contributing to redefinitions of identity and practice, as well as to shaping Tibetan medicine as a "global" alternative medicine for the international market. Craig Janes draws attention to the complexities of such phenomena through the analysis of Tibetan medicine as both a "global commodity" and a "local tradition" (2002). This is crucial to understanding what occurs in the state of Massachusetts.

The vast interest in alternative and integrative medicines has led to Tibetan *amchi* trying to corner the market, making themselves well known and available to Americans who may wish to seek their assistance. Besides the presence of organizations like the Shang Shung Institute, Tibetan *amchi* themselves make contact with and provide educational services to Americans, contributing to the presence and impact of Tibetan medicine in the US. In addition to conducting formal courses at such places as the Shang Shung Institute, *amchi* also benefit from the support of private sponsors, which allows them to give independent public talks, seminars, and courses on Tibetan medicine in educational institutions, dharma centers, and institutes, such as the New England School of Acupuncture. Some have also opened their own centers in several states. Through such activities, Tibetan *amchi* are significant contributors to both the proliferation and the commoditization of Tibetan medicine.

A good example of these high-profile Tibetan *amchi* is Menba Yangdron Kalzang, a resident of Tibetan medicine at the Five Branches Institute (Tibetan wellness and healing center) in Santa Cruz, California. She has given numerous presentations at American institutions and engaged in a research study with the anthropologist Vincanne Adams on the maternal health of Tibetan women (Adams 2001: 222–246). Her talks at the New England School of Acupuncture and the Shang Shung Institute draw a diverse clientele, from TCM practitioners to Western physicians who are interested in integrative medicine.

Another *amchi* who is making her presence known is Keyzom Bhutti, who is the clinical director of her own center, Traditional Tibetan Healing Inc., in Somerville, Massachusetts. Born in 1951 in the *Sa skya* region of Tibet, she emigrated to India at the age of 6. In 1972, Bhutti became one of the first female Tibetan physicians to complete the rigorous medical training at the Tibetan Medical and Astrological Institute in Dharamsala, India. Her training was supported by the fourteenth Dalai Lama and the Tibetan government-in-exile, plus a sponsor from abroad. In 1988, she received the *menrampa* (*Sman pa 'bum rams pa*) degree. She also served as chief physician at the Tibetan Medical Astrological Clinic in Darjeeling for twenty-five years.

Widely traveled in the US and Europe, both alone and in the company of the Dalai Lama's senior personal physician, Tenzin Choedrak, Bhutti is renowned for her service in the medical profession and has received several prestigious awards.[9] In 1998, she opened a center in Massachusetts, together with Eric Jacobson[10] and Regina Pellicano (a student of Tibetan Buddhist dharma practice with a background in Tibetan medicine). She eventually branched out on her own and founded Traditional Tibetan Healing Inc.

In an interview conducted in spring 2001 at Harvard University, and during informal discussions held in 2003, Bhutti commented on her experiences and her encounters with both Western and Tibetan patients. As part of her practice she makes "traditional Tibetan herbal massage oils" which she states "balance physical and mental energies, promoting relaxation and free flow of energies. It also helps improve memory." Bhutti's use of the term "energies" for Tibetan medical aggregates and elements (such as the three *nyes pa* and the five elements that form a person's constitution or *rang bshin*), her use of oils, and her description of their effects are all atypical of Tibetan medicine in Tibet or elsewhere in the Himalayas. They reflect her understanding of the local demand, her appropriation of modern Western terminologies, and the correspondent adaptation of both her rhetoric and her practice. Such transformations illustrate the flexibility of Tibetan medicine and the ways through which it can be made more familiar to the Western palate in order to better market its "products."

Such adaptation occurs in a variety of contexts, such as in the doctor–patient relationship. Bhutti noted that there is a critical difference between patients in the US and those in India. For Bhutti, patients in India tend to have complete faith in their doctors, taking whatever medicine is given to them, often without noticing the effects and never complaining. In contrast, she sees patients in the US as active participants in their treatment, being "just as powerful as the doctors" so that doctors "have to be very careful about how to treat them." The American patients who opt to see a medical practitioner like Bhutti are often those who seek alternative or complementary models to the passive role played by patients in the biomedical system[11] and to replace it with a more empowered and consumerist relationship. This "consumer-patient" is often armed with a laundry list of complaints and frustrations that have not been adequately addressed by the mainstream health system. In order to answer these demands from patients, whom Bhutti describes as "expressing their emotional problems," the doctor tends to psychologize her medicine.

Bhutti's comments about the doctor–patient relationship have much to do with issues of exoteric and esoteric knowledge. Among Tibetans, Tibetan medicine thrives on the fact that the "conceptual space" concerning healing and disease is shared by both the *amchi* and the patient (apart from the more advanced knowledge that the *amchi* gains through medical education). In other words, diagnosis and treatment are more obvious to, and accepted by, the patient, who is accustomed to ideas about diet, *nyes pa*, karma, seasonal changes, and so forth.[12] In contrast, the *amchi* must create a new space of understanding in a new cultural context, where the conceptual space is not so readily shared. In this regard, it is necessary both to bring adequate answers to the questions posed by the patients and to legitimate these answers, for in the West the Tibetan medical system is located on the fringes of the mainstream medical realm and of a society which challenges its credibility and therapeutic efficacy.

The exotic nature of Tibetan medicine in the eyes of the consumer may also create barriers to communication. However, as with a Chinese person performing TCM in the past, a Tibetan healer adds to the "authenticity" of the practice and renders it more credible. The Tibetan *amchi*, the new "exotic" healer, has taken center stage. The Tibetan medical system can thus be better marketed, but under which conditions?

As far as Tibetan pharmacopoeia is concerned, Bhutti recognizes that people in the US who seek "alternative" medicine are open to new views of treatment. According to her, the same "supplements" can be used in the US as in India and Tibet. However, the *amchi* would certainly utilize the term "medicines" in the East and thus the use of the term "supplement" reflects another accommodation that Tibetan medicine is undergoing in the Western context. Because of legal pressures and Food and Drug Administration (FDA) regulations, Tibetan medicine cannot be acquired in the USA as a "medicine" through a prescription provided by a Western-trained medical official. It can only be legally obtained from a practitioner or via a website, where it is sold as a "dietary supplement," thus relegating Tibetan medicine to the realm of "the alternative."

The effects of this change in status are seen in numerous ways. For example, Rhosavin 100, an adaptogen herb grown organically in Siberia and used in Tibetan regions, is widely distributed as a "dietary supplement" on the internet and claims to benefit those with symptoms including depression, sexual dysfunction, hearing impairment, hormonal imbalance, memory problems, and fatigue. The use of biomedical terminology to describe the effects of the "supplements," rather than Tibetan medical conceptual frameworks, reflects a further form of transformation that Tibetan medicine must undergo to meet the demands of Western consumers.

According to the internet site tibetanherb.com,[13] "herbal supplements [such as Rhosavin 100] that are combined to create particular properties and effects . . . are given for any imbalances that are found and to remove impediments to energetic flow". The site herbalchemy.com goes even further into reinventing Tibetan medicine, clearly framing it within "New Age" circles, alongside color therapy, science, and love.[14] Such distorted understanding and amalgamations of Tibetan medicine are also drawn from academic publications, when authors such as Steiner state: "The first priority in Tibetan medicine is to restore harmony to each person in the context of his or her life experiences" (2003: 95). Perhaps the first priority of Tibetan medicine, as a Himalayan *amchi* would put it, is simply to cure patients.

The number of websites devoted to Tibetan medicine in the US, Europe, and the PRC shows how widely disseminated Tibetan medicine is today. They clearly articulate its *scientization* (through the use of biomedical idioms) and its parallel entry into the realm of "energy medicine," as we have seen above. The Tibetan-medicine-as-a-supplement business has cornered a considerable part of what is today a highly lucrative market.

Getting Tibetan medicine integrated: strategies and prospects at Harvard University

Individuals and institutions in Massachusetts have recognized the value of Tibetan medicine, while also challenging and imposing some compromises upon it. One such individual, namely Eric Jacobson, is a member of the Department of Social Medicine at Harvard Medical School and is exemplary in this regard. Jacobson is a wealth of information on Tibetan medicine[15] and has been a key actor in the "integration" of this healing tradition in the US.

In his home-based office in Arlington, Massachusetts, Jacobson has a wall lined with shelves of herb-filled bottles with Tibetan labels on them, relics of an earlier collaboration with Regina Pellicano and Keyzom Bhutti (who provided a Tibetan language formulary for these bottles). The profile of Jacobson offers telling insights into his personal integrative approach: he is a Tibetan scholar and medical anthropologist, rolfer,[16] craniosacral therapist,[17] psychotherapist, and long-time practitioner of Tibetan Buddhism. Building upon his early interests in science and religion, Jacobson embarked on a number of practices and scholarly trainings throughout his life, from gestalt psychotherapy and transcendental meditation (specifically that of Maharishi Mahesh Yogi) to sitting under the tutelage of Tibetan teachers like Chogyam Trungpa, Tulku Thondup, and Dodrupchen Rinpoche (the lineage holder of Long Chen Nyingtig). According to him, Tibetan teachers especially attracted him because of their being "completely present. . . completely calm," unlike anything he had experienced in other teachers. He also continues to be a part of the Mahasiddha Nyingma Center in Western Massachusetts. Jacobson's practice is a reflection of the modern Westerner trained in Tibetan medicine and religion who is also operating within a Western consumer market.[18]

His interest in the "medical" aspects of Tibetan Buddhism led him to complete a doctoral degree in medical anthropology at Harvard University. Throughout his dissertation research in Kathmandu, Nepal, and Dharamsala, Darjeeling, Gangtok, and others areas of India in the late 1980s and early 1990s, he trained in Tibetan medicine under Keyzom Bhutti and other Tibetan medical practitioners at a time when few Westerners were engaging in such study. In his research, he took life histories of patients and made formal diagnostic studies, often working with depressed and anxious patients. In the time he spent in these areas, he pieced together all the things Tibetans use to construct a clinical encounter.

The cultural differences in what constitutes health and illness are of utmost importance in determining medical efficacy in any context. Jacobson pointed out to me in 2000 that the general outcome of recent psychiatric anthropology in Asia, Africa, and South America is that "there are more somatic symptoms in Third World countries that do not have psychological idioms." Therefore, in terms of Tibetan culture, he noted that the "threshold of what counts as an illness is higher in Tibetan society" than in Western society. In this context, a person is not considered sick "unless [he is] severely dysfunctional . . . This is not true in the US; once you feel bad, you are a patient."

Jacobson focused attention on the "holistic" approach of Tibetan medicine[19] and the Tibetan view that the body contains the physical, mental, and psychical or cosmological, rather than following a Cartesian dichotomy of body versus mind. He notes the perceived relationship between the body as the microcosm and the environment (i.e. the universe) as the macrocosm in Tibetan medicine. Rather than focusing on health as the absence of disease, as reflected in Western biomedical theory, Jacobson highlighted the fact that the Tibetan medical model conceives the body as being in constant flux: disease arising when one of the many elements and aggregates (especially the *nyes pa*) that constitute the "body" predominate, thus creating imbalance. This is linked to the idea that Tibetan medicine focuses on the occurrence of disease as a particular event (an imbalance that may lead to other imbalances) and that such imbalances may have multiple causes. This is clearly in opposition to Western biomedical approaches, which focus on diseases as generic entities which must therefore have "a" cause. Jacobson highlights the fact that Tibetan medical treatments are focused on the body's relationship to nature and not its opposition to it.

Although Jacobson certainly has his own and particular approach, understanding, and practice of Tibetan medicine, he also voiced his concerns over Western misperceptions of the Tibetan medical tradition. For him, "one of the major errors Westerners have made was to psychologize Tibetan Buddhism."[20] He also added that the idea of "psychosomatic" as it is understood today in the Western context is not an appropriate one to apply to Tibetan medicine. The reason he gave me in 2004 was that Tibetan medicine "views psychological and physiological systems as integrated, so that both 'psychosocial' and 'biological' 'circumstantial causes' impact the same system, and give rise to illnesses that have both psychic and somatic symptoms." For Jacobson, Tibetan Buddhism and medicine are about "physical transformation more than about psychological transformation." He sees alchemy underlying Tibetan religion, which, in turn, is a crucial element for medical understanding. According to him, within an alchemical framework, imaging the exchange of bodily fluids with sacred beings and ingesting sacred substances trigger neurochemical changes in the body.[21] This shows again the shift into a new interpretative framework, where biological science meets theories of fluids, energies, and the sacred.

As a faculty member at the Department of Social Medicine at Harvard Medical School, Jacobson collaborates with other scholars and physicians, especially within the Healing and Placebo Research Group, a section of the Division for Research and Education in Complementary and Integrative Medical Therapies (the Osher Institute). Both the director of the Institute, David Eisenberg, and faculty member

Ted Kaptchuk are trained in Chinese medical techniques and have encouraged the integration of such training and techniques at area hospitals. The primary function of the division is to coordinate research and evaluation of alternative and complementary remedies at Harvard Medical School.[22]

At the Institute, Jacobson works as a co-investigator on clinical studies of the placebo effect. He is also conducting pilot studies of Tibetan clinical reasoning. Jacobson noted:

> the pilot is to develop a system of documenting Tibetan clinical reasoning, which will be used to record the diagnostic and treatment planning of Tibetan doctors in future clinical trials. This follows the example of the same strategy leading to "ecologically valid clinical trials" of acupuncture for depression.

I will not go into details explaining what is meant by "ecologically valid clinical trials," but basically such research aims to conform, as far as possible, to the conceptual framework of the medical system in question and thus to minimize distortion of the studied medicine.[23] However this research is framed, it still ultimately operates within the Western biomedical research paradigm.

Future planning: Tibetan medicine in the USA

The Massachusetts case study points to a much larger phenomenon surrounding Tibetan medicine unfolding in the US today. On July 12–21, 2002, under the direction of Tibetan scholar Robert Thurman, Nena Thurman, and Kimberly Johnson, a short conference entitled "The Future of Tibetan Medicine" took place at Tibet House USA Menla Institute, the Asclepius Foundation in Phoenicia, New York. The purpose of this meeting – to establish the teaching and practice of Tibetan medicine in the US – appears quite straightforward but was in fact far more ambitious and complex. According to some of the participants, the conference hoped to lead Tibetan medicine to a "harmonious integration with Acupuncture, Ayurvedic, other Western and Eastern alternative traditions as well as with the Western cosmopolitan medical tradition."[24] This preliminary gathering consisted primarily of about fourteen Tibetan physicians (most of whom were trained in Tibet and India and today reside and/or practice in the US); several Western physicians; various scholars in the field of Buddhist and Tibet studies; lawyers; and other interested individuals. Jon Kabat-Zinn, who attended the gathering, is himself the retired founder of the Center for Mindfulness, Medicine, Healthcare and Society at the University of Massachusetts Medical Center in Worcester. The foundation of his stress reduction and relaxation program is the medicine of dharma practice and meditation.[25]

The participants attempted to engage in open dialogue regarding the implantation of Tibetan medicine in the US, the preservation of the Tibetan medical tradition, religious considerations, and methods and theories of Tibetan medicine. The conference reiterated the Tibetan medical focus on balance and the mind–body–spirit connection. For the organizers of the conference, Tibetan medicine, as an integrated system of health care employing a unique theory and system of practice, offers the West a different perspective on health. They stressed that it must be understood in its own terms, as well as in the context of "objective investigation." This notion has been formulated, and in various contexts attempted, but it has never been effectively put into practice: The biomedical paradigm has systematically shown its hegemony, thereby undermining the first half of the proposition. According to Eric Jacobson,[26] the conference was fruitful, as it focused on the "four areas of professionalization," that is "how to get Tibetan doctors licensed, education, research, and dialogue." He added that the "prospects look good for some serious research on Tibetan medical efficacy."

Nevertheless, Jacobson noted that often Tibetans and Westerners "ultimately do not understand each other [in respect to] medicine and pharmacological theories." He reiterated that "there has to be cross-education," so as to resolve some of the existing conflicts. For instance, there is a general mistrust of Westerners on the part of Tibetan medical practitioners and institutes, who feel they may be taken advantage of, and an overall sense of uneasiness surrounding the transmission of Tibetan medicine on Western soil. For Jacobson, "it is difficult for Tibetans to realize that, not only can they not control who practices Tibetan medicine, it is not legal. You cannot control a commercial practice." He later stated, in autumn 2004:

> The other problem is that most Tibetan practitioners and bureaucrats do not appreciate the potential expansion of the market for Tibetan medicine in the US and Europe, that is, anything that Western scientists or practitioners do to increase the public visibility or scientific credibility of their medical tradition will result in more demand for their services. They tend to react as though any recognition that Westerners get for their knowledge of Tibetan medicine is at their expense, rather than an aid in expanding that market.

The key issues that have apparently been chosen for the future of Tibetan medicine by the Western agents of its development are thus clinical research, market growth under the complementary and alternative medicine (CAM) industry, and a revised form of Tibetan medical practice and rhetoric. Given this context one might well question the extent to which the expansion of the Tibetan medical market can be seen to be a positive thing in the long run.

Such orientations were exemplary during the International Congress on Tibetan Medicine, which took place in Washington, DC, in November 2003 and was sponsored by Pro-Cultura, the Continuum Center for Health and Healing at Beth Israel Medical Center, and a host of other organizations.[27] Several of the issues outlined above were discussed and expanded upon, and workshops were held on the following: breakthroughs in mind–body medicine and neuroscience research; Tibetan theoretical and practical techniques; mental health; meditation; yoga; mantras; the exploration of Tibetan philosophical and practical concerns; Tara Rokpa therapy to treat cancer; and Tibetan and Western approaches to HIV/AIDS. Tibetan and Western scholars and medical practitioners presented papers on the effects of Tibetan medicine on physiological and psychological functions and on regulatory concerns, and new films on Tibetan healing were promoted. Venerable Tulku Thondup even conducted a couple of meditation sessions to a large, eager audience of listeners and practitioners.

The transformation of Tibetan medicine in Massachusetts shows the capacity this healing tradition has to mold itself to new social, cultural, and economic contexts. It is currently being reshaped as a medical system within which practitioners' discourses and practices increasingly differ from those of their Himalayan homologs. The situation depicted in this chapter is indicative of a wider trend surrounding anything Tibetan, which seems to be inevitably accommodated so as to thrive in the US. Indeed, the Dalai Lama, while seemingly advocating a "Buddhist modernism" and a universal religion, also advocates the adaptation of Tibetan Buddhism and medicine to the Western world (1997). This illustrates the predominance of the Western model and its requirements that externally originating systems must transform themselves in order to gain Western support – requirements which clearly apply in regard to support for the Tibetan political cause, or assistance in the commoditization of Tibetan medical "products." Donald Lopez further remarks that, "when elements of Buddhist cosmology conflict with the findings of Western science, the Buddhist views can be dispensed with" (1998: 186). The same applies to certain theoretical and practical aspects of Tibetan medicine, such as the explanatory model of disease causation which involves evil spirits, and the use of an adapted form of "Tibetan massage." Tibetan medicine has taken on a distinctly Western form, in which it fits Western ideas and ideals about the East, on the one hand, while on the other hand it still struggles to meet the scientific requirements that would afford greater credibility to its theories (whether revised or not) and thus enable even further expansion.

There is a growing concern among American citizens for alternative or complementary medical techniques, and Western doctors are increasingly interested in expanding their theories of the mind–body connection. Certain aspects of Tibetan medicine are being adapted to correspond with elements of "New Age" ideology, which is a cultural and economic growth area in the contemporary American context. The various forces that are working towards the promotion of Tibetan medicine as a commodity within the CAM industry, and the considerable effects of this process, are also well noted. This study, although focused on the state of Massachusetts, mirrors the accomplishments and transformations of Tibetan medicine that are evident in other parts of the US, especially in New York and California, where many Tibetan *amchi* reside. Tibetan medicine is evolving in a challenging environment, in which further struggles, distortions, and revisions will surely take place so as to satisfy the objective of its supporters: for this medical system to continue to implant itself and grow more widely in the North American setting.

Acknowledgements

This study was originally funded by Harvard University Center for the Study of World Religions' Religion, Health, and Healing Initiative in 2002, a research grant focusing on the interface between religion and healing, and revised in subsequent years. I would like to thank all the *amchi*, Western medical practitioners in Massachusetts, staff at Shang Shung Institute, Tibetan and Western scholars, and Tibetan practitioners for all their assistance in making this study possible. Special gratitude goes to Linda Barnes at Boston University Hospital for all her insight and Venerable Tulku Thondup for his guidance. My greatest debt goes to Eric Jacobson for always being available, informative, and entertaining.

Notes

1 This case study was initially conducted for the Harvard University Center for the Study of World Religions' Religion, Health, and Healing Initiative, 2002. Data was collected for three years from 2000 to 2004, and interviews were conducted from 2002 to 2004.

2 See Pordié (2003, 2007) regarding a discussion about medicine being differentiated from religion although the former has been established in a Buddhist religious environment.

3 Malcolm Smith and Phuntsog Wangmo were interviewed in March 2003.

4 In Tibetan Buddhism, rinpoche (*rin po che*) is a title of respect usually reserved for tulku (*sprul sku*), which is a term descriptive of certain masters (*bla ma*) who are thought to reincarnate deliberately and with perfect mastery for the benefit of other beings.

5 The practice of *bsku mnye*, although mentioned in some classical medical texts, does not consist of massage as it is widely understood in the West. It is seldom used in the Tibetan cultural area and concerns the application of butter, and more rarely sesame oil, to certain areas of the body. Furthermore, it is generally applied by the patient to him/herself (Laurent Pordié, personal communication).

6 A description of all their current activities can be found at http://www.tsegyalgar.org/community/ssi.html.

7 For example, such statements were made by both *amchi* Wangmo and Kalzang during a workshop on *bsku mnye*.

8 The emphasis on the religious aspects of Tibetan medicine has been shown to be largely a political strategy in the Indian Himalayas (cf. Pordié 2003). Although the political ramifications of such processes on Western soil are not the main subject of the current study, the move of Tibetan medicine toward becoming a religious healing practice may indeed be partially political, in relation to the wider arena of the supplements and vitamin industry. Tibetan medicine may thus escape the lobby of pharmaceutical companies, which are pressuring American politicians to limit or close down the aforementioned industry.

9 These awards include the Award of Excellence for her dedicated service in the field of Tibetan medicine for over twenty-five years by the Tibetan Medical and Astrological Institute, the Shiromani Award in 1995, and the Award of Excellence in 1997 by the Indian Board of Alternative Medicines at the International Congress of Alternative Medicines in Calcutta, India.

10 Jacobson is a prominent actor in the Tibetan medical scene in the US, and his influence is explored in detail later in this chapter.

11 Although contemporary research has shown that patients are becoming increasingly active in the conventional system, their role remains much more passive than in "alternative" therapies.

12 This is quite distinct from Western biomedicine, which operates on a model of hierarchy that privileges "esoteric" knowledge acquired through medical training and not known by ordinary patients who have not undergone such training. That is not to say, however, that all Tibetans have a detailed knowledge of the body and its functions and dysfunctions in Tibetan medical theory, but simply that they may grasp it with less difficulties than

a Western patient. For an interesting article on the comparison between modern medicine and so-called alternative medicines, see Bates (2000).

13 It is described as offering "traditional herbal remedies for modern ailments." See http://www.tibetanherbs.com/abouttibetanmedicine.html.

14 See http://herbalchemy.com/index.htm.

15 See Jacobson (2000) for the author's previous research work at Harvard University on Tibetan medicine and psychiatry.

16 A rolfer is a practitioner of Rolfing or Rolf Therapy. This therapeutic method was originated by American biochemist Ida P. Rolf (1896–1979) in the 1930s. It is generally described as the manipulation or deep tissue massage of the body's connective tissue and muscles, in order to realign and balance the body's structure. It is believed to improve posture, function, and general physical and emotional health.

17 This is sometimes presented as cranial osteopathy in the West.

18 This is a market attracted to the integration or use of alternative methods of Asian medicine as complementary to existing Western models, and Western psychological and manipulation techniques.

19 See Samuel for some reflections on how Tibetan medicine is increasingly made holistic in India (Dalhousie), to meet the market demand (2001).

20 However, we have seen earlier that this may also be, as was the case earlier for TCM, an adaptation to particular and recurring clinical contexts (emotional expression of the patients) made by Tibetan *amchi*, and certainly by American *amchi*.

21 He may refer here first to some tantric practices ("exchange of bodily fluids") and second to the ingestion of certain medications that are ritually potentialized ("sacred substances").

22 For a thorough analysis of evaluative research conducted in clinical settings in the US, including the criminalization of Tibetan medicine and Tibetan medical practitioners who participate in the global pharmaceutical pursuit of new medical products, see the work of Adams (2002). See also Pordié (2005) for a critical analysis of the global market for the evaluation of "traditional" medicines and its social consequences in terms of health coverage.

23 In the future, Jacobson hopes also to engage in Tibetan medical research at the Institute and he plans to have Tibetan *amchi* take part in this research. See also Tokar (Chapter 10) for an American national Tibetan medical practitioner's concerns about revisiting research on Tibetan medicine.

24 Although I was not able to attend the conference, Eric Jacobson and Jon Kabat-Zinn informed me of the planning and results of the conference.

25 For information on Kabat-Zinn's Center, see http://www.umassmed.edu/cfm/.

26 Here interviewed two days after the conference, on 23 July 2002.

27 The other organizations included Alternative Medicine Foundation, Capital University of Integrative Medicine, Center of Mind–Body Medicine, George Washington Center for Integrative Medicine, Herbo Tibet, Medicine Buddha Healing Center, Menla Mountain Retreat Center, New Yuthok Institute for Tibetan Medicine (Italy), PADMA Inc., Richard and Hinda Rosenthal Center for Complementary and Alternative Medicine, and Tibet House USA.

References

Adams, V. (2001). Particularizing Modernity: Tibetan Medical Theorizing of Women's Health in Lhasa, Tibet. In L. H. Connor and G. Samuel (eds.), *Healing Powers and Modernity: Traditional Medicine, Shamanism and Science in Asian Societies*, Westport, CT: Bergin & Garvey.

Adams, V. (2002). Randomized Controlled Crime: Postcolonial Sciences in Alternative Medicine Research, *Social Studies of Science* 3, 32(5–6): 659–690.

Bates, D. G. (2000). Why Not Call Modern Medicine "Alternative"?, *PBM* 43(4): 502–518.

Dalai Lama (1997). *The Heart of Compassion: A Practical Approach to a Meaningful Life*, Wisconsin: Lotus Press.

Holmes, K. (1995). Portrait of a Tibetan Doctor: Khenpo Troru Tsenam. In J. V. Alphen and A. Aris (eds.), *Oriental Medicine: An Illustrated Guide to the Asian Arts of Healing*, London: Serindia Publications (re-edited by Shambhala Publications, Boston, MA, 1997).

Jacobson, E. (2000). Situated Knowledge in Classical Tibetan Medicine: Psychiatric Aspects, Ph.D. dissertation, Harvard University.

Janes, C. (2002). Buddhism, Science and the Market: The Globalization of Tibetan Medicine, *Anthropology and Medicine* 9(3): 267–289.

Lopez, D. S. (1998). *Prisoners of Shangri-La: Tibetan Buddhism and the West*, Chicago, IL: University of Chicago.

Pordié, L. (2003). *The Expression of Religion in Tibetan Medicine: Ideal Conceptions, Contemporary Practices and Political Use*, PPSS Series 29, Pondicherry: FIP.

Pordié, L. (2005). Emergence et avatars du marché de l'évaluation thérapeutique des autres médecines. In L. Pordié (ed.), *Panser le monde, penser les médecines: Traditions médicales et développement sanitaire*, Paris: Karthala.

Pordié, L. (2007). Buddhism in the Everyday Medical Practice of the Ladakhi *Amchi*, *Indian Anthropologist* 37(1), January: 93–116.

Samuel, G. (2001). Tibetan Medicine in Contemporary India, Theory and Practice. In L. H. Connor and G. Samuel (eds.), *Healing Powers and Modernity: Traditional Medicine, Shamanism and Science in Asian Societies*, Westport, CT: Bergin & Garvey.

Steiner, R. W. P. (2003). Cultural Perspective on Traditional Tibetan Medicine. In H. Selin (ed.), *Medicine across Cultures: History and Practice of Medicine in Non-Western Cultures*, London: Kluwer Academic Publishers.

10 An ancient medicine in a new world

A Tibetan medicine doctor's reflections from "inside"

Eliot Tokar

In 1998, my first Tibetan medicine teacher, Yeshi Dhonden, gave a lecture at Columbia Presbyterian Hospital in New York City. The invitation that was extended to Dr Dhonden by the hospital represented a growing trend in some large American hospitals where in-house complementary and alternative medicine units sponsor lectures by practitioners of non-biomedical systems. The intention of such programs is to create some understanding among the hospital's personnel regarding so-called "complementary and alternative" medical systems. Unfortunately, the audiences of biomedical physicians and allied medical professionals who attend such presentations rarely have the background required for them to understand the concepts and the terminology of the presenter. This made for some difficulty, because Dr Dhonden, who is recognized as one of the great living experts on Tibetan medicine, was speaking fully in terms of his own discipline. In his lecture Dr Dhonden discussed a broad range of issues of medical, psychological, eco-logical, and spiritual matters as seen from the perspective of Tibetan medicine and Tibetan Buddhism. Despite what the hospital's organizer later described to me as a general lack of understanding by the assembled group of hospital personnel, the audience was polite, and Dr Dhonden held sway with his lecture and his considerable charisma for more than an hour.

At the conclusion of the lecture there was a question-and-answer period. During the exchange someone put forth the following query: "Dr Dhonden, you have said that the texts of Tibetan medicine are very ancient. Given that, how can Tibetan medicine possibly deal with new diseases which clearly did not exist centuries ago?" Dr Dhonden responded by saying:

> Why should this be a problem? Are we not all still living on the planet Earth? We are not after all speaking about some other unknown galaxy. The physical realities that exist here now are explained in Tibetan medicine's theory of the five elements that are the basis for all material phenomena, and they are the same as in ancient times.

He explained: "Based on our understanding of the three principles of function of the body and mind (*nyes-pa*), *rlung*, *mkhris-pa* and *bad-kan*, that are comprised of those elements, we are able to diagnose disease." He proceeded to explain how, by using Tibetan medicine's physics of the five elements, as well as its unique theory regarding physiology and pathology, Tibetan doctors have the ability to research modern diseases and then develop clinical approaches for them.

When viewed discriminatingly, Dr Dhonden's question to his audience, "Are we not all still living on the planet Earth?", and the underlying assumptions that it implied, brings to light many of the epistemological, social, political, ecological, and economic questions that come into play in any meaningful discussion of "traditional" culture in the modern context. Those questions have become even more crucial in the past two decades. To a much greater degree than ever before we must seriously consider how people of various cultures, values, and experiences can best live together on this planet (Forero 2003). New global cultural, scientific, and economic ideologies have begun to affect many aspects of our lives, including the way in which we think about health and disease.

We are living in an age where globalism and globalization are respectively the ideology and the reality upon which the policies and the economies of a majority of nations are being based. Some say that this trend spells only promise (Friedman 1999). They assert that the ability to take advantage of the quantity of all existent information and markets will unleash the true potential of the vast diversities existing on our planet. Meanwhile, others warn that globalization has the potential to threaten the very existence of cultural and ecological diversity by reducing everything to a lowest common denominator of consumerism dictated by those for whom business economics is the a priori basis of all social as well as economic value (Goldsmith and Mander 2001). In this context, medicine and health care are increasingly being regarded in industrial terms, within technologically developed and developing nations. The United States is a primary example of this trend. The People's Republic of China, which had established health care as a right under its formerly communist system, is privatizing medical care. In the new European Union the privatization of medical insurance is increasing in response to ballooning medical costs. As medicine continues to adopt a business model, it is vital that we examine the extent to which it can retain its character as a unique discipline with its traditional emphasis on humanistic principles and on the relieving of human suffering. As biomedicine continues to exert enormous hegemony over health care worldwide we must try to understand how this affects the panorama of non-Western and non-technological approaches to medicine and health care.[1] It is also important to plan how to best study and utilize traditional natural medicine[2] systems in a manner that leads to greater understanding, while avoiding cultural and ecological exploitation and the spread of cross-cultural misunderstanding.

Centuries before the Information Age and the internet, the clinical practice of Tibetan medicine was disseminated successfully throughout Asia and Central Asia. In recent years the Tibetan medical system has attracted greater interest in the West owing in large part to the exile of many thousands of Tibetans from their country in the middle of the twentieth century. As a result of the Tibetan Diaspora, very extensive contact has taken place between Tibetans, their culture and the West for almost a half-century. In both Europe and North America there exist many Tibetan Buddhist centers, universities with courses in Tibetology, and political groups involved with the Tibetan political and refugee issues. Movies are being made about Tibetan cultural and historical subjects, and there are numerous businesses publishing books or selling products concerning Tibetan culture, religion, etc. Given that this extensive contact has at times led to mutual misunderstanding – owing to romanticism, ethnocentrism, diffusion of various ideologies, politics, or simply lack of substantial knowledge about the Other – it is essential to finally begin the work necessary to create true cross-cultural communication. Such a process is the minimum required for the West to properly understand and utilize the investigation that the Tibetans made into the nature of physical (and spiritual) phenomena and the work they did to successfully correlate that knowledge with an understanding of human health. It is also imperative if the Tibetans are to better negotiate their "medical encounter" with the West.

By exploring all of these issues it is possible to discover whether one of the underlying assumptions that can be drawn from Dr Dhonden's question is correct. That is, we can see if we do in fact live together on this planet in some integrally harmonious sense. Based upon over twenty-five years as both a student and a practitioner of Tibetan medicine, I will share some reflections on how and to what extent Tibetan medicine can provide valuable answers for solving problems facing modern health care. Finally, I will define the challenges that are posed to those of us who are "inside" Tibetan medicine and more generally to a centuries-old medical tradition as it strives to develop in a "traditional" manner in our modern global society, characterized by the dominance of biomedicine and the econometrics of modern medical industrial systems.

Tibetan medicine understood in modern health care

My clinical practice in New York City and various conversations I have had with both Tibetans and Westerners in a variety of contexts have informed me about a central priority for the opening of Tibetan medicine to the West: the need for practitioners to clearly explain its unique theory regarding health and disease to Western people. That understanding may be considered as the true gold of Tibetan medicine. It is the basis for its diagnostic system and its therapeutic approaches, including its herbal tradition that many mistakenly assume to be its greatest asset.

Tibetan medical principles in the West

When I began my studies in Tibetan medicine I was uncertain as to whether I could eventually become a practitioner. I started studying Tibetan medicine in 1983 with Dr Yeshi Dhonden, and began my studies with my "root" teacher, the late Dr Trogawa Rinpoche, in 1986. I also commenced practicing the Buddhist sadhana of Sangye Menla (*Sangs rgyas sman bla*), the Buddha of Medicine. However, even as I meditated, visualizing myself as the Buddha of Medicine, as a Westerner attempting to study Tibetan medicine I sometimes felt more like Sisyphus or Don Quixote. No matter what direction my studies ultimately took I nevertheless believed that grounding myself in Tibetan medicine's ecological view of health and disease, its understanding of the interdependence of body and mind, and its spiritual view of suffering would benefit me greatly.

When Western people attempt to understand non-Western systems of knowledge, we too often do so in an incorrect manner. In encountering new ideas we frequently assume that we can simply make them conform to that which we already know. We feel that if something appears to us to be similar to that which we are already familiar with then it must be essentially the same, and so then we can afford to take shortcuts. I have seen many people fall short in their desire to understand Tibetan medicine because they try to merely graft it onto their training in biomedicine, Chinese medicine, or other medical systems.

Another mistake that is commonly made is when we try to merely expropriate components of Tibetan medicine's therapeutic approaches and substitute them for the depth of the whole system. In considering our Western scientific tradition no serious scientist would, for example, ignore Einstein's broad body of work, giving value solely to the utility of relativity theory in the development of nuclear fission. We would also never think that only theoretical physicists should find value in the full range of Einstein's scientific achievements. Yet Westerners with an interest in Tibetan medicine rarely appreciate the full value of the system's understanding of the nature of health and the causes of disease. Nowadays even some Tibetans devalue Tibetan medicine's theoretical foundation in the face of Western (as well as other) cultural, social, and economic influences (Janes 1995).

The bedrock of Tibetan medicine value lies in its physics of the five elements, which explains the basis for the interrelationships among all physical phenomena. This perspective provides us with a host of information about our world that is often very different than that which is observed by modern science. Traditional science understood through experience, research, and contemplation that the basic forces of nature were directly correlated with and thereby influenced the functioning of the human organism. The physics of Tibetan medicine utilizes a qualitatively based system of analysis and categorization to define the basic forces of the natural world in their theory of the five elements. Once defined these elements are named for their most easily identifiable manifestations: earth, water, fire, wind, and space. The characteristics and therefore the nature of all matter then result from the qualities of these elements individually or in combination.

From this theory, Tibetan medicine is able to deduce the way in which health is directly affected by all aspects of behavior in its various physical, psychological, and spiritual forms. The theory of the elements also gives rise to Tibetan medicine's ability to evaluate the specific effects of diet on health. It creates a means to analyze the qualities of foods relative to their characteristics, such as their tastes, and to correlate them with the functioning of the three principles of physiological and mental function, the *nyes-pa*, which are themselves composed of specific combinations of the selfsame elements. The same is true regarding Tibetan medicine's ability to comprehend and evaluate the medical significance of regional and seasonal climates.

Tibetan medical pathology also describes certain "super-physical" environmental influences that Tibetans believe can become pathogenic to humans when the places in which they reside become polluted or spiritually "disturbed" (for a variety of reasons, including ritual pollution, spirits, etc.) or are not treated with a proper adherence to nature (Clifford 1990). People in the West do not need to believe in the types of influences depicted in this aspect of Tibetan medical theory to benefit from the ideas presented therein. Developing an appreciation for traditional beliefs regarding the sensitivity of our environment and our interdependence with nature could aid us in lessening the public health threat posed by pollution and an unbridled manipulation of nature by an insufficiently regulated biotechnology industry.

A central aspect of Tibetan medical theory is the *nyes-pa*, which are the expressions of the elements that most primarily determine physical and mental function. Understanding their meaning helps us comprehend physiologic principles that are the basis of the complex interdependence that exists between our mind and our body. Our *nyes-pa* develop as a direct result of an interaction between our mind's developmental process and the five physical elements at various stages of development in the womb. Tibetan medicine's description of that genesis provides a model that explains how consciousness begins to play a direct role in physical function from the very early stages of embryologic development. The *nyes-pa* introduce to us the concept that there are specific principles that underlie the functioning of our body's organs, systems, and substances.

Theories regarding such principles are common to many systems of traditional natural medicine (e.g. *qi* in Chinese medicine or the three *doṣa* in Ayurvedic medicine). The recognition of the existence of these principles clearly distinguishes the perspective of traditional natural medicine systems from that of biomedicine. Traditional natural medicine places great emphasis upon understanding the role of such principle systems in the creation and maintenance of the functions of the body. The recognition of these principles and their primary role in physiology allows for the detailed definition of health. A disequilibrium occurring in these physiologic systems is understood to lead to dysfunction and, if not treated, to illness. Therefore, the theories regarding such principles of function provide the basis upon which discovering the causes of illness becomes the central consideration in the diagnosis and treatment of disease.

As a clinician, I have found that educating my patients concerning these principles contributes to their empowerment regarding preventative medical care, for which a detailed ecologic and qualitative view of health is essential.

Understanding is not merely a matter of words

There are three distinct processes of study that I have undertaken in my work in Tibetan medicine. Like my Tibetan colleagues I have, first and foremost, sought to develop a clear understanding of the theory and fluency in the practice of my discipline. Second, as a Westerner, encountering an alternative perspective on reality, it has been essential for me to gain direct experience of the actuality of Tibetan medical concepts and then to internalize my resulting new understanding. Third, because my goal is to foster cross-cultural comprehension I have needed to continually find ways to meaningfully and faithfully interpret the significance of Tibetan medicine into English.

A crucial issue facing all forms of indigenous medicine that are being utilized globally is the proper translation and interpretation of their ideas into other languages. This is an essential task that is too often not adequately accomplished. It is, for example, not always possible for Tibetan medical ideas to be translated into English because of the limitations inherent to languages. In many instances words should only be transliterated and accompanied by an appropriate explanation. It is also vital to not improperly utilize biomedical language, because its respective medical paradigm is wholly different.

In the translation of Tibetan medicine the use of antiquated and inaccurate translations of terms such as "humor" for *nyes-pa*, "bile" for *mkhris-pa* and "phlegm" for *bad-kan*, should be discontinued.[3] The common excuse for the repeated use of such incorrect translations is that they have become conventions. Yet, if Tibetan medicine is to make progress outside of its indigenous context, proper approaches to the translation and interpretation of its texts need to be established.

Terms that express concepts unique to Tibetan medicine are best expressed in the Tibetan language. The word *nyes-pa*, for example, expresses an idea that simply does not exist in biomedicine. The existence of three distinct categories of principles that maintain the proper functioning of our mind, and of our body's organs, systems, and substances, is a new concept for modern science. Further complexity lies in the fact that these principles are explained as having their genesis, in the embryo-logical stage of development, through an interaction between our consciousness and the aforementioned physical elements that constitute all matter. The *nyes-pa* have an additional esoteric meaning. Ignorance (of spiritual truth) is said to play a specific role in the creation of the *nyes-pa* which, when negatively affected by psychological or behavioral expressions of materialism, aggression, and nescience, then result in the dysfunctions that are the causes of disease. The word "humor" has an etymological meaning that defines it essentially as a fluid, and no complete description of the *nyes-pa* would result in such a definition. Insofar as the *nyes-pa* are the primary focus of Tibetan medical nosology, their proper explanation is key to understanding Tibetan medicine. Similar concepts in Chinese and Sanskrit, such as, respectively, *qi* and *doṣa*, have been properly left in their original language. Utilizing original Tibetan terms, like *nyes-pa*, will allow us to create complex definitions of those terms that depict their true meaning.

Some say that abandoning terms such as "humor," "bile," and "phlegm" will confuse patients, students, scholars, and researchers. It is my clinical experience, however, that patients are aided by precise language when trying to understand new ideas regarding their health. Students need accurate translations of Tibetan medical terms and concepts if they are to form a proper understanding of our system. Finally, inaccurate translations and interpretations of Tibetan medical texts have been a central cause for confusion among scholars and researchers who try to study Tibetan medicine.

When a term does exist in other languages whose use is clearly similar to a term used in Tibetan medicine, they should be used for translation. The Tibetan word *grag*, for example, can be properly translated as "blood" and the word *mkal ma* as "kidney." Having translated terms as such, we must then explain the complex of functions and influences that, for example, the blood or the kidneys have in Tibetan medical physiology and pathology that are different from those depicted in biomedicine.

Biomedical disease designations such as "cancer," however, should never be used to name the disease syndromes uniquely described in Tibetan medical texts.[4] It is an error for translators to think that it is vital to consult with biomedical physicians regarding the translation of Tibetan medicine's diagnostic terminology. Both biomedical and Tibetan medical terms are defined in a very precise manner. To use biomedical disease names to more or less approximate Tibetan nosological concepts might seem a convenient communication device but leads directly to misunderstanding and misinterpretation by biomedical doctors, scientists, and patients.

To properly translate Tibetan medical texts will require the use of a variety of experts. Although this huge enterprise may face a variety of technical, political, and ideological obstacles, would require good and equitable coordination, and will require a good amount of time and funding, it remains very important insofar as medicine is an applied science and not merely an abstract scholarly field or, like religion, based on a centrally shared belief system.

The place of Buddhism

In the context of translation and interpretation it is important to properly frame the meaning and significance of Buddhism in relation to Tibetan medicine. Unfortunately, the role of Buddhist spirituality in relation to Tibetan medicine is not well understood in the West and as a result it has often been fetishized and/or propagandized. The tendency to inappropriately materialize or spiritualize Tibetan medicine or, for example, to think that its practitioners have a standardized approach is a misunderstanding still often exhibited in the West.

Faith and belief do have a meaningful and practical role in medical systems that freely acknowledge and understand their importance. Tibetan Buddhist spiritual beliefs and practices have traditionally been a vehicle through which Tibetan medicine practitioners inform their practice of medicine. Spiritual discipline powerfully focuses doctors on a compassionate view of their patients and impels them to develop a pure intention. It also acts as a cognitive tool enhancing the intellectual and intuitive aspects of a doctor's approach to understanding, interpreting, and practicing Tibetan medicine. For those suffering with illness the spiritual component of medicine allows them to understand and heal their suffering while they pursue a cure for their disease.

In the West, though, people often make the mistake of thinking of Tibetan medicine as a spiritual healing system, rather than seeing it correctly, as a system of medical science. Tibetan medicine and Buddhism are, in fact, not isolated but differentiated systems (Pordié 2007). To facilitate understanding by laypeople and/or Western audiences, His Holiness the Dalai Lama has explained repeatedly that Tibetan medicine and Buddhism are separate in the way that "the fingers are separate from the hand." So what is the influence of Buddhism on Tibetan medicine?

In describing how he works as a physician, Dr Trogawa Rinpoche remarked, "my external activity is the practice of medicine, and in my inner thoughts I meditate on the Buddha of Medicine" (Trogawa 1992). Traditionally, or ideally, speaking, a doctor's clinical work becomes a vehicle for his or her ongoing practice toward spiritual development and its resultant awareness. It is true that the actual extent to which *amchi* engage in spiritual study and practice, or do not, varies. There are certainly *amchi* who lack a spiritual view, and there are those for whom Buddhism is largely a cultural religious observance. Still, the classical principle of Tibetan medicine is that the bedrock of a doctor's approach to medical practice is the maintenance of a spiritual attitude.

Buddhist teachings are meant to help define a doctor's self-image, the doctor's view of his or her patients, and the doctor–patient relationship. Buddhism's central teachings and practices place great emphasis on: 1) understanding and discovering the nature of one's mind; 2) developing a practice of compassion toward all other conscious beings; and 3) developing a sense of equanimity. If a Tibetan medicine doctor aspires toward such a view there should be no psychological or professional dilemma for him or her in identifying with his or her patients. This, because it is important for doctors to understand the nature of suffering – both the patient's and the doctor's – and that our relationship to the patient has both a professional and a spiritual significance.

The Tibetan Buddhist tradition provides the basic cosmology of the Tibetan medical system. It also provides the conceptual context through which conception, embryological development, birth, life, the interdependence of mind and body, suffering and illness, and death are understood. Tibetan Buddhist rituals and practices play a role in clinical practice to a greater or lesser degree depending upon the perspective, knowledge, and experience of individual Tibetan medicine doctors and upon the specific diagnosis of a patient and the patient's personal beliefs.

For Buddhists, study and practice upon the Buddha of Medicine is traditionally meant to bring into focus the spiritual meaning of the suffering of illness. It allows an individual to utilize the healing process as a metaphor for spiritual growth. Such an approach helps patients avoid falling into the trap of defining themselves by – and doctors defining their patients based upon – their health circumstances. For many people, especially those suffering from chronic disease, identifying themselves in terms of their medical diagnosis or the pain they are suffering is all too common and can be psychologically debilitating. Conversely, achieving an understanding about the nature of health and/or about the impermanence of physical phenomena, such as disease, can be empowering for those trying to heal. Patients who are suffering from disorders that affect the mind (i.e. psychological disorders) or that are affected by it (e.g. stress-related or psychosomatic disorders) can often benefit from an organized system that allows them to work contemplatively with specific components of emotion, perception, and/or cognition. Even rudimentary meditative practices can be used as a meaningful part of a person's treatment or preventive health regime (Benson *et al.* 1974; Kabat-Zinn 1982).

Divergent needs: patients, healers, and industrialized medicine

The complementary and alternative medicines integration scenario

After attending the Tibetan medicine conference held in Washington, DC, in 1998, a Tibetan medicine doctor from northwestern India insisted on delineating for me the priorities of native practitioners as he viewed them. The *amchi* said that he was doing so in order to differentiate those needs from the list of "Western priorities" that he had heard at the conference. The *amchi* stated that the practice and preservation of his tradition depended on five essential factors. They were: 1) creating access to Tibetan medical education for doctors and medical students, through formal institutional education, apprenticeship training, and the transfer of tradition through family lineages; 2) creating an ecologically sustainable supply of herbal ingredients; 3) maintaining sufficient stores of high-quality medicinal herbal compounds that could be regularly replenished to meet clinical needs; 4) preserving the traditional approach to the Tibetan medical system, notwithstanding its requisite modern development; 5) providing adequate levels of availability of doctors and affordable medicines so that people could choose Tibetan medicine as a primary method of health care.

The *amchi* felt that these five items were at odds with the priorities regarding Tibetan medicine that he had heard emphasized at the conference we had just attended. Those Western priorities, he said, had included research studies, the interpretation of Tibetan medical ideas in terms of biomedicine, and the development of commercial nutriceutical products. This cross-cultural event was telling. The management team of the company that organized the aforementioned conference did not include any practitioners of Tibetan medicine or of any other field of natural medicine. They were approaching Tibetan medicine largely from a perspective congruent with that of the complementary and alternative medicine (CAM) industry.

In America the term CAM is now being used by the government, universities, and the biomedical industry to describe an enormous variety of traditional and modern natural medical systems and therapies, as well as some alternative biomedical approaches.[5] The use of such "alternative" health care modalities has been expanding in the US since the 1960s, owing to a grassroot alternative medicine movement. The fact that Tibetan medicine came to be practiced in the US is as a direct result of that movement. The CAM industry only came into being in the early 1990s when the existing medical industrial complex discovered that millions of Americans were spending an increasingly large amount of money on alternative medical services through an article that appeared in the *New England Journal of Medicine* and that was featured in newspapers nationwide (Eisenberg *et al.* 1993).

This new industry places primary value on creating a field of so-called "integrative" medicine (Wolpe 1999). Integrative medicine emphasizes the incorporating into biomedicine of individual CAM therapies that have been validated through biomedical research, with an emphasis on randomized controlled trials (Adams

2002). The CAM industry has expanded the availability of certain natural therapies, with, for example, some hospitals giving their patients access to treatments including certain massage, meditation, and Chinese acupuncture techniques (Now 2002; Garner-Wizard 2003). Where these approaches aid patients they are clearly worthwhile; however, these procedures usually do not represent the full value of the traditional natural medical systems from which they have been appropriated.

CAM has sought to introduce into the field of natural medicine many of the aspects of commerce and hierarchy that are typical within the American medical industry. Biomedical physicians, government bureaucrats, and medical insurance and nutriceutical industry personnel largely dominate the assumed leadership hierarchy of the CAM industry, and university-based researchers. Typical requirements for status in this hierarchy include biomedical credentials, a doctorate degree in a field of Western science. Unfortunately, this excludes the vast majority of natural medicine practitioners in the US, who are non-licensed, largely ignores input from patients and Western scholars with substantial training in cross-cultural issues, and instead includes many health professionals who lack substantial training in natural health care.

Conferences that stem from a CAM industry perspective are not necessarily organized to foster progress in a given medical system through the interaction of experts, but rather are too often focused on advancing the commercialization and/or biomedicalization of a given discipline.[6] They often serve largely to promote market recognition of alternative health modalities, increase funding potential for those whose research relates to the field(s) being addressed, and provide a trade show for companies trying to market their products. Audiences might include Western medical professionals, CAM industry activists, nutriceutical company personnel, and interested laypeople. When indigenous doctors are suddenly thrust as actors into such public relations events there is a great potential created for misunderstanding and at times even exploitation.

The costs of Tibetan medicine commoditization

Addressing the Second International Conference of the Central Council of Tibetan Medicine in Dharamsala in January of 2006, Tibetan prime minister in exile Samdhong Rinpoche told the assembled audience of Tibetan doctors that "Commercialization is the greatest threat to the preservation of tradition." He went on to say that Tibetan medicine doctors "should serve the people by having a compassionate mind towards those individuals who are fighting against disease. And, they should not become commercialized medical professionals" (Chauhan 2007). A few years ago, a colleague reported to me that Penor Rinpoche, one of Tibetan Buddhism's highest-ranking lamas, had confided in him that he was worried that current trends in the practice of Tibetan medicine might not be sufficiently observing traditional clinical approaches. The lama felt that too many *amchi* have begun to place undue emphasis on "selling medicines." He observed that this led them to neglect proper clinical follow-ups (especially in the West) and as a result to insufficiently utilize appropriate treatment protocols.

Dr Trogawa Rinpoche expressed similar concerns to me. Rinpoche taught that *amchi* needed to place proper emphasis upon relating to individual patients by always conducting a satisfactory clinical interview. He believed that *amchi* who de-emphasized the importance of this interaction were devising treatment protocols based upon a technical diagnosis chiefly arrived at through urinalysis and pulse analysis which Rinpoche felt was generally insufficient for optimal patient care. It was also important, Rinpoche said, for *amchi* to not overemphasize the use of herbal medicines and instead use the full range of other treatment methods. Rinpoche was the first Tibetan doctor whom I saw treat patients in the fashion described in the medical texts, with behavioral modification alone if it was adequate, additionally with dietary therapies where needed, and only then with medicines and physical therapies where appropriate. He felt that *amchi* needed to strive to write herbal prescriptions that were theoretically consistent with their diagnoses and thereby aimed at treating the cause of a disease, and were not merely geared towards symptomatic treatment.

The gravest issue facing Tibetan medical herbology, however, is not the overuse of Tibetan herbal compounds by *amchi*. Rather it is the ravenous interest in these compounds and their ingredients by Western and Asian pharmaceutical and nutriceutical companies. In Europe and America corporations have already begun marketing nutriceutical products that are questionably labeled as being "Tibetan" medicines.[7] Tibetan herbal supplements produced by Chinese companies based in Tibet have been hailed in that country as one potential economic "pillar" in the new Chinese economy. But the promotion of lines of Tibetan herbal products for sale in shops[8] and healthfood stores or to licensed health professionals not qualified in Tibetan medicine encourages their improper use (Adams 2002). Unlike Chinese medicine there is no tradition of patent medicines in the Tibetan tradition, and the use of herbal treatments normally follows a proper diagnosis and prescription by a practitioner of Tibetan medicine.

The nutriceutical industry's emphasis on standardization is also in direct opposition to the individualized diagnosis and treatment of disease to which the traditional science of medical herbalism is dedicated.[9] The voracious need for raw materials that the mass marketing of Tibetan medicines requires also puts a great strain on the ecology of the plants that are required for their manufacture. While in Lhasa, in 2000, I was told by Tibetan colleagues that Tibetan medicine factories, which were privately held by non-Tibetan-owned Chinese companies, were using untrained nomadic peoples – as workers or in lieu of taxation – to pick medicinal herbs,[10] and that as a result some species of plants had begun to diminish.

As herbal resources are used, and as the packaging and marketing of Tibetan medicines are designed to emphasize sales to consumer markets in the West and throughout Asia, the cost of Tibetan medicine can rise precipitously. As a result it will be increasingly difficult for Himalayan people to afford to gain access to herbal medicines and to utilize their own indigenous medical system. Signs of this cost crisis can already be seen in Tibet. Such problems will multiply as the international demand for Himalayan herbs increasingly impinges upon the ecological sustainability of such plants.[11]

The price of ownership

There is an even more insidious issue that is affecting Tibetan medicine and herbalism. With the new standards that modern globalization is introducing to the world, the manner in which ideas are exchanged is increasingly being relegated into the form of a commercial enterprise. Evidence of this can be seen in the way in which researchers and industries have tried to promote urgency regarding the attainment of intellectual property rights (IPRs) on traditional Tibetan medicinal formulas to both the Tibetan refugee and indigenous Tibetan medical communities.

Schemes that encourage various individuals, institutions, and companies to pursue such patents are increasingly being advocated by those in the East and in the West who seek to be the arbiters of Tibetan medicine's development. This encourages those in Asia who see traditional natural medical systems as primarily a potentially lucrative source of export revenue. Most importantly, with the advent of the principle that knowledge should be thought of and owned as property, the free-flowing medical pluralism, the process of external contacts and reciprocal sharing, is being undermined.

Perpetrators of bioprospecting who see Tibetan medicine as merely a storehouse of potentially profitable ethnobotanical data are often considered to present a real danger (Dorsey 2001; Shiva 2001). People living in various regions of the Himalayas must act if they are to prevent Western and Asian pharmaceutical and nutriceutical firms from exploiting and patenting their traditional medical knowledge. Native *amchi* must protect their intellectual heritage – although this does not necessarily imply the use of the IPRs apparatus[12] – if they are to be able to continue to have the necessary free access to raw materials. However, if indigenous Himalayan people adopt the patenting ethic of global corporations, so as not to become victimized by it, a potentially devastating problem will arise, as Laurent Pordié notes in the case of intellectual property rights:

> The healers' neo-traditional elite and institutional representatives of medical traditions, in the Himalayas at least, tend today to accept the cultural authority of IPRs. . . [and] their international definition, despite defending indigenous agendas which generally aim to counter the above domination. This process ultimately justifies and consolidates the relevance of IPRs in both the international and local contexts, and maintains traditional knowledge as a subaltern form of knowledge.
>
> (Pordié 2005: 398)

The central goal of patenting is to give an individual or corporation an exclusive economic or legal claim to that which is being patented. Patenting assumes that there is merit in exclusive use, which is a value of business. The manner in which indigenous people "possess" or protect herbal knowledge has an entirely different meaning and sense of values. There indeed are "ownership, proprietary systems and property rights [that] do exist in a variety of forms in most, if not all, societies" but "the logic of patenting and intellectual property, as a generic form, is not the logic of most of the local communities" (Pordié 2005: 397).

Despite these facts, Himalayan people and their institutions face serious and destabilizing issues created by new global patenting laws. When I was in Tibet in 2000, I was told that one Tibetan medicine factory had become involved in a lawsuit with a competitor regarding who owned the patent for a very important traditional formula, Rinchen Mangjor Chenmo. I was told that, thankfully, the Chinese courts had ruled in this case that no company could properly claim ownership over a traditional formula. With China's participation in the World Trade Organization, however, they will have to conform to its edicts regarding intellectual property and patenting. Therefore, it is by no means certain that future lawsuits will be decided in a manner that is equally favorable to the preservation of traditional knowledge.

On biomedical research

The divergence between the needs of traditional healers and biomedicine is once again being expressed as doctors of traditional natural medicine (including *amchi*) are increasingly being told that they must prove the safety and efficacy of their work through the application of biomedical research. The American CAM industry, for example, has uncritically embraced the ideology of evidence-based medicine (EBM) and in doing so has tended to perpetuate the inaccuracy that randomized controlled trials (RCTs) are the "gold standard" for all legitimate medical practice (COTA 1978; Trachtenberg 1997). Natural medicine practitioners are being asked to accept such a definition of research in the hopes that it will serve as a vehicle for attaining legitimacy within the medical industrial complex. However, the proliferation of inappropriately designed research studies force complex natural medicine systems into the nosologic categories of biomedicine and do little to inform us about these systems or their efficacy (Adams 2002; Wolpe n.d.). In the end science and scholarship, as well as real concerns about health care reform, humanism, cultural diversity, and ecology, take a back seat to commercial priorities. This trend creates a roadblock for the development of new research models appropriate for the study of complex traditional natural medicine systems.

EBM, with its artificial emphasis on RCTs, is not merely a neutral scientific movement meant to enhance the availability of data in medicine. While the movement towards EBM is burgeoning in medical research, many biomedical doctors recognize it as a tool of those, such as medical insurance companies and policy makers, who are seeking to introduce an increasingly econometric approach to clinical decision-making. Despite what its early advocates might have hoped for, EBM is increasingly being used to weaken the clinical autonomy of doctors and infringe upon the doctor–patient relationship (Allsop and Mulcahy 1996; Bensing 2000; Denny n.d.; Djulbegovic *et al.* 2000; Feinstein and Horowitz 1997; Harrison 1998; Timmermans and Berg 1997; Tonelli 1998; Wolpe n.d.).

Tibetan medicine doctors are increasingly having their traditional medical approaches undermined or ignored in both the East and the West. An example of this occurring in Tibet is noted by Craig Janes:

> Tibetan medicine is becoming fully modern in its social structure and cultural content; that is . . . it is becoming . . . reconstituted as part of a centralized system of technical accomplishment and professional expertise, which in turn is expected to conform to the pervasive and powerful cultural standards of rational science and biomedicine . . . As has been documented elsewhere in the anthropological literature, when ethnomedicines are sanctioned and supported by the state, the resulting pluralism is orchestrated by institutions and structures built out of the culture of biomedicine and, therefore, entails a transformation of medical care and training so that it is consistent with the epistemological, symbolic and sociologic attributes of biomedicine . . . The modernization of ethnomedicines in such a fashion is represented by shifts in epistemology and practice that favor a standardized and radically materialistic perspective on the body, and objectification and thus desocialization (decontextualization) of disease; and transformations in the social relations of healing that put emphasis on professionalism, contribute to asymmetries of power in healing encounters and objectify/reify the patient.
>
> (Janes 1995: 24–25)

We can see that process of transformation beginning in the US, for example, in the recent research study on Tibetan medicine and breast cancer conducted at the University of California, San Francisco (Adams 2002). Most research on Tibetan medicine and generally on traditional natural medicine does not seek to engage those disciplines in a dialogue but to reduce them to mechanisms of treatment for biomedical disease pathologies. Traditional doctors are increasingly the object of modern scientific research, but almost never have control over what is studied or how studies are designed.

Modern scientific research can potentially be one valuable tool for us to use to explain and develop Tibetan medicine. However, in order to create proper research protocols, practitioners of Tibetan medicine certainly need to work directly with researchers, sharing a primary role in the design and implementation, and in the interpretation, of studies. It is vital for *amchi* to achieve a much more sophisticated understanding of the nature and actual uses of biomedical research so that a proper policy could be defined from a Tibetan medicine perspective.

Concluding remarks: toward true pluralism and collaboration?

Modern science and technology have created enormous advancements in many aspects of society. Like any taxonomy of knowledge, though, science is naturally constrained by the model with which it views the world. Our perspective is enhanced by its great insights but limited by the scope of its comprehension. It is inappropriate, therefore, for modern science to take an exclusive position as the sole determinant of scientific truth. The dangerous rise of opposing reactionary ideologies results in part from the absolutist role of Western scientific materialism in determining the path of development for modern society.

The twenty-first century should not be defined by a struggle between opposing forms of absolutism. Nor should the priority be the creation of a singular integrative approach to epistemology or science. One potential benefit of the Information Age is that we have the ability to begin to fully acknowledge and appreciate the pluralism of knowledge that has been developed by many cultures throughout the centuries. This provides us with the opportunity to achieve a panoramic view of what exists "between heaven and earth." But such insight cannot be achieved by absolutism, the fetishizing and marketing of non-Western culture and spirituality such as occurs in New Age movements, or the market fundamentalism of some globalists, or through the industrial and commercial objectives of technologists.

To truly advance health sciences into the twenty-first century it is advisable to seek to understand the full breadth of scientific knowledge contained in ancient medical traditions and expand our definition of science.

> Science is the expression of human creativity, both individual and collective. Since creativity has diverse expressions, I see science as a pluralistic enterprise that refers to different "ways of knowing". For me it is not restricted to Modern Western science, but includes knowledge systems of diverse cultures in different periods of history . . . Indigenous knowledge systems are by and large ecological, while the dominant model of scientific knowledge, characterized by reductionism and fragmentation, is not equipped to take the complexity of interrelationships in nature fully into account. This inadequacy becomes most significant in the domain of life sciences . . . The recognition of . . . diverse creativities [in the life sciences] is essential for the conservation of biodiversity as well as for the conservation of intellectual diversity.
>
> (Shiva 1997)

Creating the possibility for co-equal and collegial relationships between practitioners of traditional natural medicine and Western and Eastern biomedical doctors and scientists would be one important step. I am aware that achieving such a goal will not be easy, but such cooperation is necessary to encourage the development of true medical pluralism. Such progress will require that we Tibetan medicine doctors, for example, should make our system ripe for positive interaction with the West. This can only be achieved by ensuring that Tibetan medicine is properly understood in the West, providing a means by which all *amchi* can achieve a high standard of practice despite differences in nationality or manner of study, attempting to evolve our system so that it fully addresses the unique health problems that exist in technologically developed countries, and most importantly by cooperating together within our field.

Dr Trogawa Rinpoche used to express great concern over the insufficient cooperation between *amchi*. He felt that this negative habit constituted a significant weakness for Tibetan medicine as it comes in contact with the wider world. In a conversation regarding my intentions to organize *amchi* living in America, a former Men-Tsee-Khang official told me that he thought that such progress would not be possible because of the relatively anti-collegial attitude of many Tibetan doctors.

He said that only if there was individual and immediate benefit to be gained by cooperation might I be able to get my colleagues to organize.

A meeting organized in 1998 by an India-based Tibetan colleague and myself to help create an international *amchi* organization was negatively affected by internecine conflict. One prominent Dharamsala Men-Tsee-Khang *amchi* stood up at the beginning of the meeting and spoke to all of the non-Tibetan *amchi* from Asia (e.g. Mongolian, Ladakhi, Bhutanese, etc.) who were in attendance. He said that as far as he was concerned it was uncertain to him as to whether or not they were even practicing Tibetan medicine, especially since they were not doing so under the auspices of his institution. Most of the *amchi* that he affronted then proceeded to leave, and the meeting was effectively derailed as a result.

In a recent discussion an ethnic Tibetan colleague bemoaned the tendency he perceived among his fellow *amchi* of lacking clear goals regarding the development of Tibetan medicine. He felt that this tendency left them in a perpetually reactive position when individuals unqualified in Tibetan medicine sought to influence our field for good or ill. He told me that, although he also had tried to organize young *amchi* living in America, his efforts had effectively failed.

Given the dilemmas faced by the South Asian and Tibet-based Tibetan medical communities it is understandable that they have not come to a clear consensus regarding the extent to which and in what manner Tibetan medical knowledge should be shared with the West and with Westerners. In this vacuum, Western and Asian pharmaceutical and nutriceutical firms, Chinese authorities, CAM activists, Western doctors, and Western (Tibetan culture) impresarios, among others, have tried to control the progress of the globalization of Tibetan medicine. As a result, misinformation regarding international cultural, legal, and health care issues abounds in the Tibetan medical community.

One illustration of this phenomenon occurred at the 2000 International Academic Conference on Tibetan Medicine, held in Lhasa. At that meeting a German neurologist urged the assembled *amchi* to change their centuries-old approach to the formulation of their herbal compounds. He recommended that they give greatest priority to Western importation laws, which, he inaccurately informed them, all uniformly restricted the importation of traditional Tibetan herbal medicines. I stood up during the question-and-answer period in order to inform my German colleague and the assembled *amchi* that in fact Western laws concerning the importation of herbals still showed some meaningful diversity, with America, for example, having minimal restrictions and thereby being much more progressive for now than the EU. A day later, this physician told me that, although he was personally devoted to studying about Tibetan medicine, he doubted whether it was actually an effective medical system.

In reaction to the current circumstances, some Tibetan medical institutions have assumed the impossible goal of achieving a controlling influence over Tibetan medicine. They would be well advised to abandon subjective institutional agendas and instead fill the vacuum for progressive leadership. Shortsighted approaches by such institutions serve to enhance competition and suspicion, leave many independent doctors without a way to achieve positive goals, perpetuate ethnic prejudices among *amchi*, and deny Tibetan medicine appropriate arbiters for those big issues it currently faces. Too many young *amchi* coming to the West to find success can fall victim to the perception that they need to "sell" their loyalties to any special interest or individual who will sponsor them. It is difficult for such young people to establish a truly independent and inclusive voice for Tibetan medicine here. Tibetan medicine doctors rightly feel concerned about the positive diffusion, as well as the co-optation and exploitation, of their discipline. Many *amchi* I have spoken with in America, Asia, and Europe have important insights regarding these matters. Still, there needs to be a way in which we can reach a consensus on a properly organized and progressive way to deal with the legitimate issues that we face.

The vacuum of leadership needs to be filled with a spirit of trust and collegiality between Tibetan medicine practitioners. Those of us practicing Tibetan medicine in the West must learn to work with each other, avoiding the ethnic conflicts that can occur between the diverse Asian and Western practitioners in the field. We must try to avoid the kinds of ethnic antagonisms between native and Western practitioners that, for example, negatively affected the development of Chinese medicine in America. It is only through collaboration that we can make true progress. We need to understand that, in order to establish ourselves in the West, integrity within our profession is our most significant asset.

Whether the change in the negative habit Dr Trogawa insightfully diagnosed is likely to happen is, however, difficult to predict.

Notes

1 See, for example, Adams (2002), Adams and Li (Chapter 5), Blythman (2002), Dumoff (2003), and Janes (1995).
2 Although Tibetan medicine can be properly termed as "traditional medicine," in the United States this can be confusing insofar as many Americans understand that term to refer to Western biomedicine. As such, systems of so-called "alternative medicine" that are not congeneric with biomedicine will be generally termed "natural medicine" and indigenous systems of medicine such as Tibetan medicine will be referred to as "traditional natural medicine."
3 *Rlung* also means "wind." However, an important complexity arises because many terms can actually be polysemous. *Rlung* means the wind that makes the leaves dance, but also the medical *rlung* as well as many other things. As such, in the case of Tibetan medicine, for example, it is more clear to utilize the Tibetan term *rlung*.
4 Western diagnoses such as irritable bowel syndrome, cancer, and diabetes are in fact not diseases; rather, they are conceptual descriptions of the etiology of disease with related treatment protocols. They are based upon clinical experience, with currently validated data about and research on the treatment of a disease from a biomedical perspective. In summary, a tumor is a thing whereas cancer is solely a concept. When we appreciate this fact, the diagnostic concepts of Tibetan medicine or any other system of medicine can be considered on equal terms with the nosological categories of Western biomedicine. If we can achieve such parity we can begin to create a language that enables meaningful dialogue between different medical systems (Tokar 1998).
5 See for detail the official website of the US government on CAM: http://nccam. nih.gov/health/whatiscam/.
6 This fact was made most evident at the 2003 International Congress on Tibetan Medicine, held in Washington, DC, as a follow-up to the above-mentioned 1998 conference. The

conference's producer, Procultura Inc., decided to not include the majority of Tibetan medicine practitioners who have worked to develop Tibetan medicine's clinical practice in North America as speakers. Procultura's director replied to individuals who advocated for greater intellectual freedom at the conference (including two members of the conference's planning committee, and its speakers coordinator, who are professors doing scholarly work on Tibetan medicine, as well as the Dalai Lama's representative in the USA) by stating that the conference was in fact intentionally not meant "to be inclusive." To prove her point she specifically listed a number of Tibetans and Westerners, e.g. Shakya Dorje, Tashi Rabten, Barry Clark, Dickie Paldon Nyerongsha, etc. (Keyzom Bhutti was also not in attendance), who along with myself would not appear as speakers. Tibetan doctors from South Asia were, similarly, not invited to speak at the 2000 International Academic Conference on Tibetan Medicine held in Lhasa, Tibet, but one might have hoped for a greater degree of freedom of speech at an American meeting.

7 See, for example, http://www.padma.ch/en/, http://www.sabinsa.com/ and http://www. china-guide.com/Merchant2/merchant.mvc?Screen=CTGY&Store_Code=C& Category_Code=TF.

8 In 2000 I traveled to Tibet and to my surprise found Tibetan "jewel pills" (*rin chen ril bu*) on sale in the Lhasa airport gift shops along with the requisite postcards, candy, alcohol, cigarettes, and yak dolls.

9 The establishing of standards of *purity* and *quality* of herbal compounds would, however, greatly benefit native manufacturers of Tibetan medicine.

10 The director of one of Lhasa's largest Tibetan medicine factories confirmed the use of nomadic laborers in the picking of medicinal herbs. He claimed that such people have generations of training in herb gathering, an assertion that my informants from the Tibetan nomadic communities insisted was inaccurate.

11 See Hofer (2006) for an excellent illustration of this phenomenon.

12 Specific guidelines for such an approach have been laid out in Tibetan and English by L. Pordié and V. Brisard in the *Trans-Himalayan Amchi Medical Education Newsletter*, special issue on IPRs (THAME 2002).

References

Adams, V. (2002). Randomized Controlled Crime: Postcolonial Sciences in Alternative Medicine Research, *Social Studies of Science* 3, 32(5–6): 659–690.

Allsop, J. and Mulcahy, L. (1996). *Regulating Medical Work: Formal and Informal Controls*, Buckingham: Open University Press.

Bensing, J. B. (2000). Bridging the Gap: The Separate Worlds of Evidence-Based Medicine and Patient-Centered Medicine, *Patient Education and Counseling* 39(1): 17–25.

Benson, H., Beary, J. F. and Carol, M. P. (1974). The Relaxation Response, *Psychiatry* 37: 37–46.

Blythman, J. (2002). Health Supplements: R.I.P., *Guardian*, September 14.

Chauhan, H. (2007). Don't Commercialise Tibetan Medicines, Says PM in Exile, *dailyindia. com*, January 7, http://www.dailyindia.com/show/100705.php/Dont-commercialise-Tibetan-medicines-says-PM-in-exile (today at http://www.tibet.ca/en/wtnarchive/2007/1/8_2.html).

Clifford, T. (1990). *Tibetan Buddhist Medicine and Psychiatry: The Diamond Healing*, Maine: Samuel Weiser.

COTA (Congressional Office of Technology Assessment) (1978). *Assessing the Efficacy and Safety of Medical Technologies*, Washington, DC: Congressional Office of Technology Assessment, p. 7.

Denny, K. (n.d.). *Imperatives and the Politics of Evidentiary Discourse in Medicine*, Toronto: University Health Network, Toronto Western Hospital.

Djulbegovic, B., Morris, L. and Lyman, G. H. (2000). Evidentiary Challenges to Evidence-Based Medicine, *Journal of Evaluation in Clinical Practice* 6(2): 99–109.

Dorsey, M. K. (2001). Shams, Shamans and the Commercialization of Biodiversity. In B. Tokar (ed.), *Redesigning Life?*, London: Zed Books.

Dumoff, A. (2003). ACM: An International Perspective, *Alternative/Complementary Therapies* 9(1): 45–48.

Eisenberg, D. M., Kessler, R. C., Foster, C., Norlock, F. E., Calkins, D. R. and Delbanco, T. L. (1993). Unconventional Medicine in the United States: Prevalence, Costs and Patterns of Use, *New England Journal of Medicine* 328(4): 246–252.

Feinstein, A. R. and Horowitz, R. I. (1997). Problems in the "Evidence" of Evidence-Based Medicine, *American Journal of Medicine* 103(6): 529–535.

Forero, J. (2003). Seeking Balance: Growth vs. Culture in Amazon, *New York Times*, December 10.

Friedman, T. L. (1999). *The Lexus and the Olive Tree: Understanding Globalization*, New York: Farrar, Straus & Giroux.

Garner-Wizard, M. (2003). Newsweek Runs Cover Story on Alternative Medicine, *Herbclip*, July 31, HC 020531.

Goldsmith, E. and Mander, J. (eds.) (2001). *The Case against the Global Economy*, London: Earthscan Publications.

Harrison, S. (1998). The Politics of Evidence-Based Medicine in the United Kingdom, *Policy and Politics* 26(1): 15–31.

Hofer, T. (2006). Transmission and Transition of Sowa Rigpa in Ngamring, Tibet Autonomous Region, Paper given at 6th International Congress on Traditional Asian Medicine (ICTAM VI) of the International Association for the Study of Traditional Asian Medicine (IASTAM), University of Texas at Austin, April 27–30.

Janes, C. R. (1995). The Transformations of Tibetan Medicine, *Medical Anthropology Quarterly* 9(1): 6–39.

Kabat-Zinn, J. (1982). An Outpatient Program in Behavioral Medicine for Chronic Pain Patients Based on the Practice of Mindfulness Meditation: Theoretical Considerations and Preliminary Results, *General Hospital Psychiatry* 4: 33–47.

Now, G. C. (2002). Integrative Care, *Newsweek*, December 2.

Pordié, L. (2005). Claims for Intellectual Property Rights and the Illusion of Conservation: A Brief Anthropological Unpacking of a "Development" Failure. In Y. Aumeeruddy-Thomas, M. Karki, D. Parajuli and K. Gurung (eds.), *Himalayan Medicinal and Aromatic Plants: Balancing Use and Conservation*, Kathmandu: IDRC Canada, WWF Nepal, UNESCO/WWF People and Plants Initiative.

Pordié, L. (2007). Buddhism in the Everyday Medical Practice of the Ladakhi *Amchi*, *Indian Anthropologist* 37(1), January: 93–116.

Shiva, V. (1997). *Biopiracy: The Plunder of Nature and Knowledge*, Toronto: Between the Lines.

Shiva, V. (2001). Biopiracy: The Theft of Knowledge and Resources. In B. Tokar (ed.), *Redesigning Life?*, London: Zed Books.

THAME (2002). Special issue on IPRs, *Trans-Himalayan Amchi Medical Education Newsletter* 5.

Timmermans, S. and Berg, M. (1997) Standardization in Action: Achieving Local Universality through Medical Protocols, *Social Studies of Science* 27(2): 273–305.

Tokar, E. (1998). A Tibetan Medical Perspective on Irritable Bowel Syndrome, *Alternative and Complementary Therapies* 1(5): 343–349.

Tonelli, M. R. (1998). The Philosophical Limits of Evidence-Based Medicine, *Academic Medicine* 73(12): 1234–1240.

Trachtenberg, A. (1997). American Acupuncture: Primary Care, Public Health and Policy. In *NIH Consensus Development Conference on Acupuncture*, Continuing Medical Education 137, Bethesda, MD: National Institutes of Health.

Trogawa, R. (1992). *Ven. Dr. Trogawa Rinpoche: In His Own Words*, Boulder, CO: Chakpori.

Wolpe, P. R. (1999). From Quackery to "Integrated Care": Power, Politics, and Alternative Medicine, *Frontier Science* 8(1): 10–12.

Wolpe, P. R. (n.d.). *The Challenge of Complementary and Alternative Medicine to Evidence-Based Medicine: A Call for Medical Pluralism*, Philadelphia: Center for Bioethics, University of Pennsylvania.

Conclusion

11 The politics of Tibetan medicine and the constitution of an object of study

Some comments

Geoffrey Samuel

The chapters of this book give a different and much more varied picture of Tibetan medicine than most previous Western writing on the subject. Even the recent growth of anthropological writing on Tibetan medical practice has rarely ventured into the complex and often fraught issues of the politics of Tibetan medical practice and the social context of Tibetan medicine considered here. The material in this volume is striking in its variety: we have studies of 'Tibetan medicine' in Tibet, Mongolia, Nepal, Ladakh, the UK and the USA, from a number of at times quite strongly contrasted viewpoints. The chapters by Janes and Hilliard (Chapter 2) and Adams and Li (Chapter 5) show us aspects of the formal systems of 'traditional medicine' in Tibet and Mongolia coming to terms with biomedically dominated medical pluralism and post-socialist 'economic liberalisation'. Those by Craig (Chapter 3) and Aumeeruddy-Thomas and Yeshi Lama (Chapter 7), along with Pordié's Ladakh study (Chapter 6), show us groups of *amchi* in more marginal situations in Nepal and India negotiating and manoeuvring to establish themselves as valid bearers of 'traditional knowledge', a process in which, as Aumeeruddy-Thomas and Yeshi Lama point out, this 'traditional knowledge' can easily be replaced by a kind of simulacrum of itself. Millard (Chapter 8) and Vargas (Chapter 9) examine practitioners of 'Tibetan medicine' as they attempt to develop a viable role within two Western societies, the United Kingdom and the United States.

While these studies are all more or less within the general perspective of medical anthropology, they are quite divergent in their approaches. Two further chapters sit outside this frame: Chen Hua's contribution (Chapter 4) is a descriptive account of the institutionalisation of Tibetan medicine in modern China, while Eliot Tokar's (Chapter 10) is the perspective of a Westerner trained as a Tibetan doctor on the development of Tibetan medicine in the USA. Several of the more anthropological chapters also give us extended presentations of the perspectives of indigenous practitioners. Here too we have many voices, and they are by no means speaking in unison.

The present volume does not include a study of the Dharamsala Men-Tsee-Khang and its political role in defining and shaping Tibetan medicine.[1] However, even without a direct study of the Men-Tsee-Khang, we see its presence off-stage throughout the book: as potential competition for the Ladakhi *amchi* in Pordié's chapter (Chapter 6), as threatening to delegitimise *amchi* not trained at Dharamsala in Tokar's contribution Chapter 10) and, perhaps most significantly, as feeding into the American interest in Tibetan medicine in Vargas's piece (Chapter 9). One might note that the Men-Tsee-Khang has contributed greatly to the Western image of Tibetan medicine as a more or less uniform system whose nature can be discovered in the pages of the *Rgyud bzhi*, supplemented perhaps by the classic commentary of Sangye Gyamtso (*Sde-srid Sangs-rgyas rgya-mtsho*), the *Vaiḍūrya sngon po* or 'Blue Beryl' Treatise.

Another presence only slightly off-stage is that of the pharmaceutical companies and the international politics of drug certification and approval. Pordié suggests that the threat of biopiracy in Ladakh is mainly a scare story used by Ladakhi *amchi* activists for political purposes, but 'Big Pharma' and its associated institutions have undoubtedly had an enormous impact on how 'Tibetan medicine' and related traditions are practised today (cf. Adams 2002). The manufacture of Tibetan medicine in Chinese-controlled Tibet is being restructured in terms of regulations for general manufacturing practices (GMP), requiring mass production of standardised ingredients and the elimination of many of the specific procedures required by traditional Tibetan pharmacy (Craig 2006). The Dharamsala Men-Tsee-Khang has also changed its manufacturing procedures to allow for mass production and to eliminate ingredients now seen as problematic.[2] All this is part of the global context within which 'Tibetan medicine' now operates (cf. also Janes 2002).

If the Western image of Tibetan medicine tends to be of a coherent body of practices handed down from the past, the material in this volume may lead us to ask, by contrast, whether there is such a thing as 'Tibetan medicine' at all in the contemporary situation. We note that a range of designations are used in the book for the healing tradition being practised, and that practitioners in Ladakh and Nepal specifically avoid referring to their practice as 'Tibetan medicine' (the same is true for Bhutan). Several of the chapters stress the syncretistic nature of the healing practices they describe, and emphasise how they have been constituted through a complex relationship between local healing traditions and the Western-derived tradition of biomedicine. Mongolian medicine as portrayed in Janes and Hilliard's chapter (Chapter 2) is particularly heterogeneous, having gone through a process of revival or reinvention in which it incorporated Chinese-style acupuncture and other healing techniques. Mongolian medicine in the past is regarded as having a close linkage with Tibetan medicine; it seems that 'Mongolian medicine' today can be much more complex and varied.[3]

Is 'traditional Tibetan medicine' today as illusory a construct as the 'traditional Chinese medicine' (or TCM) that, as Volker Scheid and others have demonstrated, is a largely modern product of the interaction between historical Chinese healing practices and biomedicine (Scheid 2002, 2006)? If so, do the chapters in this book even have a common object of enquiry? When Eliot Tokar talks about the need to assert the unique theoretical basis of Tibetan medicine and the distinctiveness of its theoretical concepts, is he really talking about the same thing as the Ladakhi *amchi* campaigning to have Westerners interested in Tibetan medicine expelled from Ladakh as spies for pharmaceutical companies, or the speaker from the Dharamsala Men-Tsee-Khang asserting that the Ladakhi village *amchi* are not even legitimate practitioners of Tibetan medicine? Clearly all three are engaged in taking up a political position of some kind, but what has all this to do with Tibetan medicine as a meaningful object of study?

It is worth reminding ourselves that 'Tibetan medicine' has always been a syncretic body of healing techniques, deriving from multiple sources (including, at the very least, Ayurvedic medicine, the Galenic–Islamic medical tradition, Chinese medicine, and indigenous healing practices). The *Rgyud bzhi* itself includes elements from all these sources, and, despite its enormous prestige, even the *Rgyud bzhi* is far from definitive of the total body of healing techniques practised in the past by *amchi* throughout Tibet and the Himalayas. Tibetan medicine is a practical art, and even *amchi* who know the *Rgyud bzhi* by heart still need to learn through apprenticeship how to apply its principles in practice. Many *amchi* in the past as in recent times would have owed their knowledge to practical apprenticeship, often in a family lineage context, rather than to a medical college in Lhasa or elsewhere. Tibetan medicine, like other pre-modern medical traditions, was not a uniform craft practised in precisely the same way by all its practitioners. For that matter, neither is biomedicine.

In fact my intention is not so much to deconstruct the idea of Tibetan medicine as to try to sketch the global system that connects the various manifestations presented in the book. Before we get to sketching this overall network, I discuss some other issues, and to begin with it is worth saying a little more about the relationship between anthropology and Tibetan medicine, since, despite the variety of studies in this volume, the dominant discourse is undoubtedly that of medical anthropology.

Medical anthropology and Tibetan medicine

I will begin by returning to the question of the identity of Tibetan medicine: if the studies in this book appear to undermine an assumed unity within Tibetan medical practice, this is in part because Tibetan medicine is far from having the overwhelming institutional presence and authority that biomedicine has established in today's world. This authority is such that no number of unhygienic third world hospitals, quack doctors with fake biomedical degrees or – for that matter – high-tech hospital facilities inaccessible to most of the population of the countries they supposedly serve would seem to dent the status and prestige of biomedicine. Nor does the less-than-straightforward relationship between medical research and medical practice within biomedicine serve to weaken the demands that non-biomedical forms of practice be assessed by the current standards of evidence-based medicine and the randomised double-blind control trial. As Eliot Tokar points out in his chapter, most current biomedical practice does not meet these requirements either.

The overwhelming presence of biomedicine is doubtless one reason why it has been fashionable to see Tibetan medicine as a tightly organised and internally coherent system of ideas, as defined by the *Rgyud bzhi* and the *Vaiḍūrya sngon po*. How much stress one places on these undoubtedly significant and central texts is partly a question of perspective, and we have to bear in mind that there is a substantial body of indigenous medical practitioners for whom this textual basis is precisely what defines the tradition. Yet for medical anthropology, what matters is not the formal textual basis but medical practice as a social reality; the texts are only significant in as far as they are themselves an important factor in that social reality. This creates a certain tension between anthropology and its subjects, particularly when, as here, anthropologists are studying a literate and sophisticated tradition whose representatives are increasingly part of the same academic context as the anthropologists themselves.

This point emerged rather graphically at a conference of the International Association of Tibetan Studies, in Königswinter in Germany, in September 2006. In a meeting at the end of two large sessions on 'Tibetan medicine' it became clear that most of the Tibetan participants had very different assumptions about appropriate scholarly work from the majority of the Western participants, who were mostly anthropologists. Several of the Tibetans observed that the detailed studies of medical anthropologists of Tibetan medicine as actually delivered in villages in Tibet or Nepal were, as far as they were concerned, a complete waste of time. Why bother to study what was going on in these remote villages, where poorly trained local practitioners were doing the best they could to meet local health needs on the basis of scraps of knowledge from family traditions or from a couple of years' study in the city? What was the point of detailing the social factors that shaped the practical delivery of village-level health care at the village level? For these Tibetans, studies of Tibetan medicine meant studies of the history, theory and efficacy of the 'formal' tradition defined by the *Rgyud bzhi* and constituted within urban medical colleges. For them, perhaps, all that was really worth saying about the village situation was that the population was not receiving proper medical care, Tibetan or biomedical, and they knew this well enough to start with.

Medical anthropology has had a similarly complex relationship with biomedicine in the Western context over the last thirty or so years. While medical anthropology has now achieved acceptance as a valid academic discipline, with at least some biomedical scholars and health authorities seeing it as a useful supplement to more conventional biomedical modes of support, there continue to be large parts of the biomedical profession for whom medical anthropology (and medical social science more generally) is of little or no value. Such people remain focused on the technical questions of how biomedicine operates and how to make it operate more efficiently and effectively within its own terms.

Most medical anthropologists would nevertheless see their discipline as doing more than providing a supplement, which enables biomedical practitioners to deliver their healing techniques a little more effectively. Medical anthropology's techniques and approaches allow it to develop its own critique of the constitution of biomedical knowledge in practice, as something different from the biomedicine taught in medical schools or enshrined in medical textbooks. Medical anthropology is after all a social science, and social science's favourite mode is that of social critique. Thus medical anthropologists may fairly naturally find themselves studying biomedicine in practice – in Western or Asian societies, and particularly perhaps among the poor and disadvantaged – and demonstrating that what is being delivered hardly lives up to the claims made in biomedicine's name. Understandably, the message is not always a welcome one.

Something of the same can happen when medical anthropologists study Tibetan medicine too, as the confrontation at Königswinter demonstrated. For the Tibetan doctors and scholars, 'Tibetan medicine' was something to be developed in the urban college and medical research facility, not something to study ethnographically in the village. They did not want to be told that the reality of the delivery of Tibetan medicine might be quite different.

The anthropologists in this problematic dialogue might deplore this failure to see the value of their work. They were also mostly aware, however, that Tibetan medicine is not in the same situation as biomedicine. It is itself under constant threat of assimilation and critique by biomedicine, a process of which the chapters of this book themselves provide abundant evidence. If medical anthropology provides a critique of the practice of 'traditional Tibetan medicine' and demonstrates that its delivery in practice is often some distance from the way in which it is presented on the basis of the *Rgyud bzhi* by the Lhasa College of Tibetan Medicine and Astrology (*Sman-rtsis-khang*) or the Dharamsala Men-Tsee-Khang, this is therefore not quite the same as the role of medical anthropology in developing a critique of biomedicine. In the latter case medical anthropologists are still, for the most part, gnats striking at an elephant; in the former, the power relationship is different, and the inequality in the opposite direction.

This is something that I was very conscious of myself when I wrote my concluding chapter in the 2001 *Healing Powers* volume, which is referred to by a number of the contributors in this volume (Samuel 2001). That study demonstrated the distance between Tibetan medicine as delivered at a small Men-Tsee-Khang clinic in North India and the official presentation of Tibetan medicine, of which the Dharamsala Men-Tsee-Khang was one of the main purveyors and promoters. I felt that what I was seeing was important, but I also tried to write it up in a way that maintained the reader's respect for the healing practice being described. Other writers have approached this issue differently, but it is hard for anyone to ignore it in the current era of post-colonial scholarship, and it is surely a good thing that this is the case. That it can make for difficult and complex relationships with the people we study is also undoubtedly true.

All this serves however to make the point; Tibetan medicine is not a straight-forward or unproblematic matter, and the issues raised in these chapters often go directly to the question of what there is for us to study, and how we might make sense of it. Laurent Pordié's opening chapter raises many of these issues in relation to the practical politics of Tibetan medicine and its constitution as a social object within the field situations in which it is encountered. His approach, which borrows from Bourdieu's writing on the constitution of the scientific field, seems to me apposite and insightful. The category of neo-traditionalism which he uses to capture the character of such practitioners as the international jet-setting *amchi* also seems to me to capture some important aspects of the situation. What I shall try to do here is to take up some of the wider issues raised by the material, with the intention of moving, as I noted above, to a more global perspective on the situation.

The contexts of Tibetan medicine

We might start by returning once more to the question of how we might identify 'Tibetan medicine', our problematic object of enquiry. The problem here is not really how the particular medical tradition is labelled. In fact, *amchi* throughout the region would accept that they are engaged in a common healing tradition. The real point about Tibetan medicine as an object of enquiry is a deeper level, which is that of the constitution of the healing system itself or, to put it in another way, the plausibility of extracting Tibetan medicine as an object from its context and treating it as an atemporal and ahistorical isolate.

Labels such as 'Tibetan medicine', '*amchi* medicine', 'traditional Mongolian medicine' and 'Sowa Rigpa' are produced historically within specific social contexts and derive their meaning and application from these contexts. As scholars, part of our job is to trace the process of constitution of these labels, and the ways in which they come to have meaning and to be employed in human social life. We are also interested, doubtless, both professionally and perhaps personally, in the efficacy of the healing processes taking place within this field, but that, for the most part, lies outside the compass of the material within the present volume.

One might ask, though, just what it is about the undoubtedly fluid and complex situation that leads to 'Tibetan medicine' and its equivalent terms being produced in particular, often quite divergent, ways, and this is where we come to the attempt to put together a global picture of Tibetan medicine today. I start with the Western context, not because it has priority in any particular sense but because it has received less examination. Here it seems to me that we can see a number of components:

Popular Western literature on Tibetan medicine

One of the most striking aspects of Tibetan medicine in the Western context[4] is its literary aspect. There must be by now at least twenty or thirty popular presentations of Tibetan medicine in English and the other major European languages, and virtually all of those which I have seen do the same thing: they summarise the *Rgyud bzhi*, particularly, often almost exclusively, the first two books with their general-ising and theoretical statements about the three *nyes pa*, their basis in the three roots of *saṃsāra* (desire, hatred and confusion), and the 'systematic' basis of Tibetan medicine in general (e.g. Clifford 1989; Dhonden 1986; Dummer 1988).

One wonders a little who reads these books, since Colin Millard notes in his chapter that most people who go to a Tibetan doctor know little or nothing about Tibetan medicine. That may suggest that there is a sizeable group of people who are at least as interested in *reading* about Tibetan medicine as in applying it in their own lives. Indeed, these books do not, in many cases, offer much in the way of advice for self-medication. What they do for the most part is to present descriptions of Tibetan medicine as part of Tibetan culture, as an ancient, self-contained, spiritually based healing system with close affinities to Tibetan Buddhism.

This is also what Eliot Tokar (Chapter 10) feels is most necessary in the Western presentation of Tibetan medicine, though he rightly takes issue with the naïve equations between Western and Tibetan terminology found in some of this literature. Tokar argues that it is only through presenting Tibetan medicine as a coherent system which has its own integrity that it can be defended against piecemeal incorporation of specific drugs and other elements by Western biomedical and pharmaceutical interests. Here we see the other face of biomedicine, which is feared now not just for the bureaucratic obstacles that it can place in the way of the practice of Tibetan medicine, but for its ability to steal and absorb elements from Tibetan medicine into its own procedures, so destroying their integrity within their original context.

I will return to this question of the defence against biomedical assimilation, which plays a role in several of the Asian chapters as well (notably Pordié's study of Ladakhi *amchi*) but for the moment we note that there is a variety of reasons why *amchi* might wish to stress the coherence and consistency, and the specifically non-Western and non-biomedical epistemological and philosophical basis, of Tibetan medicine at this point in time.

In any case, it seems that there is an appetite in the West for *knowledge* about this particular, so far largely literary, version of 'Tibetan medicine', and there is clearly also a willingness on the part of practitioners, including both Tibetans and Westerners trained in the tradition, to produce works that meet this appetite. Here the Dharamsala Men-Tsee-Khang and Tibetan doctors associated with it have taken a leading role.

We do not need to be very cynical to see this Western appetite as part of the wider Western consumption of Tibetan spirituality, and the willingness of Tibetans to cater to it as linked to the still precarious situation of the Tibetan diaspora in India and elsewhere (cf. Samuel 2001). Others have written at some length on the mystique of Tibet (Bishop 1993; Dodin and Räther 1997; Lopez 1998) and several of the contributors to this book allude to this aspect, so I will not say more here except to note that this Western appetite for Tibetan *spirituality* – as opposed perhaps to an appetite for Tibetan medical treatment – is an important part of the field of forces within which the subject-matter of this book is constituted.[5] This appetite may also contribute to the interest of Westerners in *studying* Tibetan medicine, though I know of no systematic fieldwork on this question. Here we should note that not all of those Westerners who study Tibetan medicine, in one form or another, go on to become practitioners in any serious sense, and indeed one would have to be quite dedicated and persistent to gain the kind of clinical experience that would enable one to become an effective practitioner. There is a parallel here perhaps with Buddhism; relatively few of the Westerners who read books on Tibetan Buddhism, or even of those who attend lectures by Tibetan Buddhist teachers, may become seriously committed Buddhist practitioners (cf. Samuel 2005). Much of what is going on here can perhaps be seen as a kind of identity politics. It is different certainly from that which we have seen in Ladakh or Nepal, but it shares with those situations the fact that Tibetan medicine is perhaps more important for what it signifies than for what it might do as a healing practice.

Tibetan medicine as complementary medicine

The actual use of 'Tibetan medicine' as a healing practice in Western societies is a different matter, and the studies in our book throw some light on this as well. In these societies Tibetan medicine is so far practised only on a very small scale, and within the general ambit of middle-class consumption of complementary and alternative medicine. The use of Tibetan medicine in Beijing or Shanghai would seem to share much of this context of a middle-class luxury.

As Millard notes in his study of a Tibetan medical practice in Scotland, most of the clients seem to know little about Tibetan medicine. This leads one to suspect that Tibetan medicine here is functioning as an exotic healing technique whose attraction lies primarily in its association with Buddhist spirituality. If Tibetan medicine becomes established on a larger scale, with hundreds or thousands rather than tens of practitioners, this may change, and a situation may develop in which clients are making an informed choice to employ Tibetan medicine rather than some other healing modality. For the moment, though, 'Tibetan medicine' in this context may function as little more than an exotic label.

I am not suggesting here that practitioners of Tibetan medicine are not valued, and patients recommended to them, on the basis of their perceived competence and efficiency. My point is rather that patients are on the whole not going along to these practitioners because they are specifically in search of Tibetan medicine. Instead, the practitioners are part of a more general market for alternative medicine, within which the 'Tibetan medicine' brand name does not evoke any very specific set of expectations. Indeed practices which would seem to have little or nothing to do with Tibetan medicine or even Tibetan culture, such as the so-called Bon medicine promoted by Christopher Hansard (Hansard 2001), who claims to have been taught by an otherwise unknown Bonpo master who discovered him as a child in New Zealand, or the apparently largely fictitious 'Tibetan medicine' which Emilia Sulek found to be practised by Mongolian doctors in Poland (Sulek 2005), can flourish quite as effectively as what we might regard as the 'real thing'.

The pursuit of drugs and the international conservation scenario

Two more components of the picture are only partly Western in their sphere of operation, though their origins undoubtedly lie closer to Europe and North America than to India or China. These are the *international pharmaceutical industry*, which we have seen providing the threat of biopiracy in Pordié's chapter (Chapter 6), and the *international development and conservation industry*, which plays a significant role in the chapter by Aumeeruddy-Thomas and Yeshi Lama about the project in northern Nepal (Chapter 7).

If the threat of biopiracy is perhaps overrated, this is in part because there is not much need for biopiracy in a situation where Tibetan doctors in both India and China are all too willing to collaborate in scientific testing of Tibetan drugs and their ingredients (Adams 2002). The interactions here are nevertheless constitutive of the situation in quite an important sense, and again it would be good to know rather more.

As for development, conservation and indigenous knowledge, this again forms a vital background, particularly, I would suggest, to how both the Dharamsala Men-Tsee-Khang and *amchi* elsewhere in the Himalayas have been able to present themselves to the West. To the large formal organisations operating via the UN, WWF, UNESCO and the like we can also add a network of smaller voluntary organisations motivated by the popular Western interest in Tibetan medicine to which I referred earlier.

Both the pharmaceutical interest and the conservation agenda are concerned with 'indigenous knowledge'. In both cases, a primarily Western interest has shaped the environment within which Tibetan medical practitioners and institutions now operate, but it has not dictated any specific response. Instead, we see a variety of ways in which *amchi* as individuals and as organised groups have responded to these new factors and positioned themselves in relation to the possibilities provided by them.

Tibetan medicine in developing societies

If we move on to look at the actual practice of Tibetan medicine in its Asian contexts we find something very different. Here I am not talking about Tibetan clinics for middle-class Chinese in Beijing or Shanghai, or middle-class Indians in large Indian cities, which seem to me to belong more with the Western contexts I have already sketched. In much of the Tibetan regions of China, Nepal and India, including the refugee settlements, we find relatively impoverished populations with limited access to health care, biomedical or other, for whom some form of 'Tibetan medicine' constitutes one of the available health modalities. This is what my colleagues and I found when working among first- and second-generation Tibetan refugees in a small hill town in Northern India (Connor 1996; Rozario 1996; Samuel 1999, 2001). Other recent anthropological studies of Tibetan medicine in the TAR and elsewhere have revealed a similar picture (e.g. Besch 2007; Hofer 2005, 2006; Schrempf 2005, 2006, 2007), and this kind of situation forms the background to several of the chapters in the present volume, those referring to China, Mongolia, Ladakh and Nepal.

In one of Craig Janes's earlier articles on Tibetan medicine, he refers to the concept of the 'health transition', from human populations that are dominated by infectious disease and poor nutrition to those dominated by the chronic disease of old age (Janes 1999). Western societies, having undergone this transition, struggle to meet the spiralling costs of ageing populations with an increasing burden of chronic diseases. Much of Asia, however, still awaits these problems of medical success, and, as economic liberalism continues to devastate what is left of State medical provision in the third world, many societies are becoming even less able to deliver basic health care to their populations.

Tibetan medical practice has a different role in the two situations. In the West it serves as a complementary – or perhaps supplementary – mode of dealing with chronic disease among people with high expectations of health care provision. In the third world situations, we see it as part of health care provision within societies still dominated by poor sanitation, inadequate nutrition and epidemics of infectious diseases. In these cases, it exists as part of a situation of medical pluralism, alongside the limited and inadequate provision of biomedical health care. Patients consult *amchi* as part of a health-seeking process in which they are also using various kinds of biomedical provision, often after these have failed to deliver an effective cure.

The various contexts which I have been describing define much of the range within which contemporary Tibetan medicine exists in the contemporary world. I have presented these situations as independent, but they are of course far from independent. Tibetan medicine's ability to provide effective health care in Chinese-controlled Tibet is compromised by the attractions of the Chinese metropolitan context, just as urban, elite *amchi* elsewhere in the Himalayas are drawn to the Western world. Economic liberalisation, driven by the Western world, has led to drastic reductions in public health care provision throughout much of the developing world.

Biomedicine undoubtedly poses direct threats to Tibetan medicine. Alongside the threat of biopiracy is the reality of biomedical assimilation, as seen in many of the studies in this book, both in Asia and in the West. At the same time, I do not want to construct an idealized picture of Tibetan medicine in the past. The likelihood is that its resources were always limited and that much of the Tibetan population did not have access to the more sophisticated forms of Tibetan medical practice. The present situation also offers opportunities both to individual *amchi* and the medical colleges, both in Chinese-controlled Tibet and elsewhere. It also provides a certain degree of global support for something called 'Tibetan medicine', and this is a situation for which those of us interested in the survival and continuity of this particular set of healing traditions may be grateful.

At the same time, I think that there is a real sense in which Tibetan medicine is being impoverished as a result of the political and economic context in which it is now placed. This is most obvious, perhaps, in Chinese-controlled Tibet, where Tibetan medicine is increasingly forced to reconstitute itself in biomedical terms, or in Western countries such as the UK where the demands of certification and legitimation make adequate training virtually impossible. The situation in India and Nepal, however, is also problematic. The logic of the Dharamsala Men-Tsee-Khang's dominance over Tibetan medicine in these areas is the rapid reduction of what diversity remains within Tibetan medical practice in favour of a standardised product delivered by practitioners whose training is often quite limited in relation to the senior practitioners who set up these institutions. The level of demand here is also a problem, since for the present it considerably outstrips the rate at which the Men-Tsee-Khang and the few smaller training facilities that exist can provide trained personnel.

From this point of view the systematic nature of Tibetan medical theory is perhaps as much a problem as a virtue, since it poses a threat to the richness and complexity of Tibetan medicine as actually practised. The kind of dialectic we find in the Chinese tradition today between the skilled senior doctors and the systematised TCM tradition (as in Volker Scheid's study of Chinese medicine in contemporary China, Scheid 2002) appears absent in the Tibetan context. Perhaps, given the complexities of the Tibetan political situation, and the absence of a firm institutional base anywhere with the resources to maintain the richness and complexity of the system, this is inevitable, but it is unfortunate.

Perhaps, too, if Tibetan medicine becomes an established part of a global medical scene, some of that complexity will be recreated by future practitioners. It is not inconceivable that the current phase of creeping biomedicalisation may be succeeded by a phase in which the specific characteristics of Tibetan medical practice will be given more recognition and support. For the present, however, the various situations in which Tibetan medicine is being constituted or reconstituted all seem to have their problematic aspects, and the future is hard to predict. Of course, the problems here are not all unique to Tibetan medicine, but they take a particular form given the specific historical, political and demographic contingencies surrounding this tradition today.

We might ask in conclusion how far the problematic situation of Tibetan medicine forms a microcosm of the wider situation of Tibetan culture. Here I include Tibetan Buddhism, which would seem to be going through some rather similar processes of reduction and reconstitution in order to find its place in a new global context. And if this is the case, then what is the role of anthropological scholarship in relation to both Tibetan medicine and the wider repertoire of Tibetan culture – simply to document the diversity as it disappears, or to analyse the transition to modernity, or to find some way to intervene to maintain what is present before it is reduced to a globalised lowest common denominator?

Notes

1   Stephan Kloos has recently worked on this topic but has not yet published any of his research (cf. Kloos 2006). Audrey Prost's recent Ph.D. (Prost 2003, cf. 2006a, 2006b, forthcoming) was also based on work in Dharamsala.

2   The relationship between *amchi* and medicine has also changed. In the past, *amchi* were mostly knowledgeable about medicine preparation; many collected their own herbs and made their own medicines. The Dharamsala Men-Tsee-Khang removed training in medicine preparation from its standard medical training some years ago, so that Dharamsala-trained *amchi* today are dependent on factory-produced compounds (Barbara Gerke, personal communication).

3   One might also mention Emilia Sulek's work on Mongolian practitioners of 'Tibetan medicine' in Poland. This seems to be a mélange of various Asian medical practices (including acupuncture), along with assorted New Age healing techniques (Sulek 2005). Barbara Gerke's study of the Traditional Mongolian Centre for Liver Diseases (Gerke 2004) presents a similar picture of medical eclecticism, though she emphasises the accessibility of the centre via health insurance to the population as a whole, in some contrast to Janes and Hilliard's picture of Mongolian medicine as primarily accessed by an affluent urban clientele.

4   This is a somewhat imprecise term, but the reference here is essentially to Western and Central Europe, the USA, Canada, Australia, South Africa and New Zealand.

5   A similar appetite may be developing among the Chinese population outside and within China. Laurent Pordié has pointed to the sale of *rin chen ril bu* generally in Mainland China, and the craving for these ritually 'empowered' pills that occurred during the SARS epidemics as indications, but specific enquiries remain to be done (Laurent Pordié, personal communication).

References

Adams, Vincanne (2002). Randomized Controlled Crime: Postcolonial Sciences in Alternative Medicine Research, *Social Studies of Science* 32(5–6): 659–690.

Besch, Florian (2007). Making a Medical Living: On the Monetisation of Tibetan Medicine in Spiti. In Mona Schrempf (ed.), *Soundings in Tibetan Medicine: Anthropological and Historical Perspectives. Proceedings of the 10th Seminar of the International Association for Tibetan Studies (PIATS)*, Oxford, 6–12 September 2003, Leiden: Brill Publishers.

Bishop, Peter (1993). *Dreams of Power: Tibetan Buddhism and the Western Imagination*, London: Athlone Press.

Clifford, Terry (1989). *The Diamond Healing: Tibetan Buddhist Medicine and Psychiatry*, Wellingborough: Crucible.

Connor, Linda (1996). Underdetermining the Empirical Ground of Therapy Regimens among Tibetan Refugee Patients, Paper for the International Research Workshop, Healing Powers and Modernity in Asian Societies, University of Newcastle, Australia, December.

Craig, Sienna (2006). 'Good' Manufacturing Practices: Or, Efficacy by Whose Standards?, Paper for 11th Seminar of the International Association for Tibetan Studies, Königswinter, 27 August – 2 September.

Dhonden, Yeshi (1986). *Health through Balance: An Introduction to Tibetan Medicine*, ed. and trans. Jeffrey Hopkins, Ithaca, NY: Snow Lion Publications.

Dodin, Thierry and Räther, Heinz (eds) (1997). *Mythos Tibet: Wahrnehmungen, Projektionen, Phantasien*, Köln: DuMont.

Dummer, Tom (1988). *Tibetan Medicine and Other Holistic Health-Care Systems*, New York: Routledge.

Gerke, Barbara (2004). Tradition and Modernity in Mongolian Medicine, *Journal of Alternative and Complementary Medicine* 10: 743–749.

Hansard, Christopher (2001). *The Tibetan Art of Living: Wise Body, Wise Mind, Wise Life*, London: Hodder & Stoughton.

Hofer, Theresia (2005). Tibetan Medicine in Ngamring, Diplomarbeit zur Erlangung des Magistragrades der Philosophie an der Fakultät für Sozialwissenschaften der Universität Wien.

Hofer, Theresia (2006). Rinchen Rilbu for the Rich?, Paper for the 11th Seminar of the International Association for Tibetan Studies, Königswinter, 27 August – 2 September.

Janes, Craig R. (1999). The Health Transition, Global Modernity and the Crisis of Traditional Medicine: The Tibetan Case, *Social Science and Medicine* 48: 1803–1820.

Janes, Craig R. (2002). Buddhism, Science, and Market: The Globalisation of Tibetan Medicine, *Anthropology and Medicine* 9: 267–289.

Kloos, Stephan (2006). The Institutionalisation of Tibetan Medicine in Exile, Paper presented at the Lectures of the Societies and Medicines in South Asia (SMSA) Programme, French Institute of Pondicherry, 30 May.

Lopez, Donald S. (1998). *Prisoners of Shangri-La: Tibetan Buddhism and the West*, Chicago, IL: Chicago University Press.

Prost, Audrey G. (2003). Exile, Social Change and Medicine among Tibetans in Dharamsala (Himachal Pradesh), India, Ph.D. thesis, University College London.

Prost, Audrey G. (2006a). Causation as Strategy: Interpreting Humours among Tibetan Refugees, *Anthropology and Medicine* 13(2): 119–130.

Prost, Audrey G. (2006b). Gained in Translation: Tibetan Science between Dharamsala and Lhasa. In T. Herman (ed.), *Translating Others: Translations and Translation Theories East and West*, Manchester: St Jerome Press.

Prost, Audrey G. (forthcoming). Walking the Middle Way: Men-Tsee-Khang Physicians in Transition. In L. Pordié (ed.), *Healing at the Periphery: Ethnographies of Tibetan Medicine in India*.

Rozario, Santi (1996). 'Indian Medicine', *Drib*, and the Politics of Identity in a North Indian Tibetan Refugee Settlement, Paper for the International Research Workshop, Healing Powers and Modernity in Asian Societies, University of Newcastle, Australia, December.

Samuel, Geoffrey (1999). Religion, Health and Suffering among Contemporary Tibetans. In John R. Hinnells and Roy Porter (eds), *Religion, Health and Suffering*, London and New York: Kegan Paul International, pp. 85–110.

Samuel, Geoffrey (2001). Tibetan Medicine in Contemporary India: Theory and Practice. In Linda H. Connor and Geoffrey Samuel (eds), *Healing Powers and Modernity in Asian Societies: Traditional Medicine, Shamanism and Science*, Westport, CT: Bergin & Garvey, pp. 247–268.

Samuel, Geoffrey (2005). The Westernisation of Tibetan Buddhism. In G. Samuel, *Tantric Revisionings: New Understandings of Tibetan Buddhism and Indian Religion*, Delhi: Motilal Banarsidass; London: Ashgate, pp. 317–344.

Scheid, Volker (2002). *Chinese Medicine in Contemporary China: Plurality and Synthesis*, Durham, NC: Duke University Press.

Scheid, Volker (2006). Not Very Traditional, nor Exactly Chinese, so What Kind of Medicine Is It? TCM's Discourse on Menopause and Its Implications for Practice and Teaching, *Journal of Chinese Medicine* 82: 5–19.

Schrempf, Mona (2005). Filling the Gap in Public Health: Tibetan Lineage Doctors in Nomadic Areas of the TAR, Paper for the workshop Transcultural Interface and Local Implementations of Asian and Western Medical Systems: Transfer, Integration and Transformation between Asia and Europe, Central Asian Seminar, Institute for Asian and African Studies, Humboldt-Universität zu Berlin, 11–12 February.

Schrempf, Mona (2006). Negotiating Tibetan and Western Medical Systems: Case Studies of Tibetan Medical Practice in Qinghai, Paper for the 11th Seminar of the International Association for Tibetan Studies, Königswinter, 27 August – 2 September.

Schrempf, Mona (2007). Bon Lineage Doctors and the Local: Transmission of Knowing Medical Practice in Nagchu. In Mona Schrempf (ed.), *Soundings in Tibetan Medicine: Historical and Anthropological Perspectives. Proceedings of the 10th Seminar of the International Association for Tibetan Studies (PIATS)*, Oxford, 6–12 September 2003, Leiden: Brill Publishers.

Sulek, Emilia (2005). Mongolian Doctors and Tibetan Medicine in Poland, Paper for the workshop Transcultural Interface and Local Implementations of Asian and Western Medical Systems: Transfer, Integration and Transformation between Asia and Europe, Central Asian Seminar, Institute for Asian and African Studies, Humboldt-Universität zu Berlin, 11–12 February.

Index

Abélès, Marc 141–2
acupuncture 43, 47–8, 50, 190, 193–4, 223, 238, 252
Adams, Vincanne 20, 25n18, 105–31, 156n43, 208, 218
ADB *see* Asian Development Bank
Africa 10, 11
Agrawal, A. 180
Akong Rinpoche 189, 191
alchemy 222
Alter, J. 17
Ambaga, M. 51
amchi 6–9, 21, 62–90, 251, 260;
    apprenticeship 253; associations 178;
    botanical classification 169–73;
    certification 77–80, 84;
    commercialization 238–9; common
    healing tradition 256; conservation
    160, 161, 166–9, 177–9; cooperation
    between 243–4, 245; ethnic prejudices
    244–5; identity 140–1, 142, 143,
    145–8, 149, 180; intellectual property
    rights 132–3, 134–6, 137–40, 142–5,
    147, 150, 151–2, 240; International
    Conference of Amchi 83–4;
    knowledge sharing 169–70, 172,
    173–5; medicine preparation 261n2;
    neo-traditionalism 9–19, 255;
    professionalization of 20; Profile Data
    sheets 74–5; spiritual practice 236;
    terminological issues 23n4; Tibetan
    medicine in the United States 217,
    218, 219–20, 225; 'tradition' concept
    80–2; village 'clinics' 25n26; *see also*
    practitioners
'Amchi medicine' 4
Anderson, R. 206, 207
anthropology 4, 10, 162, 253–5
antibiotics 116, 120, 121–2, 123–4

Appadurai, A. 56, 58
appropriation 13
Asad, Talal 79
Asian Development Bank (ADB) 47
Aumeeruddy-Thomas, Yildiz 21, 160–85, 251
authenticity 76, 82, 145, 220
Ayurvedic medicine 13, 26n28, 37, 253;
    dośa 233; Ladakhi *amchi* 147, 148,
    149, 155n36; Nepalese *amchi* 76, 80;
    process model of disease 203, 204;
    treatment evaluation 207; UK
    regulation 193, 194

Baabar, B. 40–1
Balandier, Georges 141
Banerjee, M. 13
'barefoot doctors' 97, 108
Bauer, M. K. 165
Baviskar, Amita 132
Beijing Hospital of Tibetan Medicine 99
Belem Declaration (1988) 163
Bhutan 4, 24n5, 68; European
    programmes 8; integrative medicine
    26n37; International Conference of
    Amchi 83; practitioners 23n4
Bhutti, Keyzom 218–19, 220, 221
bile 116, 121–2, 234
bio-piracy 21, 22, 132, 137, 143–4, 145,
    149, 252, 258
bio-prospecting 21, 135, 136–7, 146, 151,
    240
biodiversity 84, 160, 163, 164, 165, 243
biomedicine 6, 9, 64, 241–2, 253;
    assessment models 210; assimilation
    260; Beijing Hospital of Tibetan
    Medicine 99; China 53–4, 55, 100,
    102n11; complementary and
    alternative medicines 238; devaluation

Printed in the United States
by Baker & Taylor Publisher Services